A Practical Approach to Neurology for the Small Animal Practitioner

A Practical Approach to Neurology for the Small Animal Practitioner

Paul M. Freeman MA, VetMB, Cert SAO, DipECVN, MRCVS

EBVS® European Specialist in Veterinary Neurology
RCVS Specialist in Veterinary Neurology
Queen's Veterinary School Hospital
University of Cambridge
Cambridge, UK

Edward Ives MA, VetMB, DipECVN, MRCVS

EBVS® European Specialist in Veterinary Neurology
RCVS Specialist in Veterinary Neurology
Anderson Moores Veterinary Specialists
Winchester, UK

WILEY Blackwell

This edition first published 2020
© 2020 John Wiley & Sons Ltd

The right of Paul M. Freeman and Edward Ives to be identified as the authors of this work has been asserted in accordance with law.

Registered Offices
John Wiley & Sons, Inc., 111 River Street, Hoboken, NJ 07030, USA
John Wiley & Sons Ltd, The Atrium, Southern Gate, Chichester, West Sussex, PO19 8SQ, UK

Editorial Office
9600 Garsington Road, Oxford, OX4 2DQ, UK

For details of our global editorial offices, customer services, and more information about Wiley products visit us at www.wiley.com.

Wiley also publishes its books in a variety of electronic formats and by print-on-demand. Some content that appears in standard print versions of this book may not be available in other formats.

Library of Congress Cataloging-in-Publication Data

Names: Freeman, Paul M., author. | Ives, Edward, author.
Title: A practical approach to neurology for the small animal practitioner /
    Paul M. Freeman, Edward Ives.
Other titles: Rapid reference series (John Wiley & Sons)
Description: Hoboken, NJ : Wiley-Blackwell, 2020. | Series: Rapid reference
    | Includes bibliographical references and index.
Identifiers: LCCN 2020017108 (print) | LCCN 2020017109 (ebook) | ISBN
    9781119514589 (paperback) | ISBN 9781119514664 (adobe pdf) | ISBN
    9781119514701 (epub)
Subjects: MESH: Dog Diseases | Nervous System Diseases–veterinary | Cat
    Diseases | Handbook
Classification: LCC SF992.N3 (print) | LCC SF992.N3 (ebook) | NLM SF
    992.N3 | DDC 636.089/68–dc23
LC record available at https://lccn.loc.gov/2020017108
LC ebook record available at https://lccn.loc.gov/2020017109

Cover Design: Wiley
Cover Image: Courtesy of Paul M. Freeman and Edward Ives

Set in 9.5/13pt MeridienLTStd by SPi Global, Chennai, India
Printed and bound in Singapore by Markono Print Media Pte Ltd

10 9 8 7 6 5 4 3 2 1

'To all of my teachers, past and present, and to my mother Claire Ives, the kindest teacher of all.'

Edward Ives
April 2020

Contents

Preface

Neurology is still perceived by many students as one of the more difficult areas of veterinary medicine to understand. In clinical practice, neurological cases can also cause much anxiety, particularly in regard to clinical decision making when referral is not an option. Ed and I wanted to write a book for students and general practitioners that represents the way we feel neurology should be taught and understood, and one which would simplify a complex topic. There are many wonderful textbooks on the subject already in existence, and this text is in no way designed to compete with those excellent volumes, but rather we hope that it might prove to complement them as an approachable and useful companion for those looking for a better grasp of a complex subject. We have tried to design and produce a practical book full of hints and tips taken from our personal collective experience, which would be accessible as a quick reference guide for use in general practice, as well as hopefully being an easy-to-read textbook for final-year veterinary students. We have tried to include as many photographs and diagrams as possible to illustrate and simplify some of the more complex subject areas, and we are sure that the videos on the accompanying website will aid recognition of some of the less common clinical presentations. We have also included video clips of a normal neurological examination as a reference. This has been a labour of love for us and we are indebted to the many colleagues, both past and present, who have inspired, taught, and assisted us, and are still doing so. The book represents the product of many hours of study, conversation, observation, and clinical practice, and we hope that it may be used and enjoyed by many.

Paul M. Freeman and Edward Ives

Acknowledgements

The authors are Board-certified neurologists with a combined total of more than 30 years in general practice before entering full-time specialist practice. This has given us a great insight into the needs of general practitioners when it comes to dealing with neurological cases. We have both benefited from excellent teaching through the University of Cambridge, both for our veterinary degrees and later our residency training. We would like to acknowledge the support and advice of our current and past colleagues, as well as that of family and friends.

The original drawings for the book were created by Paul's son Jack Freeman, with digital images produced by Edward himself. We are grateful also to our clients, past and present, especially those of the Queen's Veterinary School Hospital, University of Cambridge, and Anderson Moores Veterinary Specialists, whose images and videos bring this text to life.

Finally, thanks to Tick, star of the neurological examination videos and Paul's long-time but now sadly deceased Border Collie, whose presence in the neurology office in Cambridge was a source of education and comfort for students and staff alike.

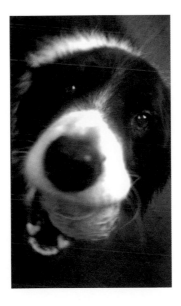

About the Companion Website

Don't forget to visit the companion website for this book:

www.wiley.com/go/freeman/neurology

There you will find valuable material designed to enhance your learning, including:

- videos of the normal neurological examination and specific disease presentations

Scan this QR code to visit the companion website.

Chapter 1 'Is it Neurological?'

Paul M. Freeman

The first step to any neurological evaluation of a veterinary patient, and probably the most common question we are asked by practitioners (in a variety of different ways), is whether the problem facing them is partially or completely neurological. In order to answer this question, it is important to understand the nature of the problem from the point of view of both the animal and the owner, and furthermore to understand what is meant by the question 'Is it neurological?'. For example, when presented with a dog that is showing signs of exercise intolerance, one possible reason may be a neuromuscular disorder, such as myasthenia gravis. However, this dog may present with a completely normal neurological examination, and the clue may be in the presenting clinical signs or medical work-up. Therefore, in such a case the initial answer may have to be 'It might be'. A dog whose problem is intermittent 'episodes' of abnormal behaviour may be having seizures, but might also be suffering from syncope, a compulsive behavioural disorder, or a movement disorder. All of these possibilities may in some way be classified as 'neurological' problems, but with very different aetiologies, treatment possibilities, and prognoses. The goal of this book is to allow practising vets to feel confident that they are approaching potentially neurological problems in a reasonable and evidence-supported way. The first step in this process is learning how to recognise when a particular presentation may be caused by a disease process somewhere within the central nervous system (CNS) or the peripheral nervous system (PNS).

1.1 What Is the Problem?

One of the key skills to be developed in general practice, as well as referral practice, is learning how to control the consultation in order to establish what the client's primary concern is, what they hope to achieve from their visit with you as the veterinarian, and how their expectations match up to their ability and/or

A Practical Approach to Neurology for the Small Animal Practitioner, First Edition. Paul M. Freeman and Edward Ives.
© 2020 John Wiley & Sons Ltd. Published 2020 by John Wiley & Sons Ltd.
Companion Website: www.wiley.com/go/freeman/neurology

willingness to afford and allow potential investigations and/or treatments to be performed. This is not an easy skill, especially for the GP vet who may have very limited time in which to carry out the initial consultation. It is, however, key to both ultimate client satisfaction and to providing the most effective service to the animal patient. Without establishing these essential facts, much time can be wasted. In the worst case the client's real concerns may not be addressed at all, meaning that they may leave the practice dissatisfied, perhaps with good reason.

Top tip: Always ask the client directly why they have come to see you today.

Don't make this mistake: Take care not to become side-tracked by a problem which may be very interesting to you, but is possibly chronic and completely unrelated to the reason for the visit!

1.2 Is this Problem Neurological?

There are many possible manifestations of neurological disease, some of which are much easier to recognise as neurological than others. There are also many non-neurological diseases which can mimic a problem involving the nervous system. In this section, we will look at the scope of neurological disease manifestations that the clinician may be presented with and we will aim to provide some clues as to the correct recognition of neurological disorders.

1.3 Neuroanatomy

When attempting to decide whether the problem is neurological, it is important to be aware of the different parts of the nervous system and how disease processes may affect them. Broadly we are concerned with the CNS (the brain and spinal cord) and the PNS (consisting of the peripheral nerves and muscles and the neuromuscular junctions between them). In the brain we can generally distinguish clinical signs referable to the forebrain, the brainstem, and the cerebellum.

The forebrain is known as the prosencephalon, and can be further divided into the telencephalon, which consists of the cerebral hemispheres, and diencephalon, containing the thalamus and the hypothalamus. The group of clinical signs which are commonly caused by lesions affecting the forebrain are sometimes referred to as a prosencephalic syndrome, and include behavioural change, central blindness, and seizure disorders in particular.

The brainstem consists of the midbrain (mesencephalon), the pons (ventral metencephalon), and the medulla (myelencephalon). Disease of the brainstem also leads to characteristic signs, which can be used to anatomically localise the problem, including proprioceptive deficits and ataxia, sometimes clusters of cranial nerve signs, vestibular syndrome, and mentation change associated with dysfunction of the ascending reticular activating system.

The third major division of the brain is the cerebellum (dorsal metencephalon), and lesions in this region can lead to some of the most recognisable abnormalities in the neurological examination, including hypermetria and intention tremor.

The medulla is contiguous with the spinal cord, which can be divided into a series of segments from which a pair of spinal nerve roots arises, one pair for each segment. For neuroanatomical localisation purposes, the spinal cord segments are grouped together according to their motor function, and whether or not they contain the cell bodies of the nerves which directly supply the skeletal muscles of the limbs (known as lower motor neurons, LMNs). In this regard, the first five cervical spinal segments (C1–C5) contain only the so-called upper motor neurons (UMNs) which run from the gait-generating centres of the cerebral cortex and brainstem to the LMNs innervating the limbs and other structures. Spinal cord lesions affecting segments in this region lead to a characteristic set of neurological examination findings involving UMN effects in all four limbs.

The sixth, seventh, and eighth cervical segments, along with the first two thoracic segments, C6–T2, contain the LMN cell bodies supplying the thoracic limbs, as well as UMNs to the pelvic limbs; lesions here cause a so-called LMN paresis or plegia (paralysis) of thoracic limbs and an UMN paresis/plegia of the pelvic limbs.

Lesions in spinal segments caudal to the second thoracic segment will generally only affect the pelvic limbs, and the division between UMN and LMN here occurs between the third and fourth lumbar segments. Hence, lesions affecting the T3–L3 spinal cord segments lead to UMN paresis of pelvic limbs, whereas lesions caudal to L3 (L4–S3) cause LMN paresis/plegia of the pelvic limbs.

As well as the descending motor tracts within the spinal cord, there are of course ascending sensory tracts including those carrying proprioceptive information from the limbs and trunk; therefore, a spinal cord disorder will usually lead to variable degrees of ataxia and proprioceptive dysfunction, as well as the paresis associated with the loss of motor function.

The final part of the nervous system within which we can make an anatomical localisation consists of the peripheral nerves, neuromuscular junctions, and muscles. Lesions affecting this neuromuscular system tend to lead to more obvious weakness and LMN paresis/plegia affecting all limbs. Therefore, syndromes such as weakness, stiffness, exercise intolerance, and collapse may all arise as a result of disease affecting this PNS.

The neurological examination and neuroanatomical localisation of specific lesions will be explored and explained in more detail in Chapters 3 and 4, but an understanding of the anatomical structures involved in neurological disorders is

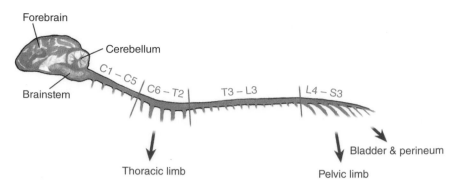

Figure 1.1 Neuroanatomical regions. The aim of the neurological examination is to localise the site of a lesion into the brain, the spinal cord, or peripheral (neuromuscular) regions. Functionally, the brain is separated into the forebrain, brainstem, and cerebellum; the spinal cord into sections containing the segments 1st cervical – 5th cervical (C1–C5), 6th cervical – 2nd thoracic (C6–T2), 3rd thoracic – 3rd lumbar (T3–L3), and 4th lumbar – sacral (L4–S3); and the peripheral nervous system consists of peripheral nerves, with the neuromuscular junctions and muscles also considered as a potential neuroanatomical localisation.

an essential part of the ability to recognise when one is facing a neurological problem (see Figure 1.1).

1.4   Manifestations of Diseases of the Nervous System

Disorders that affect different parts of the nervous system may manifest themselves in a wide variety of ways. In this section, we will briefly look at each of these, with the most important and more common problems being examined in greater detail in Chapter 6. The majority of nervous system disease will result in one or more of the following clinical presentations, some of which can be more easily defined and recognised than others. Where relevant, non-neurological disorders that can mimic or also result in these clinical presentations will also be mentioned:

- seizures
- collapse
- movement disorder/dyskinesia
- mentation change
- behaviour change
- blindness
- deafness
- tremor
- paresis/plegia
- ataxia

- abnormality of head position (head tilt/turn)
- abnormality of eye position or movements
- hypaesthesia
- lameness
- pain
- disorders of micturition/urination.

1.4.1 Seizures

For the purposes of this text, an epileptic seizure will be defined as an acute onset of excessive and hypersynchronous brain activity that results in transient visible motor activity; this description does not allow for so-called 'absence seizures', where a person may become transiently 'absent', since no motor activity is seen in such a seizure. However, such seizures, although they may occur in cats and dogs, are very difficult to diagnose without the help of an electroencephalogram (EEG).

It is rare that an affected animal will seizure during the consultation, so usually we rely on owner description and often video evidence when trying to decide if a problem is truly an epileptic seizure or some kind of seizure mimic. A generalised seizure is normally easily recognisable (see Video 1); the seizure may begin with a focal contraction of, for example, the facial muscles, but this rapidly spreads to cause loss of conscious state and tonic contraction of all the anti-gravity muscles leading to recumbency. There follows a period of tonic and clonic muscle activity causing running-like movements, and there may be vocalising, hypersalivation, jaw champing, and often urination or defecation. The tonic-clonic movements gradually subside and the animal will frequently adopt paddling movements as consciousness returns and attempts are made to stand. There will usually then follow a post-ictal period, which may last for minutes or hours, when the animal may show varying levels of altered behaviour, circling, ataxia, blindness, and other neurological abnormalities.

Focal seizures may involve simple focal muscle twitching, commonly of the orofacial muscles (see Video 2), but may also include more complex patterns of movement and/or behaviour – leading to apparent loss of consciousness and awareness. Such activity can be very difficult to distinguish from obsessive behavioural abnormalities and movement disorders for instance, but there are some key indicators which may be helpful in recognising when a problem is a true focal epileptic seizure (see below). A specific form of focal seizure is the myoclonic seizure, characterised by jerky twitches resembling the dog being fearful of a sudden stimulus, and seen especially in the genetic storage disease of Miniature Wire-haired Dachshunds, Beagles, and Bassett Hounds known as Lafora Disease (see Video 3).

Epilepsy implies a tendency for seizures to recur and can be further classified as 'reactive/metabolic', when there is an extracranial cause, 'structural', when there is an abnormality of brain structure such as an inflammatory or neoplastic lesion, and 'idiopathic', when brain structure is normal.

It is important to try to ascertain whether the abnormal event described by the owner or captured on video is an epileptic seizure or not. This is because the occurrence of true seizures implies a possible prosencephalic or forebrain lesion and dictates a certain path of investigation. The initiation of antiepileptic medication is always a subject for discussion and consideration, since all antiepileptic drugs (AEDs) can have undesirable side-effects, and their use in non-seizure disorders is usually contraindicated.

The description above contains some clues to the features of epileptic seizures that can be used in order to ascertain whether the event described is truly an epileptic seizure or represents a 'seizure mimic'. These include:

1. *Presence of post-ictal signs.* This is common and can include ataxia, blindness, polyphagia, or a temporary character change such as becoming aggressive.
2. *Presence of autonomic signs during the event.* In itself this is not necessarily pathognomonic for an epileptic seizure, but involuntary salivation, urination, and/or defecation is more common in seizure events than syncope, and is rarely observed for movement disorders.
3. *Absence of consciousness during the event.* It can be difficult to be sure about this, especially in mild focal seizures. However, the ability to rouse an animal from the behaviour, as is the case for idiopathic head-bobbing for instance, is an indication that the event is probably not a seizure.
4. *Presence of some form of tonic muscular activity, twitching, or stiffness.*

There are many other causes of paroxysmal transient events, or 'seizure mimics', and these should always be considered when trying to decide whether or not we are dealing with an epileptic seizure. These include:

- *Syncope, which may have a cardiovascular or respiratory cause.* Most cases of syncope result in a flaccid collapse, but this is again not always the case, and there is a significant 'grey zone' of signs seen with seizures and syncope which can make them difficult to distinguish. This is also the case in human medicine, with a significant percentage of people being diagnosed with epilepsy when in fact they are suffering syncopal attacks.
- *Dyskinesia or movement disorder.* These paroxysmal disorders of movement are being increasingly described, often with specific breed associations. Examples include the epileptoid cramping syndrome of Border Terriers (which has been associated with a gluten sensitivity and recently renamed paroxysmal gluten-sensitive dyskinesia, see Video 4) and episodic falling in Cavalier King Charles Spaniels (CKCSs), which has a known genetic mutation associated with it. Although these syndromes are fairly well described, the fact that the CKCS also suffers with idiopathic epilepsy can make this an even more complicated picture in this breed.

- *Behavioural events*. These are often described as obsessive compulsive or OCD behaviours, such as some cases of so-called 'fly-catching'. The latter can also be a focal seizure, and has even been associated with floating bodies within the anterior chamber of the eye, or gastrointestinal pain (see Video 5).
- *Transient vestibular events*. Perhaps associated with transient ischaemic attacks or TIAs.
- *Narcolepsy/cataplexy*. This is a rare condition with a suspected genetic basis in certain breeds, but can look very much like the so-called 'drop seizures' described in humans (see Video 6).
- *Idiopathic generalised tremor syndrome* or so-called 'little white shaker disease' (see Video 7). This is an inflammatory condition of the CNS leading to a generalised tremor. The tremor can wax and wane, worsens with excitement, and is potentially confusable with an animal suffering with a prolonged seizure or status epilepticus, such as may be seen following exposure to certain toxic substances (e.g. aflatoxins or mouldy food).
- *Episodic pain*, such as that associated with some cervical intervertebral disc herniations, may cause episodic, short-lived behavioural and physical changes. The French Bulldog in particular seems prone to such manifestations (see Video 8).
- *Episodic collapse*, which may have a neuromuscular, metabolic, or orthopaedic cause; if recovery is rapid; such events may be mistakenly diagnosed as seizures.
- *Rapid eye movement (*REM*) sleep disorder*. This is a condition where affected dogs may suffer violent episodes of paddling and limb movement during periods of REM sleep (see Video 9). It has recently been shown to have a higher incidence in dogs recovering from tetanus (Shea et al. 2018).

Top tip: Seizures can have multiple causes but also have multiple mimics.

Careful observation of video footage, together with accurate history taking, is key to defining whether the presenting problem is truly a seizure.

Ultimately, the only sure way to define a seizure (currently categorised as a Tier 3 level of diagnostic confidence for idiopathic epilepsy) is by making EEG recordings of abnormal brain activity during the abnormal event. Even in specialist referral practice this is rarely an option, and therefore we are usually working at a lower level of confidence.

1.4.2 Collapse

Collapse implies a loss of extensor motor tone, and may be either intermittent or permanent. When an owner describes a problem of collapsing, usually they are referring to episodic collapse, since a permanent collapse is immediately obvious!

Differential diagnoses for intermittent collapse include seizures, syncope, narcolepsy/cataplexy, and metabolic disorders (such as hypoglycaemia). More permanent collapse may be caused by musculoskeletal and orthopaedic problems, inflammatory conditions such as polyarthritis or polymyositis, as well as medical conditions involving weakness, anaemia, or pain. Neurological causes of loss of extensor muscle tone or strength may include brain, spinal cord, and PNS disorders. The neurological examination is therefore key to identifying, firstly, whether the problem is neurological, and then obtaining a correct neuroanatomical localisation.

Care must be taken in interpretation of the findings of the neurological examination in cases of collapse; an animal which is suffering from shock, trauma, or acute pain may well show apparent neurological deficits without any neurological disease or pathology. Examples include animals in shock which apparently have poor proprioception and spinal reflexes, lack of menace response, and even absent deep pain response. Once the shock and pain has been appropriately managed, the neurological abnormalities may disappear.

Top tip: Be careful with interpretation of the neurological examination in severely shocked or traumatised animals.

Don't make this mistake: Diagnosing severe spinal trauma due to apparent loss of deep pain perception post-trauma, especially in cats following a road traffic accident. Once stabilised, the neurological examination may change, indicating a less severe injury.

1.4.3 Movement Disorders

Movement disorders are an increasingly recognised group of conditions which affect many dog breeds. These conditions involve abnormal muscular movements, occasionally episodes of collapse, but no change of consciousness or autonomic signs that may be seen in focal epileptic seizure events (see Video 10). Well-documented examples include episodic falling in CKCSs ('Collapsing Cavaliers'), paroxysmal gluten-sensitive dyskinesia of Border Terriers (epileptoid cramping syndrome or 'Spikes disease', see Video 4), 'Scotty cramp' in Scottish Terriers and 'dancing Dobermann' disease.

Some of these conditions have a known genetic cause, and a specific test may be available (e.g. episodic falling in Cavaliers), but for many there is no specific diagnostic test. Dancing Dobermann disease is suspected to be a polyneuropathy, Spike's disease has been shown to be caused by a hypersensitivity to gluten in the diet, and it may be that some so-called movement disorders are in fact focal seizures.

In all of these conditions, the neurological examination should be normal, and in general all investigations are likely to be unremarkable (with the exception of specific genetic tests for example). The diagnosis is often one of exclusion and pattern recognition, and for many of the conditions there is no specific treatment available.

Further discussion of movement disorders and how they may present in practice can be found in Section 6.2 'Movement Disorders'.

1.4.4 Mentation and Behaviour

Observation and recognition of changes in either behaviour or mentation can be crucial in recognising that one is dealing with a neurological problem. Mentation concerns the level of general alertness and is sometimes referred to as the *level* of mentation (as opposed to the *quality* of mentation, which may be better be understood as behaviour). Mentation levels can be categorised as:

1. *Normal*
2. *Obtundation*. A generalised reduction in level of alertness or interaction with the environment; an animal which appears to show an absence of the usual anxiety and stress associated with a visit to the veterinarian, a lack of normal interaction with the owner, a 'can't be bothered' or 'couldn't care less' attitude. There can clearly be a marked difference between mild and severe obtundation, and milder levels may be variously described as lethargy or depression, although these terms should be used with caution in animal species.
3. *Stupor*. This implies a level of mentation in which the animal is basically asleep or semi-asleep, and only arousable by a noxious stimulus.
4. *Coma*. An animal which is not rousable even by a noxious stimulus.

A change in the level of mentation frequently implies neurological disease; stupor and coma are most commonly seen in moderate to severe brainstem disorders where the ascending reticular activating system is affected. This causes a reduction in sensory input to the cerebral cortex. Forebrain disease may also cause altered mentation, and in particular pituitary macroadenomas can present with obtundation as the only neurological sign.

Focal cerebrocortical lesions more rarely present with obviously altered mentation although larger lesions may, including compulsive pacing or circling behaviour. Animals with generalised encephalopathies, such as those seen in portosystemic shunting for instance, often show an altered level of mentation, sometimes intermittently. Another important observation is that raised intracranial pressure (ICP) can affect mentation, and serial observation and monitoring of mentation level in animals with suspected head trauma or with other reasons for potentially raised ICP (usually as part of the modified Glasgow Coma Scale) is extremely important in allowing recognition of a deteriorating situation/rising ICP.

> **Top tip:** Altered mentation may be the only sign of severe intracranial pathology.

It is also important to be aware that altered mentation can occur as a result of non-neurological disease. Animals which have significant medical disorders, pyrexia, anaemia, or pain may in some situations show moderate to severe obtundation without any primary neurological disease. As already mentioned, animals which have suffered significant trauma or stress, for example after a road traffic accident, may also show an apparently reduced level of mentation. In these situations, mentation may be expected to improve if the underlying problems are corrected, and this should allow a reduced suspicion of the presence of a primary neurological disorder.

Changes in behaviour or the quality of mentation usually imply involvement of the cerebral cortex. Behavioural changes can be caused by many things, including ageing, stress, change of environment or home situation, metabolic disease, chronic pain, dietary change, etc. Therefore, taking a careful clinical history is crucial in cases where a change of behaviour forms part of the presenting complaint. If a more subtle behavioural change is reported during the history-taking related to the investigation of a problem for which altered behaviour was not immediately apparent, then this may raise the level of suspicion for a possible intracranial disease.

Altered behaviour is less commonly the primary clinical sign reported for neurological disease, possibly due to our relative lack of sensitivity as veterinarians and owners in being able to identify more subtle changes. However, there are occasions when an owner will have recognised a loss of learned behaviour, or a change in demeanour or willingness to play in their pet, and this may be significant. As already stated, neurological disease leading to behavioural change usually implies a prosencephalic lesion and, in such situations, careful performance and interpretation of the neurological examination may identify other abnormalities consistent with a lesion affecting the cerebral cortex.

1.4.5 Blindness

An acute onset of blindness is usually noticed by pet owners, since it may be extremely disorientating for the affected animal, and may lead to behavioural changes as well as more obvious signs such as bumping into objects. It is often the case that vision is lost progressively rather than acutely, but in these situations owners frequently do not notice the more subtle changes brought about in their pet by a reduction in the quality of their vision, and it is only when the problem has progressed to complete or near-complete blindness that the owner becomes aware. When presented with an animal with reduced vision, it is therefore important to question the owner carefully in order to elucidate whether the visual loss may in fact have occurred progressively rather than acutely.

A blind cat or dog may be reluctant to move around, become 'clingy' or fearful in situations where they were previously relaxed and confident, and may even develop obsessive or phobic behaviours. For neuroanatomical evaluation, the important thing to establish is whether the blindness appears peripheral or central. Central blindness implies dysfunction of the central visual pathways and/or visual cortex; this is usually rare in the absence of other signs of intracranial disease. More commonly, vision may be lost in one eye as a result of a lesion affecting the contralateral visual cortex, but as vision remains normal in the other eye, the owner either may not be aware of the vision loss or may have noticed the animal bumping into objects on only one side. The menace response will be absent in the affected eye, but the pupillary light reflex (PLR) (as well as palpebral reflex and other cranial nerves) are likely to be normal. Use of the so-called 'cotton-ball' test (see Chapter 3) may also help to identify visual loss in one eye.

In general, animals that present as completely or almost completely blind with no other neurological abnormalities, will have lesions affecting either the optic nerves or the eyes themselves. In the case of ocular disease, if there are no grossly obvious abnormalities such as cataracts, then the retina is the region most likely to be affected. A fundic examination should be performed and may reveal evidence of retinal disease or detachment. In the absence of an obvious cause for sudden blindness, then the two conditions which must be considered are sudden acquired retinal degeneration syndrome (SARDS) and optic nerve disease; optic nerve disease can have a number of possible causes (see Section 6.4 'Blindness').

SARDS is a syndrome that usually presents as an apparent acute onset of complete blindness, although careful history taking may reveal evidence that vision has deteriorated over a period of weeks. There is frequently an accompanying history of polyphagia, polydipsia, and polyuria and sometimes behavioural changes. Menace responses are absent bilaterally, and PLRs are reduced although may still be present to some degree. Routine biochemistry can reveal increased alkaline phosphatase and cholesterol, and there is often a high suspicion of hyperadrenocorticism although this is rarely confirmed. Despite the problem being associated with retinal degeneration of an unknown cause, fundic examination is usually normal at least in the early stages. Diagnosis can be made with a high degree of certainty from the history, physical examination, and biochemistry findings, but confirmation requires the presence of a bilaterally abnormal electroretinogram. The prognosis for return of sight is poor, although other systemic signs may improve over time.

The optic nerves can be affected by neoplastic disease that either infiltrates the nerves, such as lymphoma, or that compresses the optic chiasm, such as pituitary macroadenomas. Inflammatory disease affecting the optic nerves is more common and can be either confined to the optic nerves as the condition 'optic neuritis', or present as part of a more generalised inflammatory condition of the CNS (such as meningoencephalitis of unknown origin, MUO). In optic neuritis cases, it is sometimes possible to visualise swollen optic nerve heads during the fundoscopic evaluation. Other neurological abnormalities may be observed in cases with MUO, such as postural reaction deficits or other cranial nerve abnormalities. Cerebrospinal fluid analysis frequently confirms the presence of inflammation.

> **Top tip:** Acute blindness with reduced or absent PLRs and no other physical or neurological abnormalities usually indicates either SARDS or optic neuritis. In both cases, the prognosis is guarded but diagnosis is worth pursuing because some cases of optic neuritis are responsive to immunosuppressive therapy.

1.4.6 Deafness

Deafness is a rare presentation in isolation, but owners may report behavioural changes which could imply that deafness or reduced hearing may be present. Bilateral hearing loss may be very significant to the lifestyle and behaviour of individual animals, and its effects should not be underestimated. Unilateral deafness is more challenging to detect and may be more debilitating than is currently thought as a result of an inability to localise the source of sounds. Deafness is a difficult neurological deficit to confirm clinically, but careful testing may lead to a high index of suspicion. As with other conditions, careful clinical history taking may provide some clues as to the origin of the deafness. Physical examination should obviously include an examination of the external ear canals. Neurological examination may reveal other abnormalities which can give clues as to the origin of the deafness (e.g. vestibular signs, facial nerve paralysis, and Horner syndrome may all be associated with otitis media/interna).

Confirmation of deafness requires electrodiagnostic evaluation through the recording of brainstem auditory evoked responses (BAER). Deafness may be either conductive, associated with abnormalities of conduction of sound waves to the receptors in the inner ear (e.g. accumulation of debris in the external ear canal or fluid accumulation in the tympanic bulla), or sensorineural, associated with a problem in the cochlea of the inner ear or the cochlear nerve itself.

1.4.7 Tremor

Tremor associated with neurological disease can be broadly divided into head tremor and whole-body tremor. Head tremor is most commonly associated with cerebellar disease (see Video 11), when it may be permanent, but tremor often becomes more severe when an affected animal attempts to perform some action involving the head, such as eating or drinking (termed an 'intention tremor'). The tremor may be very mild and subtle, and occasionally has not been appreciated by the owner. If a head tremor is observed in the consultation, then a full neurological examination should be performed, particularly to look for other signs consistent with cerebellar disease.

A slower head 'tremor' known as idiopathic head bobbing is occasionally seen, particularly in young Boxers and English Bulldogs (see Video 12). The cause is unknown, the problem is intermittent, and is generally self-limiting. All investigative and diagnostic tests tend to be normal in affected dogs, and the head-bobbing movements may be vertical ('Yes') or horizontal ('No'). Affected dogs can usually be distracted during an episode; when distracted the head bobbing will cease, and this can be used to distinguish this paroxysmal occurrence from a focal seizure.

Whole-body tremor is an uncommon presentation, but when seen can be severe and debilitating. The two most common forms of whole-body tremor are that associated with toxin ingestion (particularly tremorgenic mycotoxins found in mouldy food, metaldehyde, chocolate, and some prescription medications) and idiopathic generalised tremor syndrome (see Section 6.2 'Movement Disorders' and Video 7). Tremors resulting from toxicity usually affect the whole body, can be severe and unremitting, do not subside with recumbency, and may occasionally progress to generalised seizures. This is a neurological emergency and requires emergency treatment to prevent hyperthermia and hypoglycaemia. Diagnosis generally relies on thorough history taking and the clinical presentation.

Another type of tremor that may be encountered is orthostatic tremor. This type of tremor predominately affects the limbs in large and giant breed dogs (particularly Great Danes) and is present only when the limbs are weight-bearing (see Video 13). The condition is benign and there is no treatment. Occasionally, a limb tremor may be associated with orthopaedic disease, especially if there is significant muscle atrophy or pain. It can also occur in some older dogs, apparently as part of an ageing process, and this is termed an 'essential' or 'senile' tremor (see Video 14).

There are a few conditions affecting the myelination of axons which present as whole-body tremors in young puppies around 6–8 weeks of age. Breeds that are typically affected include the English Springer Spaniel, Chow, Samoyed, Weimaraner, and Dalmatian.

Top tip: The major differential diagnoses for an acute onset of generalised tremor in an adult dog are toxin ingestion and idiopathic generalised tremor syndrome ('little white shaker' disease); in the former the tremor is persistent and severe, in the latter it may wax and wane and disappears when the dog is at rest.

1.4.8 Paresis/Plegia

Paresis can be defined as a reduced ability to initiate or maintain motor activity. It may manifest as a reduced ability to support weight (LMN paresis) or a reduced ability to generate gait (UMN paresis). Plegia is defined as an absence of voluntary movement (i.e. paralysis). A plegic animal usually indicates that severe CNS injury has occurred, either at the level of the brainstem or neck for tetraplegia or caudal to the T2 spinal segment for paraplegia. Paraplegia, involving only the pelvic limbs, is far more common than tetraplegia, partly because any lesion in the CNS that is capable of causing tetraplegia may be accompanied by other severe effects which may include respiratory failure and death. When an animal is presented in such a condition, particularly if there is a history of possible or definite trauma, great care should be taken when moving the patient in case there is instability of the vertebral column and the potential for further spinal cord damage.

In an animal that is plegic (and only in these animals), it is necessary to include the testing of so-called 'deep pain perception' (DPP), which is the ability of the animal to recognise a noxious stimulus applied to the deep structures of the foot or toe (see Chapter 3). The loss of DPP is a poor prognostic indicator in many situations, since the sensory fibres that convey this information are carried in many tracts which are located deep within the spinal cord. Their loss may therefore indicate spinal cord damage at the deepest level. However, DPP is *not* likely to be lost in animals which have less severe spinal cord injury and remain paretic; testing for DPP therefore need not be performed in such animals.

The neurological examination is critical to being able to localise the likely anatomical location of any lesion causing paresis or plegia. This particularly includes an understanding of the spinal reflexes. It is still a common mistake to interpret the presence of a normal pedal withdrawal reflex as an indicator that DPP is present, and this can lead to overly optimistic prognosis being given to owners of animals with severe spinal cord injury (see Chapter 3 and Video 15).

Don't make this mistake: In paralysed animals, make sure you understand the difference between testing spinal reflexes and testing for deep pain perception (see Chapter 3).

Disorders affecting the PNS can present as a relatively acute onset of tetraplegia or severe tetraparesis. In this situation, the differentiation from a spinal cord lesion can usually be made by the fact that the neurological deficits cannot be explained by a single, focal CNS lesion as the spinal reflexes are reduced in all limbs. The major differentials for acute onset severe tetraparesis/tetraplegia localising to the PNS are acute canine polyradiculoneuritis, fulminant myasthenia gravis, and botulism.

Milder forms of paresis may be much more difficult to identify and a degree of paresis affecting one or more limbs may be the only sign of a neurological problem. Close observation of gait, including retrospective and slow-motion video analysis, may be helpful in identifying a reduction in the quality of movement. UMN paresis occurs when the control or initiation of movement is affected by a lesion that is affecting either the gait-generating regions of the cerebral cortex or brainstem or the spinal cord pathways containing the UMNs descending to synapse with the LMNs in the brachial or lumbosacral plexi. UMN paresis may lead to a long-strided gait, toe dragging, and postural reaction deficits, but the affected limbs retain normal spinal reflexes and are not weak. LMN paresis, by contrast, causes a paresis like that seen in PNS diseases, characterised by weakness, an inability to support weight, and a short-strided, choppy gait. For lesions affecting the C6–T2 spinal cord segments, this can lead to the so-called 'two-engine' gait, with short, choppy thoracic limbs and long-striding, ataxic pelvic limbs.

Paraparesis can be misinterpreted as bilateral pelvic limb lameness of orthopaedic origin, and vice versa. Some conditions, such as hip dysplasia and bilateral cranial cruciate ligament disease, can present in a very similar way to a paraparesis caused by a spinal cord disorder. A knowledge of orthopaedic disease and a familiarity with basic orthopaedic examination is therefore important for the neurologist to avoid unnecessary investigative procedures resulting from a failure to recognise potential orthopaedic problems. Testing of postural reactions may allow recognition of a genuine neurological problem, but significant orthopaedic disease involving pain and a reluctance to bear weight may also complicate the interpretation of postural reaction testing. When in doubt, it may be wise to consult the opinion of an orthopaedic surgeon in these cases before assuming a neurological problem.

Don't make this mistake: An acute onset of bilateral cranial cruciate ligament failure can appear surprisingly similar to an acute T3–L3 myelopathy!

1.4.9 Ataxia

Ataxia is frequently, but not always, associated with paresis. Ataxia implies some disorder of coordination of movement, and there are three recognisable forms of ataxia that each suggest a lesion involving different parts of the nervous system. The observation of ataxia is highly suggestive of a neurological problem. However, as for paresis, some non-neurological problems can mimic ataxia if they significantly interfere with an animal's gait (e.g. bilateral cruciate ligament disease). The hallmark of ataxia is an unpredictability of limb placement, which is usually different to the predictable gait abnormalities observed in cases with lameness or orthopaedic disease.

The form of ataxia that is most commonly associated with paresis is a general proprioceptive ataxia (or 'spinal' ataxia, see Video 16). This occurs when a lesion disrupts the proprioceptive pathways in the spinal cord or brainstem, and is invariably therefore seen in conjunction with paresis. It may be symmetric or asymmetric, depending on the precise location of the lesion and, as for paresis, may affect all limbs or just the pelvic limbs. Attempting to differentiating between ataxia and paresis for lesions affecting the brain or spinal cord is neither necessary nor particularly useful; the most important thing is being able to recognise mild forms of either, which may give a clue to the possibility of a neurological condition as opposed to, for instance, an orthopaedic problem.

Lesions affecting the vestibular system result in a vestibular ataxia. This has a different quality to general proprioceptive ataxia, being caused in part by a loss of extensor muscle tone on the side of the lesion due to a reduction in the level of activity in the ipsilateral vestibulospinal tracts. This leads to a tendency to collapse or fall towards the affected side, and sometimes tight circling towards that side; there is also a loss of balance associated with the vestibular disturbance, which increases the tendency to fall or lurch towards the affected side (see Video 17).

The third form of ataxia is caused by lesions of the cerebellum, resulting in a cerebellar ataxia (see Video 18). The cerebellum is intimately involved in the coordination of gait and movement, receiving proprioceptive information from the limbs and body, as well as from the vestibular system; this involves feedback loops with the gait-generating centres of the forebrain and brainstem, as well as having a significant inhibitory function on the vestibular nuclei of the brainstem. All of this explains the signs seen with cerebellar disease, including the intention tremor described above, the classical hypermetric gait, and the potential for vestibular signs. The gait of a dog with a cerebellar lesion may therefore have qualities of both vestibular and cerebellar ataxia, sometimes termed 'cerebellovestibular ataxia'. The hypermetria seen in cerebellar ataxia can affect all limbs but may also be confined to one side of the body, or even just one limb, depending on the precise location of the lesion. The other confusing aspect of cerebellar disorders, which can cause problems when trying to decide if the neurological deficits can be explained by a single lesion, is its involvement with the vestibular system; because the cerebellum receives some direct input from the peripheral vestibular system bilaterally, some cerebellar lesions will cause vestibular signs (such as a head tilt) on the same side as the lesion (ipsilateral). However, since the cerebellum itself has a primarily inhibitory influence on the vestibular nuclei of the brainstem, cerebellar lesions in specific locations may result in a so-called paradoxical vestibular syndrome, where the vestibular signs would suggest a lesion on the opposite side of the body to that of the actual lesion (see Chapter 4 and Section 6.8 'Cerebellar Dysfunction' for a fuller explanation, and Video 19). If this is not appreciated, then it may lead to the incorrect assumption that there must be a multifocal localisation, potentially suggesting a different set of differential diagnoses to a problem explained by a single (focal) lesion.

Top tip: Learn to recognise the three common forms of ataxia, as this provides a short cut to lesion localisation and assists with forming the list of differential diagnoses.

Don't make this mistake: Remember, pure cerebellar lesions may cause variable hypermetria, and either ipsilateral or contralateral vestibular signs.

1.4.10   Abnormalities of Head Position and Eyeball Position and Movement

1. Head tilt

Rotation of the head about the long axis of the body is known as a head tilt and is typically associated with disorders of the vestibular system or cerebellum (see above). The head is rotated so that the affected side is down relative to the midline, such that the ear on the affected side lies at a lower level than that of the unaffected side (see Figure 1.2). This is indicative of a reduction in the influence of the vestibular system on the affected side. This also explains the so-called paradoxical head tilt seen with certain unilateral cerebellar lesions, where the head is tilted in the opposite way due to relative increase in influence of the vestibular system on the affected side brought about by a loss of inhibitory input from the cerebellum.

2. Head turn
Some unilateral forebrain lesions can cause a phenomenon known as a head turn. This occurs when the head remains level about its central long axis, but is turned to right or left, usually towards the affected side. It may also be associated with compulsive circling in the same direction and is thought to be caused by the loss of sensory input being perceived from the contralateral environment (i.e. the animal turns and circles towards the side from which it still perceives sensory information).

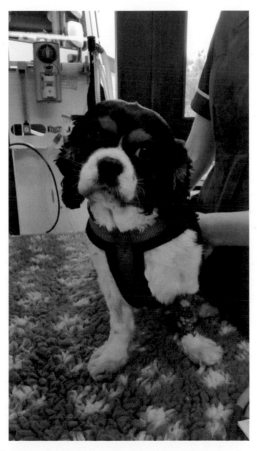

Figure 1.2 A Cavalier King Charles Spaniel with a left head tilt associated with a left peripheral vestibular syndrome caused by otitis media/interna.

3. Strabismus

This indicates an abnormal position of one or both eyes and may be either static or positional. In a static strabismus, the eye is permanently positioned incorrectly, and this indicates a lesion affecting either the extraocular muscles or one or more of the cranial nerves supplying them (III, IV, or VI, see Chapter 3). The direction of the strabismus is governed by the precise loss of muscle function. A bilateral ventrolateral strabismus (so-called 'sunset sign') is seen in certain cases of severe hydrocephalus, and is thought to occur as a result of either changes in skull morphology or pressure on the oculomotor nuclei in the midbrain.

Positional strabismus occurs when an eye moves into an abnormal position only when the head position is changed. When there is a suspicion of vestibular syndrome it is necessary to elevate the head so that the affected animal is looking directly up at the observer. In this position, the eye on the affected side often assumes an abnormal ventrolateral position. This occurs due to loss of the ability to determine the new correct position of the eye when the head has been moved (see Section 6.7 'Vestibular Syndrome' for a fuller explanation).

4. Nystagmus

This is the phenomenon of rapid involuntary eye movements. Physiological nystagmus is seen in response to head movement, and is a normal phenomenon requiring the vestibular system and extraocular muscles to all be functioning normally (see Chapter 3). Pathological nystagmus occurs most commonly when there is an imbalance between the two sides of the vestibular system. This usually implies a unilateral vestibular lesion, and in this situation the movements are commonly described as a jerk nystagmus, with fast and slow phases in opposite directions. The direction of the movements may be horizontal, rotatory, and occasionally vertical. When it is possible to define the direction of each phase, the slow phase of movement tends to be directed towards the side of the vestibular lesion (see Video 20).

Pendular nystagmus is seen in some oriental cat breeds, especially Siamese cats. Affected animals show rhythmic, usually horizontal, eye movements at rest, with no fast or slow phase. This is considered normal in these cats, and does not appear to affect their quality of life. It is thought to occur as a result of an abnormal degree of crossing over of optic nerve fibres at the optic chiasm during embryological development (see Video 21).

Top tip: Be prepared to move an affected animal's head into abnormal positions to induce nystagmus or strabismus when there is a suspicion of vestibular disease; any abnormality of eye position or movement which occurs when the head is at rest is likely to be pathological and usually indicative of vestibular dysfunction.

Don't make this mistake: Pendular nystagmus can be a 'normal' phenomenon in certain pedigree oriental cats and is not always an indicator of vestibular disease.

1.4.11   Reduced Sensation (Hypaesthesia)

The skin is supplied with sensory receptors that are sensitive to pressure and deformation (mechanoreceptors), heat (thermoreceptors), and pain (nociceptors). These are relatively specific and respond only to the source of energy for which they are adapted. Each spinal cord segment receives information from sensory neurons that enter via the dorsal horn from a region of skin known as the dermatome. Along most of the trunk, this information is carried in cutaneous nerves which arise in a largely segmental fashion and form an important part of the cutaneous trunci reflex (see Chapter 3). Skin sensation in the limbs is transmitted via sensory neurons carried in the major peripheral nerves of the limb, most of which are mixed nerves carrying both motor and sensory fibres. In the limbs, much of the skin is supplied by more than one peripheral nerve. The area of skin supplied by a single nerve is divided into overlap zones around the edges; the specific regions in the centre supplied by just that nerve are known as autonomous zones (see Figure 1.3). A knowledge of these zones is important to allow for the identification of damage to individual spinal nerves or segments, for instance in the case of brachial or lumbosacral plexus injury.

Skin sensation from the face and head is carried largely within the different branches of the trigeminal nerve (V), including from the surface of the cornea. Identification of hypaesthesia on one side of the face can be indicative of a trigeminal neuropathy, sometimes in the absence of other signs. The only exception is the skin of the outer (concave) surface of the pinna, which is supplied by the auricular branch of the facial nerve (VII).

Loss of sensation from the inner medial surface of the nose (nasal planum sensation) may be useful in recognising the presence of a focal forebrain lesion. Touching the nasal planum induces a conscious reaction in the normal dog or cat, and lesions either of the ipsilateral trigeminal nerve or of the contralateral forebrain may lead to a loss of this response (see Chapter 3).

1.4.12   Lameness

Lameness represents a reluctance to bear weight on a limb. Lameness resulting from neurological disease (neurogenic lameness) can be very difficult to distinguish from orthopaedic lameness. Monoparesis may also appear very similar to a true lameness in many cases. Clues to the lameness having a neurogenic origin may include rapid muscle atrophy, reduced proprioception, toe dragging, and reduced spinal reflexes (particularly the pedal withdrawal reflex). However, in many cases electrodiagnostic testing and imaging are required for certainty of diagnosis. Neurogenic lameness can arise from a variety of causes, such as a lateralised disc herniation, peripheral nerve sheath tumour, neuritis, nerve trauma, and degenerative lumbosacral stenosis (DLSS).

DLSS is a common condition with a variety of causes in which the nerves of the cauda equina are variably compressed by adjacent structures at the level of the lumbosacral disc and intervertebral foraminae. These structures include the intervertebral disc, bony structures, such as the articular facets, pedicle, and arch of the sacrum, and other soft tissue structures, including the interarcuate ligament and joint capsules. Because of the different functions supplied by the nerves of the cauda equina at this level, the presentations associated with DLSS can be variable and also similar to orthopaedic diseases such as hip dysplasia. Unilateral lameness may occur if there is significant foraminal stenosis leading to compression of the L7 nerve root which exits the vertebral canal at this level. Bilateral lameness, paresis, and stiffness, as well as pain, are also commonly seen. Ataxia is usually mild or non-existent in these cases.

1.4.13   Pain (Hyperaesthesia)

Pain can be very severe in neurological disease and may be the only presenting sign in some conditions. Pain is defined as the conscious awareness of a noxious stimulus, and requires a conscious response to stimulation of nociceptors. Detecting, interpreting, and localising the source of pain, even when one is reasonably certain it is present, can be a challenge. In some conditions, the pain may be focal but so severe that the animal responds to palpation in multiple regions of the body. At other times, multiple regions of the body may be genuinely painful, but this again may make the examination difficult to interpret.

In the authors' experience, when an animal presents with a history of crying or screaming in pain, a neurological cause should always be considered. There are very few conditions which will induce this reaction in an animal. Orthopaedic conditions, even including fractures, will rarely cause an animal to vocalise unless a peripheral nerve is involved in the fracture site. Visceral pain can be severe, but affected animals usually become dull and depressed rather than vocalise. The pain associated with mechanically pinching or stretching a peripheral nerve is extreme and acute, and is often associated with specific or sudden movements; this history should therefore lead to a high index of suspicion for a neurogenic origin.

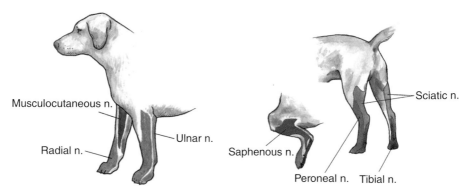

Figure 1.3 The cutaneous autonomous zones of the distal parts of the thoracic limb and the distal parts of the pelvic limb. A knowledge of these zones may assist the clinician in determining which peripheral nerves may be involved in a traumatic injury for instance.

Other potential sources of severe neurogenic pain include inflammation of the meninges, as seen in conditions such as steroid responsive meningitis arteritis (SRMA), stretching of the meninges and/or compression of the nerve roots in intervertebral disc herniation, atlantoaxial instability, certain spinal neoplastic conditions, and inflammation/infection of the intervertebral disc in discospondylitis. The nerves of the cauda equina and tail can be the source of severe pain associated with DLSS or other compressive or inflammatory lesions. In these situations, the presenting signs can be limited to behavioural change or extreme reluctance to lift the tail. An animal presenting with severe pain when defecating may have tail-base pain, which can be associated with intervertebral disc disease at this level. Severe inflammation of the epidural fat and meninges, such as in epidural empyema, may also cause severe pain.

Certain intraparenchymal spinal cord conditions such as syringohydromyelia can present with signs of intermittent crying in pain. In this situation, there appears to be an association with larger lesions and those affecting the dorsolateral horns of the spinal cord. In susceptible breeds, this diagnosis should be considered in an animal presenting with pain only.

When faced with a potentially painful animal, the physical examination becomes crucial in trying to locate the source of the pain, but as already stated this can easily be misinterpreted or misleading. Great care should be taken, and the examination initially performed gently and with minimal movements of head and/or limbs. The amount of movement and pressure applied by palpation can then gradually be increased. If a potentially painful region is identified (e.g. in the thoracolumbar region), the examination should focus on other parts of the body before returning to the suspected region in order to try to elucidate if this is really the source of the pain. Even with this approach, mistakes will be made!

Top tip: Always look for a neurogenic cause when presented with an animal with a history of vocalising in pain.

Don't make this mistake: Be prepared to repeat imaging when an animal remains persistently in pain and a cause of the pain has not been found. Non-displaced vertebral fractures can be missed!

1.4.14 Disorders of Micturition

The ability to pass urine can be affected by many neurological problems, although rarely in isolation. Spinal cord lesions (myelopathies), particularly severe lesions associated with intervertebral disc extrusion, are commonly associated with problems of micturition, and the anatomical level of the myelopathy dictates the nature of the dysfunction. It is necessary to have an understanding of the innervation of the bladder and urethral sphincters in order to appreciate why this is the case.

The bladder is innervated by the pelvic nerve which arises from the sacral spinal cord segments. This provides motor (parasympathetic) innervation to the smooth muscle of the detrusor as well as carrying sensory information from stretch receptors in the bladder wall. The external urethral sphincter (striated muscle) is supplied by the pudendal nerve arising also from S1–S3 spinal cord segments. This is also motor to the anal sphincter and carries sensory information from the perineum. These LMNs receive modulation from the UMNs arising from the micturition centre in the medulla (see Figure 1.4). Problems affecting the spinal cord segments cranial to S1 usually lead to a so-called UMN bladder, whereas problems caudal to L7 normally lead to a LMN bladder.

In the UMN bladder, loss of modulation of the LMNs leads to an increase in tone in both detrusor and external urethral sphincter. The result is a bladder which over-fills to the point at which the pressure from inside the bladder is enough to force leakage through the spastic urethral sphincter. The detrusor muscle can be stretched and, if not treated, irreversible detrusor muscle damage can occur, and this leads to irreversible incontinence.

In the LMN bladder, damage to the LMNs supplying both the detrusor and sphincter muscles leads to a flaccid bladder and sphincter, so that urine leaks out easily and the bladder remains small and flaccid. Lesions that cause this type of presentation usually also cause loss of anal tone, loss of perineal sensation, and,

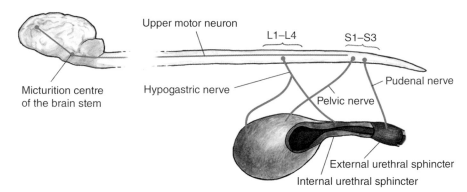

Figure 1.4 The innervation of the urinary tract. The bladder detrusor muscle is innervated mainly by the pelvic nerve (parasympathetic supply) originating in the sacral spinal cord segments (S1–S3), but also by the sympathetic nervous system via the hypogastric nerve, which originates in the lumbar spine. The pelvic nerve carries both motor fibres responsible for contraction of the detrusor muscle in micturition and sensory fibres responsible for detecting bladder wall stretching. In young animals, there is a simple reflex arc involving these fibres, meaning the bladder empties when it is full; in older animals, higher centres in the brainstem and forebrain lead to voluntary control of micturition and the possibility of 'toilet-training'. The external urethral sphincter is a skeletal muscle sphincter innervated by the pudendal nerve, arising from the sacral spinal cord (S1–S3); this nerve also receives upper motor neuron input, as well as carrying sensory information back from the sphincter. The internal urethral sphincter is a smooth muscle thickening of the urethral wall innervated by the sympathetic fibres of the hypogastric nerve.

sometimes, loss of tail function. The prognosis for return to function with this type of injury may be more guarded than for an UMN lesion. A common presentation of LMN bladder that does not always behave in this way is the so-called 'tail-pull' injury seen in cats, when a traumatic incident results in fracture/luxation of sacral or caudal vertebrae. In this situation, the bladder often becomes over-full, as in the UMN bladder, and is difficult to express. This is believed to result from on-going innervation of the internal urethral smooth muscle sphincter by the hypogastric (sympathetic) nerve which arises from more cranially in the lumbar spine. Interestingly, this phenomenon is rarely seen in dogs with fractures of the sacrum for instance.

Reflex dyssynergia is a disorder of micturition where the coordination between contraction of the detrusor muscle and relaxation of the urethral sphincters is lost. This leads to an inability to empty the bladder; the usual presentation is of an over-full bladder with no urethral obstruction and a history of straining and sometimes urine leakage or dripping. The cause of this problem is unknown, and treatment can be challenging.

1.5 Summary

It is clear that diseases of the nervous system may present in a wide variety of different ways, and this presents the first challenge to their diagnosis and treatment. Once it has been decided that a problem is likely to have a neurological origin, the next step is to use the neurological examination to decide where the lesion may be located within the CNS or PNS. It is only at this stage that further investigations should be planned. In the following chapters we shall attempt to present a logical and methodical approach to neurological disease, which should enable the practitioner to develop a good differential diagnosis list when faced with such problems. We also attempt to give sensible, practical advice to owners of animals affected by neurological conditions.

Bibliography

Amin, U. and Benbadis, S.R. (2019). The role of EEG in the erroneous diagnosis of epilepsy. *J. Clin. Neurophysiol.* 36: 294–297.

Añor, S. (2014). Acute lower motor neuron tetraparesis. *Vet. Clin. North Am. Small Anim. Pract.* 44: 1201–1222.

De Risio, L., Bhatti, S., Muñana, K. et al. (2015). International veterinary epilepsy task force consensus proposal: diagnostic approach to epilepsy in dogs. *BMC Vet. Res.* 11: 148.

De Strobel, F., Paluš, V., Vettorato, E., and Cherubini, G.B. (2019). Cervical hyperaesthesia in dogs: an epidemiological retrospective study of 185 cases. *J. Small Anim. Pract.* 60 (7): 404–410.

Díaz Espiñeira, M.M., Viehoff, F.W., and Nickel, R.F. (1998). Idiopathic detrusor-urethral dyssynergia in dogs: a retrospective analysis of 22 cases. *J. Small Anim. Pract.* 39: 264–270.

Forman, O.P., Penderis, J., Hartley, C. et al. (2012). Parallel mapping and simultaneous sequencing reveals deletions in BCAN and FAM83H associated with discrete inherited disorders in a domestic dog breed. *PLoS Genet.* 8: e1002462. https://doi.org/10.1371/journal.pgen.1002462 .Epub 2012 Jan 12.

Ives, E.J., MacKillop, E., and Olby, N.J. (2018). Saccadic oscillations in 4 dogs and 1 cat. *J. Vet. Intern. Med.* 32: 1392–1396.

Jeffery, N.D., Barker, A.K., Hu, H.Z. et al. (2016). Factors associated with recovery from paraplegia in dogs with loss of pain perception in the pelvic limbs following intervertebral disk herniation. *J. Am. Vet. Med. Assoc.* 248: 386–394.

Kitchell, R.L., Whalen, L.R., Bailey, C.S., and Lohse, C.L. (1980). Electrophysiologic studies of cutaneous nerves of the thoracic limb of the dog. *Am. J. Vet. Res.* 41: 61–76.

Komáromy, A.M., Abrams, K.L., Heckenlively, J.R. et al. (2016). Sudden acquired retinal degeneration syndrome (SARDS) – a review and proposed strategies toward a better understanding of pathogenesis, early diagnosis, and therapy. *Vet. Ophthalmol.* 19: 319–331.

Lowrie, M. and Garosi, L. (2016). Classification of involuntary movements in dogs: tremors and twitches. *Vet. J.* 214: 109–116.

Lowrie, M. and Garosi, L. (2017). Classification of involuntary movements in dogs: paroxysmal dyskinesias. *Vet. J.* 220: 65–71.

Lowrie, M., Garden, O.A., Hadjivassiliou, M. et al. (2018). Characterization of paroxysmal gluten-sensitive dyskinesia in border terriers using serological markers. *J. Vet. Intern. Med.* 32: 775–781.

Meeson, R. and Corr, S. (2011). Management of pelvic trauma: neurological damage, urinary tract disruption and pelvic fractures. *J. Feline Med. Surg.* 13: 347–361.

Platt, S.R., Radaelli, S.T., and McDonnell, J.J. (2001). The prognostic value of the modified Glasgow Coma Scale in head trauma in dogs. *J. Vet. Intern. Med.* 15: 581–584.

Rusbridge, C., Stringer, F., and Knowler, S.P. (2018). Clinical application of diagnostic imaging of Chiari-like malformation and syringomyelia. *Front. Vet. Sci.* 5: 280.

Shea, A., Hatch, A., De Risio, L. et al. (2018). Association between clinically probable REM sleep behavior disorder and tetanus in dogs. *J. Vet. Intern. Med.* 32 (6): 2029–2036.

Smith, S.M., Westermeyer, H.D., Mariani, C.L. et al. (2018). Optic neuritis in dogs: 96 cases (1983–2016). *Vet. Ophthalmol.* 21: 442–451.

Tipold, A. and Schatzberg, S.J. (2010). An update on steroid responsive meningitis-arteritis. *J. Small Anim. Pract.* 51: 150–154.

Walmsley, G.L., Herrtage, M.E., Dennis, R. et al. (2006). The relationship between clinical signs and brain herniation associated with rostrotentorial mass lesions in the dog. *Vet. J.* 172: 258–264.

Chapter 2 Clinical History and Signalment

Paul M. Freeman

The ultimate goal of the consultation in the investigation of any neurological problem is to come up with a sensible and reasonably short list of differential diagnoses. This short list can then be used to focus and direct the diagnostic approach, dependent on the client's expectations and budget. To that end, the starting point is taking an appropriate and complete clinical history. The animal's signalment can then be incorporated with this information to formulate a ranked list of differential diagnoses once the general physical and neurological examinations have been performed.

2.1   General Medical History

It is important not to neglect the general medical history when approaching a neurological case. This is particularly relevant when the problem appears to clearly represent a neurological disease, such as generalised seizures. In acute and severe presentations, where time may be important, detailed client questioning should be tempered by the need to start investigations and treatment, such as in cases of status epilepticus or suspected head or spinal trauma. However, important facts pertaining to the ultimate diagnosis may be missed if certain information is not gathered, and the clinician must always be aware of these potentially conflicting demands. Furthermore, many general practitioners will be expected to complete the consultation in a relatively short period of time. The taking of a complete general medical history as well as the specific neurological history, in addition to performing a physical and neurological examination, can therefore put severe time pressures on the consultation. In a non-emergency situation, the option of admitting the animal for a more detailed examination and to allow a longer time for client questioning should always be considered.

A Practical Approach to Neurology for the Small Animal Practitioner, First Edition. Paul M. Freeman and Edward Ives.
© 2020 John Wiley & Sons Ltd. Published 2020 by John Wiley & Sons Ltd.
Companion Website: www.wiley.com/go/freeman/neurology

Potentially important questions from the general medical history may include the following.

a. *How long has the animal in question been in the owner's possession?*
For any suspected neurological disease, one of the key factors to be looked at in the neurological history will be the onset of the problem; if an animal has been 'rescued' or has been owned for a relatively short period of time, and the problem is intermittent, it may not be possible to establish precisely how long the presenting problem has been ongoing. In a case of behavioural change, a knowledge of how this has developed may be very important, and an animal which has not been with the current owner since a puppy or a kitten may exhibit behavioural changes which are due to an alteration in environment or other factors, rather than reflecting a primary brain disorder.

b. *Vaccination status*
There are a number of viral diseases which are largely preventable by appropriate vaccination, but which may be responsible for neurological disease. Canine distemper virus (CDV) was once a major cause of neurological disease, causing a variety of signs including blindness, vestibular syndrome, seizures, and, in particular, myoclonus. In the UK, the frequency of CDV has been greatly reduced by vaccination, although cases are still seen in environments where there are a large number of unvaccinated dogs. It may also cause neurological disease in vaccinated animals, although this is unusual, and signs may be reduced in severity and often not accompanied by systemic disease. Feline leukaemia virus (FeLV) may be associated with lymphoma, which is a relatively common cause of neurological dysfunction in cats, with signs dependent on the specific lesion location. However, FeLV has also been reported to have direct neurotoxic effects, and has been associated with progressive central nervous system (CNS) signs (Hartmann 2012). Feline immunodeficiency virus (FIV) has been associated with an inflammatory encephalopathy as well as polymyositis (Hartmann 2012). Feline panleukopenia virus infection in utero can lead to a syndrome of cerebellar hypoplasia in newborn kittens and is another potential diagnosis which may be suspected simply by knowing the vaccination status.

c. *Anti-parasite treatment*
This has a specific bearing on the likelihood of vascular neurological disease associated with *Angiostrongylus vasorum* infection but may also be important due to the possibility of overdose or adverse reactions. Permethrin toxicity in cats associated with the use of proprietary 'pet-shop' antiparasiticides is well recognised, and certain dog breeds may be at significant risk of neurological signs following treatment with products containing ivermectins. Many Border Collies and some other breeds are affected with a mutation of the MDR gene, leading to a dysfunctional P-glycoprotein complex; this forms an important part of the blood–brain barrier by pumping substances out of the

CNS, and may lead to acute toxicity when such dogs are treated with ivermectins due to accumulation of drug within the CNS.

d. *Travel history (outside and within the country)*

Certain parasite-transmitted diseases that may have neurological manifestations should be included as possible differential diagnoses in animals with a known travel history to regions where these infections are common (e.g. *Ehrlichia canis*, *Leishmania* spp., and *Babesia* spp.). When the affected animal has an unknown travel history, or has been imported or 'rescued' from a country or region where such infections are endemic, their likelihood should also be considered. There is an increasing tendency in the United Kingdom (UK) for canine rehoming centres to import dogs from countries such as Spain and Romania, and these animals may be important as carriers of infectious diseases that may potentially lead to neurological syndromes.

Other diseases may be more common in certain parts of the UK. For example, the canine lungworm *Angiostrongylus vasorum*, which is transmitted through molluscs, may be present in as many as 50% of foxes in the southeast of the UK (Taylor et al. 2015), but appears less common in other parts of the country. This parasite may cause a coagulopathy in affected dogs, which can present as an acute onset of neurological signs. The tick-borne infection *Borrelia burgdorferi*, which results in the condition Lyme disease, is known to be more common in the south and southwest of England and the Scottish Highlands. Although an uncommon cause of neurological disease, exposure to the appropriate environment may increase consideration of this disease as a possible cause of certain presenting signs.

e. *Toxin exposure*

Known, suspected, or potential exposure to neurotoxins is a key part of the clinical history taking for any acute syndrome, particularly for presentations such as whole-body tremor and status epilepticus with no previous seizure history. Mouldy food may contain mycotoxins, which are a common source of tremorgenic toxicity in dogs and can lead to severe and difficult to control tremors, or even status epilepticus. Clues, such as being walked off-lead in areas where food may have been discarded or going missing for a period of time when on a walk, may increase the suspicion of such toxicity. Tremor may also be induced by other toxins including permethrins, organophosphates, hexachlorophene (used as a disinfectant), and bromethalin (a neurotoxic rodenticide). Other potential excitatory neurotoxins include chocolate, caffeine, and amphetamines. Exposure to potential human recreational drugs should also be considered, with many cases of cannabis toxicity being reported in dogs, usually resulting in depression, hypersalivation, mydriasis, and hypermetria; signs may be variable and hyperexcitability and seizures can also be seen. Bear in mind that owners may be reluctant to admit to the possession of illegal recreational drugs, and therefore this line of questioning must be carried out in a careful and sensitive manner. There are many other reported neurotoxic substances to which dogs in particular may be exposed. These include lead, metaldehyde, alphachloralose, and avermectins. The widely used antibiotic metronidazole may cause an acute onset of central vestibular signs, especially at higher or prolonged doses (see Section 6.7 'Vestibular Syndrome'). This may be overlooked if the animal is seen by a different veterinary surgeon to the individual who originally prescribed the drug, or if the animal has been taking the drug for a long period of time (e.g. for chronic diarrhoea). Diagnosis may be difficult or impossible in many cases of intoxication, and therefore careful history taking may be crucial in identifying potential cases of toxic disease.

f. *Previous and concurrent illness*

Cases of neurological disease may present with previous or concurrent systemic disease that could also predispose the animal to the development of neurological signs. Examples include hyper- and hypoadrenocorticism; the former can occasionally present as a myopathic syndrome, or can lead to hypertension and hypercoagulability, which may in turn predispose to cerebrovascular disease. Hypoadrenocorticism ('Addison's disease') may lead to a variety of clinical signs, including episodic weakness or collapse. Hypothyroidism has been linked to a variety of cranial neuropathies, polyneuropathies, and polymyopathy (Bertalan et al. 2013); however, it is frequently difficult to prove a definitive association. Chronic renal disease may lead to hypertension and/or urinary protein loss, the former predisposing to haemorrhagic stroke and the latter to thromboembolic disease, including stroke and aortic thromboembolism. Vascular diseases, such as vasculitis, systemic inflammatory conditions, and non-neurological neoplasia may all either directly or indirectly predispose to neurological disease of some kind. There are some specific, well-documented associations between certain neurological conditions and diseases affecting other body systems which clinicians should also be aware of, such as that between myasthenia gravis and the presence of a thymoma (Robat et al. 2013). In other cases, a paraneoplastic syndrome should be considered when investigating certain generalised conditions, such as a suspected polyneuropathy.

g. *Trauma*

A history of trauma will be known at the time of presentation in the majority of cases; however, this may only be suspected in outdoor cats and in some dogs the animal may have disappeared before presenting with neurological signs. Moderate to severe trauma is usually required to cause signs associated with CNS damage, since both the brain and spinal cord are well protected by the skull, vertebral column, cerebrospinal fluid, and other soft tissues. For this reason, trauma is an uncommon cause of neurological signs in animals which are confined to the house and garden. Whenever trauma is suspected, great care should be taken in moving the animal, since there may be instability of the vertebral column that could lead to further damage to the spinal cord. In cases of head trauma, there may also be a depressed fracture and/or raised intracranial pressure. Acute traumatic injury to the CNS will be considered in more detail in Chapter 7. Peripheral nerve trauma may occur in a variety of ways and should always be considered when an animal presents with a severe monoparesis or single limb neuropathy.

In humans, head trauma can lead to a delayed onset of epilepsy known as post-traumatic epilepsy, and this phenomenon is also thought to occur in dogs and cats (Steinmetz et al. 2013). It can be difficult, if not impossible, to prove a definitive association between prior trauma and a latter diagnosis of 'idiopathic' epilepsy. However, if an animal presents with a history of seizures then asking the question about whether there has been any history of head trauma in the recent or more distant past is a sensible consideration. Vertebral or appendicular trauma can, in rare cases, lead to delayed nerve root or peripheral nerve compression due to callus formation. More often, delayed or malunion limb bone fractures may lead to muscular contracture which can be very difficult to resolve.

h. *General questions regarding the household from which the animal comes from*
General questions may occasionally yield some useful pieces of information that may end up being the clue to unravelling the disease process. In a multi-cat household, viral infection is more likely; in a home with young children, inadvertent trauma may be a consideration. If an infectious disease or toxin ingestion is suspected, a knowledge of whether other animals in the household are similarly affected may be important.

2.2   Specific History of the Neurological Problem

2.2.1   Onset

'When and how did the problem begin?' is one of several key questions, the answers to which provide important information that enables the clinician to draw up the most likely differential diagnoses. Depending on the problem, this may or may not be an easy question for the owner to answer. For instance, in the case of acute onset paraplegia the owner is likely to have a good idea of the day and even the hour that the problem started. However, for other conditions it may not be so easy or so certain. In the case of seizures, the owner may not have been present when the first seizure occurred but may have a suspicion, due to returning home and finding their pet in some sort of distress, or having unusually urinated or defecated in the house. This can be significant, especially when an animal is presented after what is apparently a 'first' seizure event. If, after careful questioning, it appears likely that the event in question may not have been the first, this can affect the decision-making process (see Chapter 6). In cases with a history of mentation or behaviour change, it may be very difficult to establish the precise time of onset, since these may frequently be waxing and waning or may not be obvious until they have become quite severe. Thorough history taking could lead to the realisation that some changes may have been present for longer than the owner initially was aware. This can also be the case with an apparent acute onset of blindness where, as discussed in Chapter 1, visual deterioration may in fact have gone unnoticed until complete blindness occurred.

The nature of the onset of signs is at least as important as the timing of the onset. Disease onset may be either acute (the syndrome developed within minutes to hours), subacute (onset over a few days), or chronic (onset over several days to several weeks). Further subdivision into peracute (instantaneous onset) and acute may also be possible. Frequently, it is difficult to truly categorise the onset of a syndrome, especially when attempting to distinguish between subacute and chronic onset. However, this is less important than establishing the truly acute and peracute onset syndromes, as outlined below.

In Chapter 5, we will discuss in more detail the use of the differential diagnosis mnemonic VITAMIND or DAMNITV; these mnemonics break down potential differential diagnoses into categories of disease, where V is for vascular diseases, I is inflammatory/infectious, T is traumatic/toxic, A is anomalous, M is metabolic, I is idiopathic, N is neoplastic (and nutritional), and D is degenerative. Most diseases fit into a single category although some, such as intervertebral disc disease, may occur either as a degenerative or traumatic process. An understanding of how the different categories of disease behave is crucial in constructing the differential diagnosis list, and the information derived from this part of the history taking is specifically intended to allow certain groups of disease to be eliminated from the differential list of likely causes of the presenting syndrome.

For the categories mentioned above, vascular diseases (such as ischaemic stroke and fibrocartilaginous embolism, FCE) normally have an acute or peracute onset; an exception would be aortic thromboembolism in the dog where signs often develop in a more chronic manner. Inflammatory and infectious diseases (such as meningoencephalomyelitis of unknown origin, MUO) are normally subacute or occasionally acute in onset. Discospondylitis (intervertebral disc infection) may have a more chronic onset, and the protozoal infections of toxoplasmosis and neosporosis may also be more chronic in onset. Trauma should be peracute, and toxic diseases are usually acute in onset. The anomalous disease category includes anatomical abnormalities, both congenital and developmental, and encompasses problems such as hydrocephalus, vertebral anomalies (e.g. hemivertebrae), arachnoid space disorders (e.g. diverticuli and fibrosis), and syringohydromyelia. Onset of signs is usually subacute or chronic, but occasionally may appear to be acute. Metabolic diseases (such as portosystemic shunt, hypoglycaemia, and endocrine disorders) will usually have a subacute onset of signs, although again there can be exceptions to this such as might be the case with an insulinoma where the first sign may be one of collapse or an epileptic seizure due to hypoglycaemia. Idiopathic disease encompasses idiopathic epilepsy and some cranial neuropathies, with onset usually being acute. Neoplastic disease characteristically has a subacute or chronic onset, although spinal neoplasia is often an exception to this rule and may present acutely due to sudden decompensation or even pathological fracture. Finally, degenerative diseases (such as lysosomal storage diseases, cerebellar abiotrophy, and degenerative polyneuropathies) normally have a chronic onset of signs; the exception is Hansen type 1 intervertebral disc disease, where onset of neurological signs is often apparently acute.

2.2.2 Progression

The next key question is: 'How has the problem developed since the onset?' Assuming that the condition has been present for long enough to tell, then a distinction needs to be made between disease states which are improving, deteriorating, static, or waxing and waning. As with the disease onset, this is important for establishing which diseases or categories of disease are more or less likely in the given situation. Most owners will be able to answer this question with reasonable certainty, although differentiating between a static and slowly progressive condition or between a slowly progressive and waxing and waning condition may be more difficult. In a case of suspected seizures, the use of a seizure diary may allow a more objective analysis of disease progression, and video clips taken by the owner at different stages of the disease may also be helpful in establishing the progress of a syndrome. Some conditions may progress from affecting just one or two limbs to affecting all limbs for instance, or an animal may have progressed from paresis to plegia, or vice versa. If a condition is considered to be waxing and waning, then some discussion of the details of when the problem appears better or worse may be helpful in elucidating the underlying cause.

Vascular conditions, which, as stated above, normally have an acute onset, are usually either static or improving by the time the animal is seen by the veterinarian.

Inflammatory and infectious conditions are usually deteriorating, especially if no treatment has been instigated, and a history of acute or subacute onset and relatively rapid deterioration is typical for the inflammatory CNS diseases that are grouped under the term MUO. Some inflammatory diseases, such as steroid responsive meningitis arteritis (SRMA), however, may take a more waxing and waning course.

Traumatic conditions will usually be static or occasionally improving, but rarely deteriorating. Trauma involving either the CNS or PNS will likely produce a peracute onset of deficits which either remain static until there is some intervention, or very gradually improve due to recovery of nervous tissue. Exceptions include unstable fractures, where there may be some deterioration associated with movement, and head trauma, where deterioration may occur due to the development of haematoma and raised intracranial pressure. The so-called traumatic intervertebral disc extrusion, also known as a hydrated nucleus pulposus extrusion or acute non-compressive nucleus pulposus extrusion (ANNPE), may be improving more rapidly than would be expected for other types of traumatic spinal cord injury, and this needs to be borne in mind when considering this differential diagnosis. As will be discussed below, there are other factors that can help to distinguish between a traumatic disc extrusion and bony trauma involving the nervous system, in particular the presence or absence of pain.

Anomalous conditions may be static or deteriorating, dependent on whether they are congenital or developmental. Congenital hydrocephalus, for example, may be expected to lead to static signs, whereas syringomyelia is a progressive condition with an expected progression following diagnosis due to gradual enlargement of the syrinx within the spinal cord. These individual conditions will be discussed in more depth in Chapter 6.

Metabolic diseases often have a waxing and waning disease progression. Hepatic encephalopathy associated with a portosystemic shunt often becomes severe after eating but may improve following a period of relative starvation. Detailed questioning around paroxysmal, intermittent, or waxing and waning conditions may help to elucidate the likely underlying aetiology, or at least provide some clues. With a suspected seizure disorder, asking the owner specifically when the 'seizures' occur and whether anything appears to predispose the animal to an attack may be very important. As mentioned in Chapter 1, true epileptic seizures involve a prodrome and aura that owners may recognise. It has also recently been shown that many owners are able to identify seizure 'triggers' in epileptic dogs (Forsgård et al. 2019), and so-called feline audiogenic reflex seizures have been well described (Lowrie et al. 2016). If an animal only suffers its apparent 'seizure' when excited or exercising, it may be that the episodes are in fact cardiorespiratory syncopal attacks rather than epileptic seizures. Whilst these details are not strictly part of the disease progression, they are important in establishing likely differential diagnoses, which is the primary goal of the consultation.

Neoplastic diseases should have a deteriorating progression with a few exceptions; the only presenting sign of brain neoplasia may be seizures, with the animal being normal in between. The course of progression with CNS neoplasia can be quite rapid, with animals going downhill over a period of days in many cases.

Degenerative conditions also should usually have a progressive deteriorating disease course, although this is usually more slowly progressive over weeks to months. Once again, the exception to this rule is the Hansen type 1 intervertebral disc extrusion, where progression may be more rapid.

2.2.3 **Presence or Absence of Pain**

The identification of pain as part of the presenting syndrome is another key aspect of arriving at the definitive differential diagnosis list. The clinical and neurological examinations may allow the clinician to determine the presence/absence and potential location of any pain, but this is only part of the process. It can also be surprisingly difficult to be certain whether an animal is painful from examination alone. Dogs may have altered pain sensation when examined due to stress; they may react to palpation or head or limb movements in a way which is very inconsistent and variable, and so leave the clinician wondering whether a particular reaction was an indication of pain or not. Cats, on the other hand, tend to become depressed or even aggressive when in pain; they can be difficult or impossible to examine and making any sort of judgement about the presence of pain from the examination can be very difficult.

In these situations, the clinical history may provide important information that can suggest that the animal is in pain. Depression can be an indicator of pain, particularly head pain, in both cats and dogs. Changes in behaviour, such as a reluctance to play, increasing levels of fear and anxiety especially around other people and animals, and even uncharacteristic aggressive behaviour, may all be caused by the presence of pain. Typically, cats want to be left alone, not touched or picked up, and may scratch or bite when handling is attempted. If these sorts of behaviours are reported as a new syndrome in conjunction with the presence of potential neurological signs, then pain should always be suspected. Dogs may exhibit similar behavioural changes, but often will also vocalise when affected by neurogenic pain. Vocalising due to pain in dogs is rare except in neurological disease. Orthopaedic disease, even when severe such as in the case of fractures, luxations, and osteosarcoma, rarely leads to persistent or episodic spontaneous vocalisation. Any condition which causes inflammation or stretching of the meninges, stretching or entrapment of spinal nerve roots or peripheral nerves, or distortion of the dorsal horn of the spinal cord may result in intermittent crying or screaming in pain. An owner reporting this type of behaviour should always lead the clinician to consider the possibility of neurological disease.

When considering the categories of disease in relation to the presence/absence of pain, there are again some generalisations which can be made. Vascular conditions are in general not painful. Exceptions may be conditions such as subdural haemorrhage, where there may be meningeal stretching or inflammation, and aortic thromboembolic (ATE) disease in cats, which leads to an ischaemic neuromyopathy that can be very painful. By contrast, ATE in dogs, as mentioned previously, tends to present as a more chronic and non-painful syndrome associated with partial obstruction to blood flow in the distal aorta.

Inflammatory and infectious diseases are often associated with pain due to the presence of inflammatory cytokines and other factors. Bacterial discospondylitis is typically very painful on spinal palpation, but is less commonly associated with vocalisation because it rarely causes meningeal inflammation or nerve root entrapment. Steroid-responsive meningitis arteritis can be extremely painful, leading to a very depressed animal, although the pain may wax and wane with this condition. Inflammatory conditions of the CNS may be painful, especially when involving the spinal cord. Protozoal infections such as toxoplasmosis and neosporosis are rarely associated with obvious pain, despite the presence of oocysts in multiple tissues provoking often significant inflammation (Barber et al. 1996).

Trauma may often present with pain, as would be expected. The exception here is the acute, traumatic intervertebral disc extrusion of non-degenerate nucleus pulposus material that is not resulting in spinal cord compression. In this condition, the onset is often peracute and associated with some kind of physical activity such as jumping for a ball; the affected animal often vocalises at the time the intervertebral disc extrudes, and may exhibit some signs of pain for up to 24 hours, but beyond this usually appears relatively comfortable. Toxic disease is rarely painful, and the same is true for metabolic diseases. Anomalous conditions vary with respect to pain. Many, such as vertebral anomalies and arachnoid space disorders, may be relatively pain-free, whereas others, such as syringohydromyelia, can be associated with significant pain, discomfort, and vocalising. Atlantoaxial instability often presents with a history of significant intermittent vocalisation.

Neoplasia affecting the central or peripheral nervous systems is commonly painful. Tumours of the brain are often associated with significant depression; much of this may be due to severe headache, although this can only be extrapolated from human reports and clinical improvement following administration of analgesics and corticosteroids. Tumours of the spinal cord may be extradural (e.g. vertebral body osteosarcoma), intradural (e.g. meningioma), or intramedullary (e.g. glioma). Extradural and intradural masses are commonly painful, whereas some intramedullary tumours may not be associated with pain. Neoplasia of the peripheral nerves, such as malignant nerve sheath tumours, commonly present with lameness that is thought to result from pain. However, in these situations vocalising is rare and response to analgesics is often poor.

Degenerative conditions, with the exception of intervertebral disc disease, are rarely painful. Hansen type 1 intervertebral disc extrusions, especially in the cervical region, can be associated with significant pain and vocalisation. Hansen type 2 disc protrusions, on the other hand, may be less painful, being more associated with chronic progressive compression of the spinal cord and minimal inflammation. Unless such a protrusion is lateralised and impinging on a spinal nerve root, these disc protrusions often are accompanied by little or no apparent back pain.

2.2.4   **Response to Medication**

If an animal has previously been presented to you or another veterinary surgeon for the same presenting problem, then careful attention to the owner's reporting of their pet's response to any medications administered or prescribed may further help to refine the list of differential diagnoses. This type of questioning needs to be carried out in a thorough manner, often with reference to the patient's records. Owners may require some prompting to recollect any response to medication given historically. Furthermore, many owners will reply that a medication was not beneficial if the improvement was not permanent, even if there was an initial improvement following its administration.

A response to *analgesics* may support a suspicion that the condition is painful; however, understanding whether the apparent response was real by taking into account all of the medications that were administered and the possibility of a placebo effect is also important. A positive response to *corticosteroid* administration may indicate that the disease is inflammatory or has an inflammatory component. Many of the inflammatory diseases of the CNS already discussed may initially respond to anti-inflammatory doses of corticosteroid, even if they ultimately require immunosuppressive therapy to achieve remission. Again, it is important to remember that corticosteroids have a wide variety of effects. Temporary improvement may therefore be seen following their administration for many neoplastic conditions, where they may reduce peri-tumoural oedema or have a specific anti-neoplastic effect (e.g. lymphoma). Corticosteroids may also lead to improvement in Hansen type 2 intervertebral disc protrusion through a reduction in spinal cord oedema, and may also lead to improvement in some anomalous conditions such as hydrocephalus and syringomyelia due to their ability to reduce the rate of production of cerebrospinal fluid.

An improvement following the administration of a non-steroidal anti-inflammatory drug (NSAID) may be seen in many painful conditions, as well as for some inflammatory conditions. Conditions such as SRMA are commonly associated with pyrexia, and NSAIDs may assist in reducing the fever and thereby improving the condition of the affected animal.

Bacterial infections such as discospondylitis may show a response to antibiotic administration. A relatively common history in such cases may be of a partial response to a standard course of broad-spectrum antibiotics followed by relapse, since this condition typically requires prolonged administration of a suitable antibiotic to achieve a permanent cure.

2.2.5   **History of Asymmetry**

As for the presence or absence of pain, the presence or absence of asymmetry in the presenting neurological signs can assist with formulating the list of differential diagnoses. The neurological examination should establish whether or not the presenting animal shows asymmetry in some way and this may form part of the neuroanatomical localisation. However, it is also important to question the owner about this, as the condition may have changed and evolved with time since the onset. What we are concerned with here is whether there is a significant difference in the level of paresis, ataxia, or proprioceptive dysfunction affecting the limbs on one side of the body relative to the other, or whether there is more obvious or severe hypermetria on one side relative to the other. Many cranial nerve presentations will be asymmetrical due to them having an idiopathic or inflammatory cause. It is worth remembering that the presence of symmetrical cranial nerve deficits, in the absence of other neurological deficits such as a change in the level of mentation, tetraparesis, ataxia, or even breathing difficulties, makes a central (brainstem) lesion unlikely and makes a peripheral cranial neuropathy more likely (see Chapter 4).

The reason why the symmetry of the neurological deficits can be important is that we would generally expect toxic, metabolic, and many degenerative conditions to present with largely symmetrical signs as they do not typically target specific, lateralised regions of the nervous system. Of course, there are always exceptions to every rule, and the presence of asymmetric vestibular signs may be observed for some toxic, metabolic, or degenerative conditions.

In contrast, vascular causes of neurological dysfunction, such as FCE and stroke, usually have a markedly asymmetric presentation. This is due to the bilateral nature of the blood supply to most parts of the brain and spinal cord; it would be uncommon for an FCE to affect both left and right spinal arteries equally and, consequently, it is more common for these cases to present with a significant degree of asymmetry. Inflammatory lesions can occur anywhere in the CNS and there may be multiple lesions affecting different regions; it is therefore common for a degree of asymmetry to be present on the neurological examination for such conditions.

Intervertebral disc disease can be very variable in presentation; in general, the extruded material associated with a Hansen type 1 extrusion lies more to one side of the spinal cord than the other, and the neurological deficits will show a degree of asymmetry to reflect this (e.g. proprioceptive deficits). However, because the spinal cord injury caused by such an extrusion reflects a mixture of initial contusion followed by compression and a cascade of secondary effects, it is also common for the clinical signs to appear quite symmetrical even with a markedly asymmetric extrusion. It has also been documented that the most severely affected side on the neurological examination does not always correlate with the side of the disc extrusion (Smith et al. 1997). For Hansen type 2 disc protrusions, the clinical signs are usually fairly symmetrical because most of these protrusions are relatively midline. However, it is again possible to have a very lateralised, focal protrusion leading to markedly lateralised signs such as monoparesis or unilateral lameness.

Table 2.1 provides a summary of the information regarding the evolution and expected presentations expected with the major categories of neurological disease that are described in more detail above.

Table 2.1

	Onset	Progression	Pain	Symmetrical signs
Vascular	Acute/peracute	Static/improving	Usually no	Often marked asymmetry
Inflammatory/ infectious	Acute/subacute	Deteriorating	Usually yes	
Toxic	Acute			Usually yes
Traumatic	Peracute	Static/improving	Usually yes	
Anomalous	Usually chronic		Variable	
Metabolic	Variable	Often waxing/waning	Usually no	Usually yes
Idiopathic	Variable, often acute		Usually no	
Neoplastic	Usually chronic	Deteriorating	Variable	
Degenerative	Usually chronic	Deteriorating	Variable	

2.3   Signalment

2.3.1   Breed-specific Conditions

Many conditions have been shown to have a significant predilection for a particular breed of dog or cat, and a knowledge of these predilections may be helpful when considering potential differential diagnoses. For some problems, a definite mode of inheritance has been identified within the breed, and genetic testing to confirm the presence of a specific mutation known to predispose to the problem may be available. In other cases, there may be a known over-representation of a certain breed, but the exact cause remains unknown. Tables listing these breed predilections tend to become out of date, even by the time they are ready for production. Genetic testing is a rapidly growing area in veterinary neurology, with new tests becoming available relatively frequently. All of this information is readily available online and we have included links to some of the important genetic testing centres below. What we have attempted to include in the table in 'Appendix : Common breed-associated neurological conditions in cats and dogs' is a list of the more commonly seen problems which have a known breed predilection. This is in order to assist the general practitioner with the recognition of such problems. The list is by no means exhaustive and should not be used to rule out the possibility that a disease may be inherited; it is intended to provide a quick reference of the more common and well-recognised conditions. It is also important to remember that a specific condition should never be excluded just because it has never been reported in that particular breed.

Useful links for genetic testing:

www.ahtdnatesting.co.uk/test-category/canine#

http://www.caninegeneticdiseases.net

2.3.2 Sex-linked Conditions

There are few common neurological diseases which show a significant sex predilection. Probably the most widely known is X-linked muscular dystrophy of male golden retrievers. Feline infectious peritonitis (feline coronavirus) infection is a common cause of neurological disease in the cat, and this has a strong predilection for male cats (Crawford et al. 2017). Spinal nephroblastoma, a tumour which is found in the thoracolumbar region of the spinal cord in young dogs, appears to have a significantly higher occurrence in female dogs as opposed to males (Brewer et al. 2011). However, in general the patient's sex is unlikely to provide much help when considering the list of differential diagnoses.

2.3.3 Age

The age of an animal at presentation clearly has a bearing on the likely differential diagnoses. In general terms, younger animals are more likely to suffer with congenital and inflammatory conditions, whereas neoplastic conditions are more commonly seen in older animals. However, there are many exceptions to these rules, and the practitioner should always be aware of this.

For specific diseases and categories of disease, there are certain observations which can be made.

- *Vascular disease*
  FCE is associated with the presence of an at least partially degenerate intervertebral disc. Therefore, this will be unlikely in very young animals (less than 1 year of age). Most cases of FCE occur in middle-aged larger breeds, although the miniature schnauzer also appears to be a commonly affected breed (Bartholomew et al. 2016). Neither haemorrhagic nor ischaemic stroke has been shown to have a significant age distribution, which may be surprising considering that these conditions are often associated with underlying disease such as hypertension. Some studies have shown a breed association with Cavalier King Charles Spaniels and Greyhounds being overrepresented (Wessmann et al. 2009).
- *Inflammatory/infectious disease*
  SRMA is usually seen in younger dogs and very rarely occurs in dogs over 3 years of age. MUO is generally a disease of younger dogs, although it may be seen at any age. Infectious diseases are more common in younger animals, with feline infectious peritonitis virus being the most common cause of spinal cord disease in cats <2 years of age (Marioni-Henry et al. 2004). However, this virus can also cause neurological disease in much older cats, with the oldest being 10 years in a recent study (Crawford et al. 2017).
- *Anomalous disease*
  Congenital anomalies such as hydrocephalus usually manifest themselves early in life, as would be expected. However, occasionally a diagnosis of hydrocephalus may be made in an older animal, either due to an obstruction to the flow of cerebrospinal fluid caused by a neoplastic or inflammatory lesion, or

due to the progression of a case of congenital hydrocephalus, possibly associated with inflammation or trauma. Many other anatomical abnormalities are developmental and, as such, lead to signs later in life. In some instances, a degenerative process such as an intervertebral disc herniation may occur in association with a congenital vertebral anomaly.

- *Metabolic disease*
  Congenital portosystemic shunts usually lead to signs of hepatic encephalopathy in young, growing animals. However, portosystemic shunts may also be acquired and therefore lead to similar signs in adult dogs or cats.

- *Neoplastic disease*
  As would be expected, most neoplastic disease is seen in older animals. Exceptions include spinal cord nephroblastoma, which is seen in young dogs between 5 months and 4 years, and lymphoma in young dogs and cats (Marioni-Henry et al. 2004).

- *Degenerative disease*
  Lysosomal storage diseases are caused by genetic defects leading to abnormalities of metabolism, with CNS signs often being the earliest to present due to the inability of the CNS neurons to regenerate. As would be expected, signs are usually seen in young animals <1 year of age. However, there are also exceptions with the most significant being Lafora disease; this is a late-onset storage disease occurring in the Miniature Wire-haired Dachshund and Bassett Hound, where the onset of signs occurs later in life. Hansen type 1 intervertebral disc disease can occur at any age from 1 to 2 years, whereas Hansen type 2 disc disease typically occurs in middle-aged and older animals.

2.4 Summary

All of these signalment features are merely guides to the clinician, enabling sensible use of what is currently known from the literature and from our own experience. There will always be exceptions to any rule, and when faced with a neurological disease it is wise to keep an open mind when it comes to differential diagnoses. However, by following the basic guidelines set out in this text and combining these with the neuroanatomical localisation resulting from the neurological examination (see Chapters 3 and 4), it will usually be possible to come up with a relatively short, rational, and evidence-based list. This should then allow a sensible dialogue with the pet's owner regarding an investigation and treatment plan. The aim of this book is to provide the general practitioner with an uncomplicated and logical approach to veterinary neurology, and not a comprehensive list of disease descriptions for which much information already exists. However, many of the individual conditions mentioned above will be discussed in greater detail in Chapter 6.

Appendix: Common breed-associated neurological conditions in cats and dogs

Breed	Disease	Signs	Genetic test
Abyssinian cat	Myasthenia gravis	Weakness	No
Airedale	Cerebellar degeneration	Cerebellar signs 3 months	No
Alaskan Malamute	Hereditary polyneuropathy	Tetraparesis 11–18 months	No
Basset Hound	Cervical spondylomyelopathy (wobbler syndrome)	Progressive tetraparesis, neck pain	No
	Hansen type 1 intervertebral disc extrusion	Depends on location	No
Beagle	Idiopathic epilepsy	Seizures 6 months to 6 years	No
	Steroid responsive meningitis arteritis	Pain and pyrexia <3 years	No
	Hansen type 1 intervertebral disc extrusion	Depends on location	No
Bernese Mountain Dog	Steroid-responsive meningitis arteritis	Pain and pyrexia <3 years	No
	Degenerative myelopathy	Progressive paraparesis and ataxia >5 years	Yes
Border Collie	Idiopathic epilepsy	Seizures 6 months to 6 years	No
	Sensory neuropathy	Progressive ataxia 2–6 months	Yes
	Fibrocartilage embolism	Acute asymmetrical myelopathy	No
Border Terrier	Paroxysmal gluten-sensitive dyskinesia (Spike's disease)	Cramping +/– GI or skin signs 1–8 years	No
Boxer	Steroid-responsive meningitis arteritis	Pain and pyrexia <3 years	No
	Immune-mediated polymyositis	Generalised weakness, myalgia, atrophy	No
	Degenerative myelopathy	Progressive paraparesis and ataxia >5 years	Yes
	Idiopathic head-bobbing	Episodic head bobbing <2 years	No
	Idiopathic epilepsy	Seizures 6 months to 6 years	No
	Primary brain tumour	Depends on location	No
Cavalier King Charles Spaniel	Syringomyelia/Chiari-like malformation	Pain, pruritis 2–6 years	No
	Episodic falling	Episodic hypertonicity and collapse <1 year	Yes
	Idiopathic epilepsy	Seizures 6 months to 6 years	No
	Stroke	Acute brain signs	No
Chihuahua	Hydrocephalus	Forebrain signs, usually congenital	No
	Necrotising meningoencephalitis	Brain signs, usually young	No
	Atlantoaxial instability	Neck pain, tetraparesis, <1 year	No
Cocker Spaniel	Hansen type 1 intervertebral disc extrusion	Depends on location	No

Breed	Disease	Signs	Genetic test
Dachshund	Hansen type 1 intervertebral disc extrusion	Depends on location	No
	Idiopathic epilepsy	Seizures 6 months to 6 years	No
	Lafora disease	Progressive myoclonic seizures >3 years	Yes
	Narcolepsy/cataplexy	Sudden episodic collapse/sleep	Yes
	Congenital myasthenia gravis	Episodic weakness 1–2 months	No
Dalmatian	Congenital deafness	Deafness	No
	Cervical spondylomyelopathy (wobbler syndrome)	Progressive tetraparesis, neck pain	No
	Laryngeal paralysis polyneuropathy complex	Stridor, weakness 4–6 months	No
Dobermann	Cervical spondylomyelopathy (wobbler syndrome)	Progressive tetraparesis, neck pain	No
	Congenital deafness and vestibular disease	Deafness/vestibular syndrome	No
	Dancing Dobermann disease	Intermittent pelvic limb gait abnormality	No
English Bulldog	Vertebral malformation	Often asymptomatic	No
	Idiopathic head bobbing	Episodic head bobbing <2 years	No
	Cerebellar degeneration	Cerebellar signs 3 months	No
French Bulldog	Vertebral malformation	Paraparesis, ataxia, incontinence	No
	Hansen type 1 intervertebral disc extrusion	Depends on location	No
	Idiopathic head bobbing	Episodic head bobbing <2 years	No
German Shepherd Dog	Degenerative myelopathy	Progressive paraparesis and ataxia >5 years	Yes
	Cervical spondylomyelopathy (wobbler syndrome)	Progressive tetraparesis, neck pain	No
	Idiopathic epilepsy	Seizures 6 months to 6 years	No
	Gracilis muscle contracture	Non-painful pelvic limb lameness	No
	Immune-mediated polymyositis	Generalised weakness, myalgia, atrophy	No
	Acquired myasthenia gravis	Episodic weakness, megaoesophagus	No
	Hansen type 2 intervertebral disc herniation	Depends on location	No
Golden Retriever	Idiopathic epilepsy	Seizures 6 months to 6 years	No
	X-linked muscular dystrophy	Stiffness, muscle atrophy 2–3 months males	Yes
	Acquired myasthenia gravis	Episodic weakness, megaoesophagus	No
Gordon Setter	Cerebellar degeneration	Cerebellar signs 3 months	Yes

Breed	Disease	Signs	Genetic test
Great Dane	Cervical spondylomyelopathy (osseous wobbler syndrome)	Tetraparesis 6–18 months	No
	Orthostatic tremor	Weight-bearing tremor of limbs	No
	Inherited myopathy	Generalised weakness 6 months	No
	Distal symmetrical polyneuropathy	Paraparesis or tetraparesis 1–5 years	No
Greyhound	Steroid-responsive meningitis arteritis	Pain and pyrexia <3 years	No
	Stroke	Acute brain signs	No
Jack Russell Terrier	Hereditary (spinocerebellar) ataxia	Progressive cerebellar ataxia >2 months	Yes
Labrador Retriever	Idiopathic epilepsy	Seizures 6 months to 6 years	No
	Exercise-induced collapse	Weakness after strenuous exercise	Yes
	Acquired laryngeal paralysis/ polyneuropathy	Progressive dysphonia, stridor, cough >6 years	No
Leonberger	Inherited polyneuropathy	Tetraparesis and typical gait 1–2 years	Yes
Maltese Terrier	Idiopathic tremor ('little white shaker')	Generalised tremor	No
	Syringomyelia/Chiari-like malformation	Pain, pruritis 2–6 years	No
Miniature Schnauzer	Myotonia congenita	Stiffness and collapse	Yes
Nova Scotia Duck Tolling Retriever	Steroid-responsive meningitis arteritis	Pain and pyrexia <3 years	No
Newfoundland	Immune-mediated polymyositis	Generalised weakness, myalgia, atrophy	No
Old English Sheepdog	Cerebellar degeneration	Cerebellar signs 3 months	Yes
Pembroke Welsh Corgi	Degenerative myelopathy	Progressive paraparesis and ataxia >8 years	Yes
Poodle	Idiopathic epilepsy	Seizures 6 months to 6 years	No
	Hansen type 1 intervertebral disc extrusion	Depends on location	No
Pug	Vertebral malformation and arachnoid space disorder	Paraparesis, ataxia, incontinence	No
	Necrotising meningoencephalitis	Brain signs, usually young	No
Rottweiler	Adult onset and juvenile polyneuropathies	Weakness, tetraparesis +/− stridor	No
	Several congenital/juvenile myopathies	Weakness, stiffness, paresis	No
	Spinal arachnoid diverticulum	Progressive tetraparesis and ataxia, adult	No
St Bernard	Idiopathic epilepsy	Seizures 6 months to 6 years	No
	Polyneuropathy	Weakness, laryngeal paralysis	Yes

Breed	Disease	Signs	Genetic test
Springer Spaniel	Hypomyelination	Congenital tremor	No
Siamese cat	Congenital pendular nystagmus	Permanent pendular eye tremor	No
Staffordshire Bull Terrier	L-2-Hydroxyglutaric aciduria	Progressive ataxia, seizures, encephalopathy	Yes
Hungarian Vizsla	Idiopathic epilepsy	Seizures 6 months to 6 years	No
Weimaraner	Steroid-responsive meningitis arteritis	Pain and pyrexia <3 years	No
	Hypomyelination	Generalised tremor from 3 weeks	No
West Highland White Terrier	Idiopathic tremor ('little white shaker')	Generalised tremor	No
Yorkshire Terrier	Necrotising leukoencephalitis	Brain signs, usually young	No
	Atlantoaxial instability	Neck pain, tetraparesis, <1 year	No
	Syringomyelia/Chiari-like malformation	Pain, pruritis 2–6 years	No
	Portosystemic shunt/hepatic encephalopathy	Waxing/waning encephalopathy, young	No

Bibliography

Barber, J.S., Payne-Johnson, C.E., and Trees, A.J. (1996). Distribution of *Neospora caninum* within the central nervous system and other tissues of six dogs with clinical neosporosis. *J. Small Anim. Pract.* 37: 568–574.

Bartholomew, K.A., Stover, K.E., Olby, N.J., and Moore, S.A. (2016). Clinical characteristics of canine fibrocartilaginous embolic myelopathy (FCE): a systematic review of 393 cases (1973–2013). *Vet. Rec.* 179: 650.

Bertalan, A., Kent, M., and Glass, E. (2013). Neurologic manifestations of hypothyroidism in dogs. *Compend. Contin. Educ. Vet.* 35: E2.

Brewer, D.M., Cerda-Gonzalez, S., Dewey, C.W. et al. (2011). Spinal cord nephroblastoma in dogs: 11 cases (1985–2007). *J. Am. Vet. Med. Assoc.* 238: 618–624.

Brutlag, A. and Hommerding, H. (2018). Toxicology of marijuana, synthetic cannabinoids, and cannabidiol in dogs and cats. *Vet. Clin. North Am. Small. Anim. Pract.* 48: 1087–1102.

Cardy, T.J., De Decker, S., Kenny, P.J., and Volk, H.A. (2015). Clinical reasoning in canine spinal disease: what combination of clinical information is useful? *Vet. Rec.* 177: 171.

Crawford, A.H., Stoll, A.L., Sanchez-Masian, D. et al. (2017). Clinicopathologic features and magnetic resonance imaging findings in 24 cats with histopathologically confirmed neurologic feline infectious peritonitis. *J. Vet. Intern. Med.* 31: 1477–1486.

Forsgård, J.A., Metsähonkala, L., Kiviranta, A.M. et al. (2019). Seizure-precipitating factors in dogs with idiopathic epilepsy. *J. Vet. Intern. Med.* 33 (2): 701–707.

Garosi, L., Dawson, A., Couturier, J. et al. (2010). Necrotizing cerebellitis and cerebellar atrophy caused by *Neospora caninum* infection: magnetic resonance imaging and clinicopathologic findings in seven dogs. *J. Vet. Intern. Med.* 24: 571–578.

Giza, E.G., Płonek, M., Nicpoń, J.M., and Wrzosek, M.A. (2016). Electrodiagnostic studies in presumptive primary hypothyroidism and polyneuropathy in dogs with reevaluation during hormone replacement therapy. *Acta Vet. Scand.* 58: 32.

Gredal, H., Willesen, J.L., Jensen, H.E. et al. (2011). Acute neurological signs as the predominant clinical manifestation in four dogs with *Angiostrongylus vasorum* infections in Denmark. *Acta Vet. Scand.* 53: 43.

Hartmann, K. (2012). Clinical aspects of feline retroviruses: a review. *Viruses* 4: 2684–2710.

Lowrie, M., Bessant, C., Harvey, R.J. et al. (2016). Audiogenic reflex seizures in cats. *J. Feline Med. Surg.* 18 (4): 328–336.

Mandara, M.T., Motta, L., and Calò, P. (2016). Distribution of feline lymphoma in the central and peripheral nervous systems. *Vet. J.* 216: 109–116.

Mariani, C.L., Shelton, S.B., and Alsup, J.C. (1999). Paraneoplastic polyneuropathy and subsequent recovery following tumor removal in a dog. *J. Am. Anim. Hosp. Assoc.* 35: 302–305.

Marioni-Henry, K., Vite, C.H., Newton, A.L., and Van Winkle, T.J. (2004). Prevalence of diseases of the spinal cord of cats. *J. Vet. Intern. Med.* 18: 851–858.

Nelson, O.L., Carsten, E., Bentjen, S.A., and Mealey, K.L. (2003). Ivermectin toxicity in an Australian Shepherd dog with the MDR1 mutation associated with ivermectin sensitivity in collies. *J. Vet. Intern. Med.* 17: 354–356.

Parzefall, B., Driver, C.J., Benigni, L., and Davies, E. (2014). Magnetic resonance imaging characteristics in four dogs with central nervous system neosporosis. *Vet. Radiol. Ultrasound* 55: 539–546.

Robat, C.S., Cesario, L., Gaeta, R. et al. (2013). Clinical features, treatment options, and outcome in dogs with thymoma: 116 cases (1999–2010). *J. Am. Vet. Med. Assoc.* 243: 1448–1454.

Ryan, R., Gutierrez-Quintana, R., Ter Haar, G., and De Decker, S. (2017). Prevalence of thoracic vertebral malformations in French bulldogs, Pugs and English bulldogs with and without associated neurological deficits. *Vet. J.* 221: 25–29.

Smith, J.D., Newell, S.M., Budsberg, S.C., and Bennett, R.A. (1997). Incidence of contralateral versus ipsilateral neurological signs associated with lateralised Hansen type I disc extrusion. *J. Small Anim. Pract.* 38: 495–497.

Steinmetz, S., Tipold, A., and Löscher, W. (2013). Epilepsy after head injury in dogs: a natural model of posttraumatic epilepsy. *Epilepsia* 54: 580–588.

Taylor, C.S., Garcia Gato, R., Learmount, J. et al. (2015). Increased prevalence and geographic spread of the cardiopulmonary nematode *Angiostrongylus vasorum* in fox populations in Great Britain. *Parasitology* 142: 1190–1195.

Tipold, A. and Schatzberg, S.J. (2010). An update on steroid responsive meningitis-arteritis. *J. Small Anim. Pract.* 51: 150–154.

Wessmann, A., Chandler, K., and Garosi, L. (2009). Ischaemic and haemorrhagic stroke in the dog. *Vet. J.* 180: 290–303.

Chapter 3 The 'Stress-free' Neurological Examination

Edward Ives

The neurological examination can strike fear in the hearts of many practitioners, often due to a lack of confidence in its interpretation or the belief that it is a confusing and time-consuming process. However, the neurological examination is a simple, focused assessment that, with practice, can be approached with the same confidence as for the general clinical examination. This should make neurology more approachable and encourage you to perform repeated examinations in more animals. The primary goal of this process is to make the neurological examination as 'stress-free' as possible for the veterinarian, the owner, and the animal involved. This is particularly true for nervous or aggressive animals, when the most useful information can often be gleaned from simple observation in a calm environment.

3.1 Why Perform a Neurological Examination?

In contrast to diseases affecting other body systems, in which specific tissues and organs can be palpated, auscultated, or directly visualised, the majority of disorders affecting the nervous system can only be identified by recognising their impact on normal neurological function. This almost invariably represents abnormal, reduced neurological function, termed a neurological deficit; an exception being the excessive, involuntary movements observed during epileptic seizures or certain forms of movement disorder. In order to recognise neurological deficits, the spectrum of normal neurological function between individuals and species must be known, which underlies the importance of regularly performing a complete neurological examination.

The neurological deficits identified on examination reflect the location of the lesion and not the cause. It is therefore essential to identify this location before

A Practical Approach to Neurology for the Small Animal Practitioner, First Edition. Paul M. Freeman and Edward Ives.
© 2020 John Wiley & Sons Ltd. Published 2020 by John Wiley & Sons Ltd.
Companion Website: www.wiley.com/go/freeman/neurology

considering what type of disease process could result in a lesion at that location. The most common error is jumping straight to possible causes and planning further investigations without first performing a full neurological examination.

The aim of the neurological examination is to answer two questions:

1. *Does this animal have a disorder affecting the nervous system?*
   As discussed in Chapter 1, answering this question will ensure that conditions affecting other body systems (e.g. orthopaedic, cardiovascular, metabolic) are also considered. These conditions can mimic neurological disease and their early identification will ensure that the most appropriate further investigations are chosen in the first instance.
2. *Where is the lesion?*
   This is termed the neuroanatomic localisation. The aim is to identify the site of a single lesion that could explain all of the neurological deficits found on examination. Less commonly, diseases may present with multiple lesions scattered throughout the nervous system (e.g. inflammatory diseases), whilst others may cause diffuse and symmetrical dysfunction (e.g. toxic or metabolic disorders). The possibility of a multifocal or diffuse disease should always be considered in cases that present with a combination of neurological deficits that cannot be explained by a single, focal lesion.

The neuroanatomic localisation can then be used in combination with the clinical history (e.g. signalment, onset, and progression of the clinical signs) to achieve the following:

- *Formulate a problem list and a ranked list of differential diagnoses.* This process is discussed in Chapter 5.
- *Estimate disease severity and potential prognosis.* As clinicians we are often focused on achieving a definitive diagnosis; however, one of the most important pieces of information for an owner is the anticipated prognosis for their pet.
- *Plan and guide the most appropriate diagnostic investigations to rule in/out the differential diagnoses.* As an example, deciding whether spinal radiography would be useful prior to referral for advanced imaging (if possible) is entirely dependent upon your differential diagnoses. Spinal radiography would be an excellent choice if your lesion localises to the vertebral column and your differential diagnoses include a vertebral malformation (e.g. atlantoaxial subluxation), discospondylitis, or an osteolytic lesion (Figure 3.1). However, spinal radiography may be unrewarding if your top differential diagnoses include intervertebral disc disease or degenerative myelopathy.

The neuroanatomic localisation is also vital for deciding where to focus any subsequent diagnostic imaging. Imaging the entire spine, particularly using radiography or magnetic resonance imaging (MRI), is a time-consuming

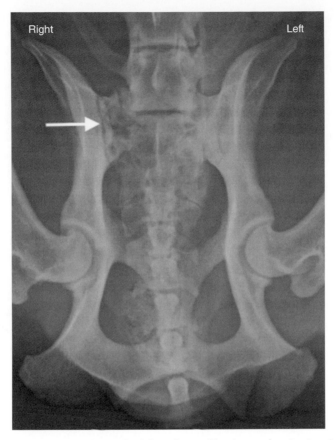

Figure 3.1 A ventrodorsal radiograph of the pelvis and lumbosacral region in a 12-year-old, male neutered Labrador retriever with a 4-week history of weight loss and progressive right pelvic limb lameness and paresis. There was marked discomfort on palpation of the lumbosacral spine and radiography demonstrated an osteolytic and proliferative lesion affecting the right side of the sacrum at the level of the sacroiliac joint (arrow). A neoplastic process was suspected in this case, but further investigations would be required to definitively characterise the lesion.

and inefficient process that is costly for the owner unless completely necessary. Focusing your imaging to the region of interest also means that it is easier to determine the clinical significance of any observed abnormalities (e.g. spondylosis deformans, in situ intervertebral disc mineralisation, or disc space narrowing).

3.2 When to Perform a Neurological Examination

A neurological examination should be performed in every animal that presents with clinical signs that could reflect a lesion affecting the nervous system. This decision may be easy in animals with a convincing history of epileptic seizures or marked neurological dysfunction (e.g. pelvic limb paralysis). However, the possibility of a neurological disorder can be overlooked in animals with conditions that mimic disorders affecting other body systems, or in those that present with subtle or vague clinical signs (e.g. lethargy, lameness, collapsing episodes).

Performing the neurological examination on a regular basis should increase your confidence in its interpretation and will assist in the appreciation of the broad spectrum of normal variation between different breeds and individuals. Therefore, taking the time to perform a full neurological examination is always valuable and should be carried out in every case if time allows. However, as one gains in confidence a smaller number of more focused examinations can often be chosen.

3.3 Where to Perform a Neurological Examination

The neurological examination should ideally be performed in a quiet, unrestricted environment that allows adequate time and space for observation of the animal's demeanour, gait, and interaction with the environment. This initial observation can usually be performed when taking the history from the owner. Other basic screening tests can be performed in the consultation room, but often this is not the ideal environment for a more thorough examination. Therefore, if the clinical history is suggestive of neurological disease, an owner should be reassured that admitting their pet into the hospital for further assessment is the most important first step and by far the best use of their money before performing other clinical investigations.

The ideal environment for a neurological examination would be an uncluttered, enclosed room that allows for unrestricted movement of the dog or cat, and that does not have potential hiding places or escape routes. A non-slip floor is most useful for assessing gait and performing proprioceptive testing but is often impractical for most hospitals in terms of hygiene and allowing deep cleaning. A roll of rubber matting can be stored for this purpose and used at the time of examinations. Observation of the gait on both smooth and non-slip surfaces can sometimes assist in the identification of more subtle proprioceptive deficits, which will be more obvious on surfaces with less grip. Black out blinds, or a room without external windows, can be useful when performing retinal examination and for the assessment of pupil abnormalities.

For dogs that present with a history of lameness, gait abnormalities, or exercise intolerance, lead walking on a concrete surface at various speeds of gait can be extremely informative. An audible 'scuff' may be heard in animals that do not flex their limbs sufficiently during protraction; this could indicate either a mechanical resistance to flexion, reluctance to flex the limb, or a proprioceptive deficit. Encouraging an animal to perform tight circles, figure-of-eight walking, or walking up and down a kerb can also reveal more subtle gait abnormalities. Stair climbing can be used to accentuate the excessive limb flexion associated with cerebellar lesions (hypermetria).

3.4   How to Perform the Neurological Examination

As previously discussed, the aim of the neurological examination is to determine whether an animal may have a neurological disorder, and the location of the lesion(s) responsible if this is the case. Performing a complete neurological examination should always be encouraged; however, this may not be possible in all animals. The choice of the most appropriate tests in an individual animal is dependent on the presenting clinical signs, the tolerance of the dog or cat to handling, and the presence of significant pain or a history of trauma that would limit the ability to perform certain tests. For example, the gag reflex or pupillary light reflex (PLR) may be difficult to perform and interpret in a stressed or aggressive animal, with the results unlikely to influence your neuroanatomic localisation in many cases.

The neurological examination can be broadly divided into a number of parts, involving assessment of:

1. mentation
2. gait and posture
3. cranial nerves
4. postural reactions (proprioceptive testing)
5. spinal reflexes
6. palpation and assessment for regions of apparent discomfort.

When performing the neurological examination, the clinician should further consider two distinct phases:

- an initial period of observation ('hands-off' assessment)
- followed by a more 'hands-on' assessment to screen different regions of the nervous system in a logical manner.

It cannot be overstated how important the initial period of observation is, but this is often overlooked in favour of immediately performing more focused tests. This initial period of observation allows for a broad assessment of the animal, time to process that information, and can reveal subtle deficits that would be missed if the animal were restrained for other tests. A preliminary neuroanatomic localisation can be formed on the basis of the history and observation of the animal alone, which can then be further interrogated by the choice of specific 'hands-on' tests. This approach allows for an efficient and rewarding examination that is as stress-free as possible for all involved.

If abnormalities are identified at any stage of the examination, then they should be added to the problem list and both neurological and non-neurological causes should be considered for each abnormality in turn.

3.4.1 Observation: 'Hands-Off' Assessment

This vital part of the examination can usually be performed whilst taking the clinical history and involves observation of the animal as it roams around the consultation room without the restriction of its lead or owner.

The key questions to consider when observing the patient are:

- Is this animal interacting with the owner and environment as expected?
- Are the limbs, head, and body held in a normal position?
- If the animal can walk, is the gait normal?
- Are there any involuntary movements or muscle contractions?
- Does the face look symmetrical?
- Can the animal blink voluntarily?

1. Level of alertness and interaction with the environment

The level of alertness or wakefulness is primarily determined by diffuse stimulation of the cerebral cortex from an extensive neuroanatomical structure residing within the brainstem called the ascending reticular activating system (ARAS). Focal lesions affecting the ARAS in the brainstem, or more diffuse lesions affecting its cortical projections via the thalamus or the cerebral cortex itself, may result in a diminished level of alertness (Box 3.1). This can range from mild obtundation to coma, dependent on the severity, extent, and location of the lesion.

- *Obtundation.* A subjectively quiet state in which the animal is less responsive to commands, interaction, or stimulation. As discussed in Chapter 1, the term 'depressed' has also been used in veterinary medicine to describe a similar reduced level of alertness. However, this term should be used with caution in

---

Box 3.1 Level of Alertness and Interaction with the Environment

- Non-neurological: primary behavioural disorder, pain, systemic disease, adverse effects of medications.
- Neurological: brainstem or forebrain lesion.

Top tip: Animals will often, but not exclusively, circle towards the side of a forebrain lesion.

Don't make this mistake: Some animals may be particularly sensitive to certain medications (e.g. methadone, buprenorphine, apomorphine). This can result in significant short-term changes in the level of mentation and mimic primary intracranial disease or a deteriorating mental status. Serial examinations are advised if this is suspected.

animal species due to its association with specific mental health conditions in human medicine.

- *Stupor.* Unconscious but responsive to painful stimuli.
- *Coma.* Unconscious and no response to painful stimuli.

Lesions affecting other regions of the forebrain, particularly those involving the limbic system, can result in various behaviour changes that appear inappropriate in a given situation or environment, such as:

- *Compulsive pacing around the consultation room.*
- *Becoming stuck in corners or confined spaces.*
- *Circling in a particular direction.* Compulsive circling often indicates a unilateral lesion affecting the forebrain or brainstem (see Video 22). It may also be seen in association with a head tilt and ataxia in cases with vestibular dysfunction. Whether the circling appears wide or tight does not appear reliable for determining the specific location of a lesion.
- *Bumping into furniture.*
- *Sleeping throughout the consultation or appearing disinterested.*
- *Reduced interaction with the owner.*

Judging how appropriate an animal's behaviour appears to be at the time of examination is complicated by the wide range of normal variation between different individuals. This will therefore always represent a subjective impression rather than an objective assessment. An owner is often the best source of information regarding their pet's normal behaviour and response to veterinary assessment, and this information can be very useful in determining the significance of a subjectively quiet or withdrawn animal.

The apparent level of alertness and interaction with the environment can also be influenced by other factors, which should always be considered when interpreting these findings:

- *visual deficits* (e.g. cataracts, progressive retinal atrophy, sudden acquired retinal degeneration, optic nerve lesions, cortical blindness)
- *pain* (e.g. abdominal, orthopaedic, spinal)
- *pyrexia or systemic disease* (e.g. hypovolaemia, sepsis)
- *cardiorespiratory disease*
- *medications* (e.g. sedatives, analgesics, anti-epileptic medications).

The behaviour of cats can be particularly difficult to interpret as many become nervous, are reluctant to walk, or seek hiding places when placed into a foreign environment. However, a general impression as to how appropriate their behaviour appears can usually be determined throughout the examination and interpreted in the light of other examination findings.

2. Abnormal posture

Abnormal postures can be divided into those affecting the head, limbs, individual joints, the entire body, spine, or tail.

a. Head position

Head tilt. This posture is characterised by rotation of the head in the transverse plane so that one ear is held lower than the other (Figure 3.2 and Box 3.2).

Head turn. This posture is characterised by a lateral turn of the head to one side with the ears remaining horizontal (Box 3.3).

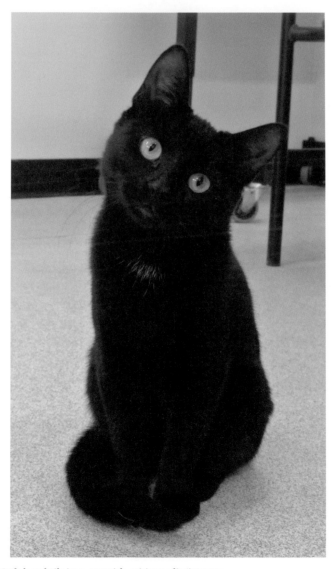

Figure 3.2 Left head tilt in a cat with otitis media/interna.

Box 3.2 Head Tilt

- Non-neurological: aural irritation, aural haematoma.
- Neurological: vestibular syndrome (central or peripheral).

Top tip: Whilst uncommon, bilateral vestibular syndrome will not result in a head tilt as the output from the vestibular nuclei on each side remains balanced. This syndrome is often characterised by wide head excursions from side to side.

Don't make this mistake: Previous episodes of vestibular syndrome may leave a residual head tilt. This has the potential to confuse future neurological examinations if this history is not available.

Box 3.3 Head Turn

- Non-neurological: paraspinal cervical mass resulting in mechanical deviation of the head.
- Neurological: forebrain lesion, vertebral malformation (scoliosis), neck pain.

Top tip: As for circling, the direction of a head turn is most commonly towards the side of a forebrain lesion.

---

b. Limb and joint position

Abnormal positioning of one or more limbs when standing, excessive joint flexion, or excessive joint extension can be the result of many different neurological and non-neurological causes (Box 3.4). A thorough general clinical examination, orthopaedic assessment, and neurological examination are therefore required to distinguish between these different causes.

Wide-based stance. Often observed secondary to lesions affecting the knowledge of where the affected limbs are in space (proprioceptive deficit), or as an attempt to correct for balance loss in cases with vestibular and/or cerebellar dysfunction.

Narrow-based stance. Animals with proprioceptive deficits may variably adopt a narrow- or wide-based stance when standing, or if they abruptly stop when walking.

Poor joint extension. An inability to extend a joint can be caused by mechanical disruption to the structures involved in maintaining joint stability (ligaments, tendons), or a weakness of the extensor muscles associated with that joint. The most commonly affected joints are the elbow (triceps muscle innervated by the radial nerve), stifle (quadriceps muscle innervated by the femoral nerve – see Figure 3.3), and hock (gastrocnemius muscle innervated by the tibial branch of the sciatic nerve).

Box 3.4 Limb and Joint Position

Poor elbow extension:

- Non-neurological: triceps tendon rupture.
- Neurological: C7–T2 spinal cord segments, C7–T2 nerve roots, radial nerve injury.

Poor stifle extension:

- Non-neurological: cruciate ligament rupture (unilateral or bilateral), patellar fracture, patellar tendon injury.
- Neurological: L4–L6 spinal cord segments, L4–L6 nerve roots, femoral nerve injury.

Poor hock extension:

- Non-neurological: Achilles tendon rupture, calcaneal fracture.
- Neurological: L6–S1 spinal cord segments, L6–S1 nerve roots, sciatic-tibial nerve injury.

Top tip: Carpal hyperextension is most commonly the result of palmar carpal ligament insufficiency (chronic or acute) rather than representing a primary neuropathy (Figure 3.4). This posture can also be observed in some dogs with congenital myopathies.

Don't make this mistake: Dogs with bilateral cruciate ligament rupture show reluctance to walk and a crouched pelvic limb posture that can be easily confused with paraparesis as a result of spinal cord disease. However, proprioception will be normal in the pelvic limbs and orthopaedic examination in these cases will reveal stifle swelling, discomfort on stifle extension, and joint instability.

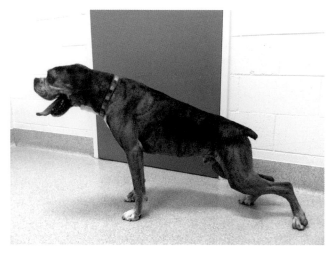

Figure 3.3 Reduced extension of the stifle joints in a 10-year-old boxer dog with chronic degenerative radiculomyelopathy (CDRM). Note also the wide-based pelvic limb stance and worn nails of both pelvic limbs, suggestive of bilateral proprioceptive dysfunction.

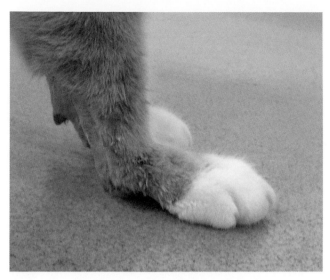

Figure 3.4 Bilateral carpal hyperextension in a cat with palmar carpal ligament insufficiency that was exacerbated after jumping out of a window.

c. Body and spinal postures

A number of terms are used to describe different body or spinal postures, some of which may help guide the neuroanatomic localisation.

Decerebrate rigidity. A body posture that is characterised by rigid extension of all limbs and extension of the neck (opisthotonus). This posture results from lesions at the level of the midbrain, or can be seen secondary to severe, diffuse forebrain lesions. Animals presenting in this posture will have a markedly reduced level of mentation (stupor or coma) and should be treated as a neurological emergency.

Decerebellate rigidity. Severe dysfunction of the rostral cerebellum can result in a posture that is similar in appearance to decerebrate rigidity; however, important differences are that the pelvic limbs are often held flexed at the hips and the animal remains alert and responsive to external stimuli (Figure 3.5).

Schiff–Sherrington posture. This posture is characterised by increased extensor muscle tone in the thoracic limbs following an acute T3–L3 spinal cord lesion, such as an intervertebral disc extrusion, fibrocartilaginous embolism (FCE), or vertebral fracture (see Video 23). The increased extensor tone is the result of interruption to *inhibitory* pathways that run from cells in the lumbar spinal cord segments (known as 'Border cells') up to the cell bodies of the nerves that innervate the thoracic limb extensor muscles. Loss of inhibition following damage to these pathways results in increased extensor muscle tone in the thoracic limbs. The increased extensor muscle tone in the thoracic limbs can restrict an animal's ability to rise into sternal recumbency, and affected animals may therefore be suspected of having a cervical spinal cord lesion. However, once these animals

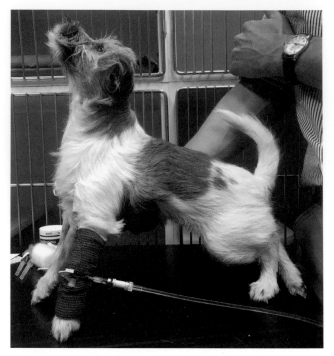

Figure 3.5 A decerebellate posture in a 2-year-old Jack Russell terrier with meningoen-cephalitis of unknown origin. Note the increased extensor muscle tone in the thoracic limbs and extended neck posture (opisthotonus). This dog remained responsive to visual and auditory stimuli.

are assisted to stand it becomes clear that voluntary movement and propriocep-tion are normal in the thoracic limbs. This would not be expected for a cervical spinal cord lesion that is severe enough to result in recumbency. It is important to remember that whilst this posture is commonly associated with extensive T3–L3 spinal cord lesions that result in non-ambulatory paraparesis or paraple-gia, it has no prognostic significance (Box 3.5).

Kyphosis. A dorsal curvature of the spine resulting in a more convex dorsal aspect.

- Non-neurological causes: intra-abdominal pain, polyarthritis resulting in joint pain and shifting of the limbs under the body to reduce loading.

Box 3.5 Schiff–Sherrington Posture

Don't make this mistake: Schiff–Sherrington posture is most commonly associated with acute, severe T3–L3 spinal cord lesions that result in non-ambulatory paraparesis or paraplegia. However, this posture has no prognostic significance and should not be used to guide an owner as to the prognosis for return of pelvic limb function.

- Neurological causes: spinal pain, vertebral malformation, neuromuscular weakness.

Lordosis. A ventral curvature of the spine resulting in a more concave dorsal aspect.

- Non-neurological causes: intra-abdominal pain (prayer positioning).
- Neurological causes: spinal pain, vertebral malformation, neuromuscular weakness.

Scoliosis. A lateral curvature or twisting of the spine.

- Non-neurological causes: mechanical deviation by a paraspinal mass.
- Neurological causes: vertebral malformation, damage to spinal cord dorsal horn (e.g. syringomyelia).

d. Tail postures

Elevated tail posture. Many dogs and some cats may have a naturally elevated tail carriage or adopt this posture appropriately during excitement or greeting. However, cats with vestibular dysfunction will often elevate their tails to assist with balance (Figure 3.6).

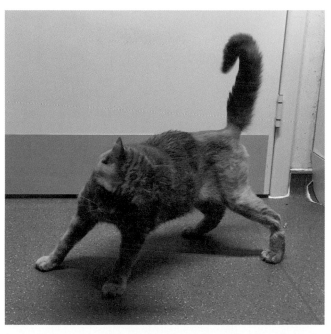

Figure 3.6 Elevated tail posture in a cat with left-sided peripheral vestibular dysfunction. Note also the wide-based stance, left head tilt, and leaning to the left side displayed by this cat.

Low tail carriage. A low tail carriage may simply reflect the nervous demeanour of an animal, or a reluctance to elevate the tail as a result of pain in the region of the tail base (e.g. coccygeal intervertebral disc disease, acute caudal myopathy, cat bite abscess, neoplasia). The tail tone should be normal in these cases and a degree of voluntary movement will be present. In contrast, lesions affecting the caudal spinal cord segments or caudal nerves will result in a flaccid tail with minimal or no voluntary movement (Box 3.6). The adjacent sacral spinal cord segments or nerve roots (S1–S3) may also be affected, resulting in deficits in anal tone, bladder tone, and/or a poor perineal reflex.

3. Gait

Disorders affecting many different regions of the nervous system can result in an abnormal gait and careful gait analysis is vital to ensure an accurate neuroanatomic localisation. Objective methods for gait analysis are increasingly reported; however, these techniques are time consuming and impractical for general practice. Therefore, a logical approach to subjective gait analysis is important, together with careful consideration of non-neurological conditions that may also affect gait. Choice of the most appropriate further tests can then be made to identify the underlying cause for an abnormal gait and to refine the differential diagnoses (e.g. cardiac auscultation, focused orthopaedic examination, hands-on neurological assessment).

A number of specific terms are used to describe gait abnormalities (e.g. ataxia, paresis, hypermetria); however, the authors recommend simply describing what appears to be abnormal about the way the limbs are moving, before reaching for a specific term. This will help to avoid making incorrect assumptions about a particular gait that may result in mislocalisation and an inappropriate choice of further investigations.

The key points to consider when assessing the gait are:

- How many limbs are affected?
- What is the stride length in the affected limbs?
- Is the limb placement predictable on each stride?
- Does the animal appear exercise intolerant or is the gait abnormality exacerbated by exercise?

Box 3.6 Aortic Thromboembolism in Cats

Aortic thromboembolism is a common cause of acute pelvic limb paralysis in cats and can sometimes be mistaken for a spinal cord lesion. However, a spinal cord lesion that is severe enough to cause pelvic limb paralysis would also be expected to affect the voluntary motor function of the tail. The tail function may be normal in cats with aortic thromboembolism, as the blood supply to the muscles and nerves of the tail can be preserved.

How many limbs are affected?

- All limbs
- Thoracic limbs only
- Pelvic limbs only
- Thoracic and pelvic limbs on one side of the body
- Single thoracic or single pelvic limb

Stride length of the affected limbs
- A short stride length suggests that the animal is either prematurely shifting weight away from a *painful* limb (i.e. a reluctance to weight bear on the limb) or is shifting weight away from a *weak* limb to avoid collapsing through the affected limb.
- A long stride length is most commonly seen in association with disruption to the spinal cord upper motor neuron (UMN) tracts that run from the motor centres in the brain to the cell bodies of the peripheral motor neurons that directly innervate the limb muscles. These UMN tracts are involved in the initiation and termination of the stride. Disruption to these messages will therefore delay both the onset and termination of limb movements, resulting in a long or 'over-reaching' stride.

Is the limb placement predictable for each stride?
When evaluating the gait of a dog or cat it is important to assess whether the placement of a limb (or limbs) is predictable with each stride, as a limb may be placed into an abnormal position for numerous reasons. If this abnormal placement is identical for every stride, then a mechanical cause (e.g. orthopaedic disease) should always be considered before assuming a neurological deficit. If limb placement is erratic and unpredictable then a neurological disorder is more likely; the term 'ataxia' is often used to describe this incoordination (see below). Further tests during the 'hands-on' assessment can be used to provide support for this initial impression (e.g. proprioceptive testing).

Exercise intolerance
If there is an apparent deterioration of the gait as an animal is exercised, then conditions affecting oxygen delivery to the muscles (e.g. cardiorespiratory disease, anaemia, polycythaemia, thromboembolic disease [Box 3.7]), the neuromuscular junction, or the muscles themselves (e.g. myopathies) should be considered. This will often present as an increasingly short-strided gait, or the animal choosing to sit or lie down during exercise. Spinal cord disorders typically result in static clinical signs that are not influenced by exercise unless there is significant discomfort or vertebral instability.

Specific terminology
Specific terms that can be used to describe gait abnormalities include 'ataxia' and 'paresis'. The correct use of these terms and understanding their meaning is

---

Box 3.7 Aortic Thromboembolism in Dogs

Aortic thromboembolism may also occur in dogs (see Video 24). In contrast to the acute embolisation seen in cats, this more commonly presents as a chronic aortic thrombosis resulting in progressive pelvic limb weakness. Affected dogs may present with marked exercise intolerance as the blood flow becomes insufficient to meet the increased muscle demand during exercise, and this can mimic spinal cord disease or myasthenia gravis. Taking time to feel for adequate femoral pulses in any dog presenting with a pelvic limb gait abnormality will ensure that this unusual but easily diagnosed condition is not overlooked.

---

important, particularly when describing an animal's gait in the clinical records or to another clinician.

a. Ataxia

This term is used to describe an incoordination of limb movement and placement that is secondary to dysfunction of the complex neurological pathways and structures involved in gait coordination. These structures include the proprioceptive receptors in the joints and muscles, the spinal cord proprioceptive tracts, the vestibular system, and the cerebellum. Lesions affecting these components will result in forms of ataxia with different characteristics. Recognition of ataxia on examination is useful to support the presence of a neurological disorder. However, the distinction between these different forms of ataxia can be difficult and should not be used to form a definitive neuroanatomic localisation without considering the presence of other consistent deficits.

Spinal (or proprioceptive ataxia). This form of ataxia is characterised by unpredictable limb placement when walking, crossing of the affected limbs, scuffing of the dorsal aspect of the nails or paws, and circumduction of the affected limbs during the swing phase of the stride (see Video 16). All limbs, the limbs on one side, or only the pelvic limbs may be affected, dependent on the lesion location and distribution along the spinal cord.

Vestibular ataxia. Animals with vestibular dysfunction may drift or fall to one side when walking or may stumble after sudden changes in head position (e.g. turning to look upwards, shaking of the head) (see Video 17). All limbs will be affected by disorders of the vestibular system, but the pelvic limbs may appear more noticeably affected as they lie further away from the centre of gravity.

Cerebellar ataxia. This gait abnormality is characterised by an abnormal rate, range, and force of movement. This is clinically apparent as excessive flexion of all limbs during the swing phase of the stride ('hypermetria'), erratic limb placement, and rapid limb extension at the time of placement resulting in a 'bouncing' nature to the gait (see Video 18). Dependent upon the precise location of the lesion within the cerebellum, it is possible for just the thoracic and pelvic limbs on the side of the lesion to be affected, and occasionally even just a single limb.

Components of the central vestibular system also reside within the cerebellum; therefore, a gait with a vestibular nature, or a combination of vestibular and cerebellar characteristics, may also be observed in cerebellar disorders.

b. Paresis

The use of this term can cause much confusion and does not simply relate to 'muscle weakness'. It should be used more broadly to suggest an inability to generate normal voluntary movements, and therefore a normal gait. This can be the result either of the skeletal muscles being too weak to support the weight of the body against gravity and to perform voluntary movements, or disruption to the messages from the brainstem motor centres, via the descending spinal cord UMN tracts, to the peripheral motor nerves that innervate the limbs.

Paretic animals may therefore present with a long-strided gait if the lesion responsible is affecting the brainstem motor centres or spinal cord UMN tracts (e.g. in all four limbs for a C1–C5 spinal cord lesion). This gait results from a delay in the onset and termination of the stride. Limb strength will be preserved, as the peripheral motor nerves to the limb muscles and the limb muscles themselves are unaffected. This is termed 'upper motor neuron paresis' and is usually accompanied by concurrent ataxia, as any pathology affecting the spinal cord UMNs will commonly affect the adjacent, ascending spinal proprioceptive tracts.

If a lesion involves the cell bodies or axons of the peripheral motor nerves, the neuromuscular junction, or the limb muscles themselves then the UMN messages for initiation and termination of the stride will be unaffected. However, the muscles of the affected limb(s) will be less able to support the animal's weight against the effects of gravity. This will be clinically apparent as a short-strided gait due to shifting of weight away from a 'weak' limb to avoid collapse.

If an animal is reluctant or unable to walk at all, then gait evaluation is obviously not possible. However, it is still very important to determine why the animal is unable to walk, and to assess the degree of any voluntary movement that is present in the affected limbs. A diminished degree of voluntary movement is termed 'paresis' and an absence of voluntary movement is termed 'plegia' or 'paralysis'.

4. Involuntary movements

Spontaneous muscle contractions that result in involuntary movements of the limbs, face, or body are more commonly reported by owners as part of the clinical history than they are directly observed in the consultation. As previously discussed in Chapters 1 and 2, it is essential to obtain a detailed description of these movements from an owner as the nature of such movements may be misinterpreted by owners, potentially resulting in the incorrect use of terms such as 'seizure' or 'fit'. Access to video footage of any abnormal events observed in the home environment can be extremely useful for further classification of involuntary movements or episodes of collapse, guiding the choice of the most appropriate diagnostic investigations.

Involuntary movements arise from the spontaneous contraction of skeletal muscles, with the nature and appearance dependent on their origin and the number and location of muscles involved. These spontaneous muscle contractions can arise secondary to disorders affecting the skeletal muscles, the peripheral motor nerves, the spinal cord, or motor centres within the brain (including the motor cortex, basal nuclei, and cerebellum). Therefore, a number of possible neuroanatomic localisations need to be considered when presented with an animal showing involuntary movements. Disorders of involuntary movement, including seizures, tremors, peripheral nerve hyperexcitability, myoclonus, and dyskinesias, are further discussed in Chapter 6.

5. Basic cranial nerve functions

A number of basic cranial nerve functions can be assessed during the 'hands-off' assessment, before a more-focused cranial nerve examination is performed during the 'hands-on' assessment. This is particularly useful in animals that will not tolerate handling.

a. Facial asymmetry

Non-neurological causes to consider for facial asymmetry include congenital skull malformations, cranial neoplasia, nasal disease, and abscesses/cellulitis.

Dysfunction of the facial (VII) nerve will result in loss of tone to the muscles of facial expression on the same side as the affected nerve. Clinical signs of facial paralysis include drooping of the ipsilateral lip, an inability to retract the lip commissure when panting, deviation of the nasal philtrum (initially away from the affected side in acute cases, and then towards the affected side following atrophy and fibrosis of the affected muscles in chronic cases), a narrow palpebral fissure on the affected side, or an inability to move the auricular cartilage (Figure 3.7).

b. Voluntary blinking

The absence of voluntary blinking in one or both eyes is consistent with dysfunction of the facial (VII) nerve. Animals with facial paralysis will still protract the third eyelid across the globe, which is often commented on by owners as appearing unusual.

c. Strabismus

Strabismus is the term used to describe an abnormal position of the eyeball within the orbit. A resting strabismus (i.e. when the head is in a normal position) can be caused by:

- mechanical deviation or distortion of the eyeball (e.g. retrobulbar abscess, retrobulbar mass, intra-ocular mass)
- imbalance in the tone of the extra-ocular muscles responsible for maintaining a normal eyeball position.

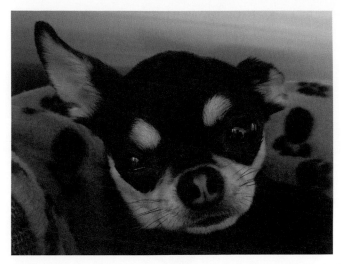

Figure 3.7 Right-sided facial paralysis in a Chihuahua with inflammatory brain disease. Note the narrow palpebral fissure on the right side and the inability to voluntarily retract the right ear against the head compared to the normal left side. The palpebral reflex and menace response were absent on the right side, but the vision and facial sensation remained normal.

The position and movement of each eye is determined by six extra-ocular muscles that act as three agonist–antagonist pairs:

- lateral rectus (LR) and medial rectus (MR) for movement in the horizontal plane
- dorsal rectus (DR) and ventral rectus (VR) for the vertical plane
- dorsal oblique (DO) and ventral oblique (VO) for torsional movements (Figure 3.8).

These muscles are innervated by motor neurons of three separate cranial nerves: the oculomotor (III) nerve innervating the MR, DR, VR, and VO, the trochlear (IV) nerve innervating the DO, and the abducent (VI) nerve innervating the LR. The muscles are innervated in yoked pairs to allow conjugate movements of the eyeballs (e.g. right MR and left LR, left DO and right VO). Denervation of one or more of the extra-ocular muscles will result in loss of tone in the affected muscles and deviation of the eyeball by unopposed contraction of the unaffected muscle(s).

- Oculomotor (III) nerve dysfunction results in denervation of the MR, DR, VR, and VO. Unopposed contraction of the LR and DO will result in a lateral or ventrolateral strabismus.
- Trochlear (IV) nerve dysfunction is rarely seen in isolation but would result in loss of tone in the DO and rotation of the eyeball secondary to unopposed contraction of the VO muscle. This is clinically apparent in the cat as the verti-

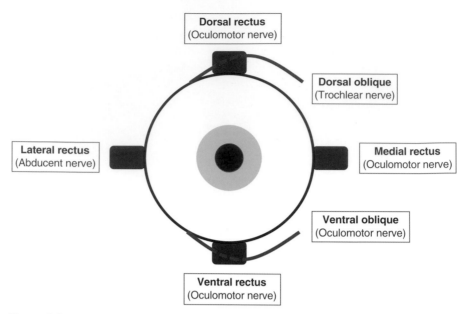

Figure 3.8 The extraocular muscles and their innervation in the right eye of a dog.

cally orientated, slit-shaped pupil becomes diagonally orientated, with lateral deviation of the dorsal aspect of the pupil away from the nose. The presence of a round pupil in dogs means that this is not immediately appreciable; however, retinal examination reveals lateral deviation of the dorsal retinal vein away from its normal vertical position.

- Abducent (VI) nerve dysfunction results in denervation of the LR and a medial strabismus in the affected eye secondary to unopposed contraction of the MR.

d. Jaw tone and position

Reduced jaw tone is clinically apparent as an inability to close the mouth ('dropped jaw'). This results from dysfunction of the motor axons in the mandibular branches of *both* trigeminal (V) nerves.

> **Top tip:** A unilateral lesion affecting the motor component of one trigeminal (V) nerve will not result in a dropped jaw, as sufficient muscle strength will be present on the unaffected side to maintain a normal jaw position and function.

An important differential diagnosis to consider for an *inability* to close the mouth is a *reluctance* to close the mouth. This can be seen with temporomandibular joint disease or intraoral lesions. However, in contrast to cases with bilateral trigeminal neuropathy, evidence of discomfort is frequently found on clinical examination in these cases.

e. Tongue symmetry and tone

This can be assessed if a dog is panting or licks its nose in the consultation. Deviation of the tongue to one side, tongue atrophy, or reduced tone of the tongue suggests dysfunction of the hypoglossal (XII) nerve and/or its nucleus in the caudal brainstem. Acute lesions result in deviation of the tongue away from the affected side as a result of unopposed contraction of muscles on the unaffected side. With time, denervation atrophy of the affected tongue muscles will slowly deviate the tongue back towards the affected side.

3.4.2 'Hands-On' Assessment

The 'hands-on' part of the neurological examination involves performing specific tests to screen certain regions or components of the nervous system. A wide array of different tests is described and it is important to appreciate that some of these tests simply represent different ways to screen the same components of the nervous system, whilst others may not add further information to that already acquired from the clinical history and simple observation of demeanour, gait, and posture.

It is always important to perform a number of basic tests in every case to ensure that neurological deficits are not missed, particularly those that could suggest the presence of more than one lesion (e.g. concurrent disease processes or multifocal disease). Familiarity with performing and interpreting these different tests is vital as there is a wide range of normal variation that can only be appreciated with practice and experience. However, once a practitioner gains in confidence a selection of 'hands-on' tests can often be chosen, tailored to each case, to refine the preliminary neuroanatomic localisation based upon the clinical history and 'hands-off' assessment.

A number of the tests performed during the 'hands-on' assessment involve the application of a tactile stimulus to the skin of a specific region of the body, followed by observation of an appropriate response. This is most commonly in the form of a reflexive muscle contraction resulting in movement of a body part. An abnormal test result can therefore be the result of an inability to detect or transmit the initial sensory information and/or an inability to perform the appropriate motor response. For example, the corneal reflex involves gently touching the surface of the cornea and observing for an appropriate blink in response. The absence of an appropriate blink could therefore result from:

- An inability to feel the stimulus following the application of topical local anaesthetic drops.
- A lesion affecting the ophthalmic branch of the trigeminal nerve, resulting in an inability to detect and transmit the sensory information to the level of the brainstem.
- Damage to connections between the trigeminal sensory nucleus in the brainstem and the motor nucleus of the facial nerve, or damage to the nuclei themselves.

- Dysfunction of the facial nerve innervating the periocular muscles required for blinking.
- A disorder affecting the neuromuscular junction or periocular muscles, resulting in reduced muscle tone and facial paresis.

If each test that you perform is approached in a similar manner, from start to finish in terms of its sensory and motor arms, then the interpretation of each test should hopefully be more logical and approachable. Combinations of tests that share common sensory or motor pathways can then be used to determine the most likely reason for an abnormal test result.

The 'hands-on' part of the examination can be divided into the following parts:

1. Cranial nerve examination
2. Limb palpation
3. Assessment of postural reactions (proprioceptive testing)
4. Spinal reflex testing
5. Spinal palpation and neck manipulation
6. Testing for pain perception (nociception)

1. Cranial nerve examination

The cranial nerve examination can be approached in an efficient and logical manner if it is separated into different parts according to the regions of the head being assessed. This also means that several tests can be performed concurrently to provide complementary information and assist in determining the neuroanatomic localisation (e.g. the palpebral reflex and menace response).

a. Eyes

With the animal sitting or standing to face you, use the fingers of one hand to gently hold the muzzle and stabilise the head. The following tests can then be performed:

- Palpebral reflex and menace response testing
- Assessment of pupil size and symmetry
- Observation of any abnormal spontaneous eye movements (e.g. nystagmus)
- Elevation of the head towards the ceiling to look for a positional strabismus or positional nystagmus
- Vestibulo-ocular reflex testing
- Pupillary light reflexes and dazzle reflexes

Palpebral reflex testing. Gently cover one of the animal's eyes with the fingers of one hand (i.e. cover the right eye with your left hand) and touch the medial canthus of the exposed eye (see Video 1a). This should induce a reflex contraction of the muscles of the upper and lower eyelids, resulting in a blink. This test screens the integrity of the sensory fibres in the ophthalmic branch of the trigeminal nerve, the motor fibres in the facial nerve, and the interneurons in the brainstem that connect the sensory nucleus of the trigeminal nerve to the motor nucleus of the facial nerve. Touching the lateral canthus of the eye will stimulate sensory nerves in the maxillary branch of the trigeminal nerve, with the remainder of the pathway being the same as described for medial canthus stimulation.

An abnormal palpebral reflex therefore implies one or more of the following:

- ipsilateral trigeminal (sensory) nerve lesion resulting in an inability to feel the stimulus
- ipsilateral facial (motor) nerve lesion resulting in an inability to blink (i.e. facial paresis/paralysis)
- brainstem lesion
- mechanical inability to blink (e.g. marked exophthalmos)

The precise cause for the abnormal reflex can be determined by considering the following:

- A trigeminal nerve lesion should result in loss of sensation to other regions of the face innervated by the branch affected (e.g. nasal septum for the ophthalmic branch or lateral muzzle for the maxillary branch). Concurrent involvement of the motor fibres residing in the mandibular branch of the trigeminal nerve would result in masticatory muscle atrophy on the affected side.
- A facial nerve lesion will result in an inability to voluntarily blink on the affected side or blink in response to a menacing gesture (absent menace response). In these cases, the animal will still be able to retract the eyeball and protract the third eyelid when performing the palpebral reflex, confirming an intact sensory arm of the reflex.
- A brainstem lesion that results in an abnormal palpebral reflex will commonly affect adjacent neuroanatomical structures in addition to the trigeminal and/ or facial nuclei. This will result in other neurological deficits on examination, which will be dependent on the structure or tract affected: altered mentation (ARAS), paresis (descending UMN tracts), proprioceptive deficits (ascending proprioceptive tracts), other cranial nerve deficits (other cranial nerve nuclei).

Menace response. The menace response can be performed concurrently with the palpebral reflex by alternately touching the medial canthus of the eye and moving your hand towards the eye in a 'menacing gesture' (see Video 1a). This provides a visual stimulus for blinking, but care should be taken to avoiding creating a waft of air when moving your hand towards the face as this could also provide a tactile stimulus. This is to ensure that only visual stimulation for blinking is tested by the menace response. Alternating between actually touching the face (palpebral reflex testing) and performing a menacing gesture can be particularly useful when testing the menace response of cats. The nature of this species means that they may not blink in response to a visual stimulus unless they think that it may actually touch their face! A study assessing the menace response in 50 neurologically and ophthalmologically healthy cats concluded that the majority of cats showed a strong menace response when the untested eye remained uncovered, but 40% failed to show a complete menace response when the contralateral eye was covered (Quitt et al. 2018). The most reliable examination appeared to be achieved when the examiner was positioned behind the cat and each eye was tested without covering the contralateral eye.

As the name suggests, the menace response is not a true reflex and is classified as a 'response' because the pathway tested includes areas of the cerebral cortex. This is a learned response that is absent in dogs and cats before about 12 weeks of age. The sensory arm of the pathway involves recognition of an object approaching the eye via the retina, optic nerve, optic chiasm, optic tracts, and central visual pathways (thalamus, contralateral visual cortex in the occipital lobe). Initiation and coordination of an appropriate blink in response to this visual information involves the cerebral motor cortex, cerebellum, brainstem, and facial nerve (Figure 3.9). Therefore, there are several lesion locations that can result in an absent menace response:

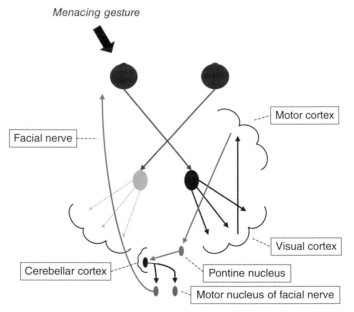

Figure 3.9 The menace response. An object approaching the eye is interpreted as a potential threat to the health of the eye by the brain, resulting in a coordinated response to blink and protect the surface of the eye (see Video 1a).

- *Ipsilateral retina or optic nerve.* The direct PLR may be absent in the affected eye. If vision is intact in the opposite eye, then the pupil of the affected eye will passively dilate if the visual eye is covered.
- *Contralateral visual and/or motor cortex.* The PLR will be normal in the affected eye.
- *Ipsilateral cerebellar lesion (rare).* Vision will be normal in both eyes and other signs of cerebellar disease will usually be present (e.g. ataxia, intention tremor, hypermetria, head tilt).
- *Ipsilateral facial nerve lesion resulting in an inability to blink (facial paresis/paralysis).* The palpebral reflex will also be absent but eyeball retraction in response to the menacing gesture will still occur if vision is present in the eye being tested.

As the palpebral reflex and menace response both require normal function of the facial nerve, they are complementary tests that can be used to screen for potential lesions involving the trigeminal (sensory) nerve, facial nerve, and visual pathways. For example, the most likely reason for the following neurological deficits would be:

- *intact palpebral reflex, absent menace response* – visual deficit in the affected eye
- *absent palpebral reflex, intact menace response* – absent facial sensation (trigeminal nerve lesion)
- *absent palpebral reflex, absent menace response* – facial paralysis (facial nerve lesion) or multiple cranial nerve deficits (e.g. blindness and absent facial sensation).

Pupil size and symmetry. Pupil size is determined by two main factors:

1. The external light levels
2. The emotional status of the animal.

Pupil size is controlled to ensure optimum vision; the brighter the light level, the more constricted the pupil will become to avoid becoming dazzled. Light is detected by the retina, and this information is transmitted to the parasympathetic nucleus of the oculomotor nerve in the brainstem to reflexively control pupil constriction. This is the pathway that is tested by the PLR. The pupil will passively dilate as the light levels fall to ensure that enough light enters the eye for optimum vision.

The emotional status of the animal is determined by the sympathetic nervous system, with stimulation of the sympathetic nervous system ('fight or flight' response) resulting in active pupil dilation.

Abnormal or excessive pupil dilation is termed 'mydriasis', and abnormal or excessive pupil constriction is termed 'miosis'. Asymmetry of pupil size is termed 'anisocoria' and may result from unilateral autonomic lesions affecting the ability of the pupil to either dilate or constrict on the affected side. Application of topical medications and non-neurological diseases are also common causes for anisocoria and should always be considered before neurological disease. Further discussion on the approach to pupil abnormalities can be found in Chapter 6.

Top tip: Always consider stress during examination as a common cause for apparent bilateral mydriasis: the PLR may also appear reduced due to sympathetic stimulation. However, vision should be normal in both eyes and the menace responses will be intact bilaterally.

Spontaneous eye movements. If the head is in a static position and the animal is not tracking objects in their visual field or attempting to look for their owner, then the eyeballs should be stationary within the orbits and pointing in the same direction as the head.

The presence of abnormal, spontaneous eye movements is most commonly encountered in the form of rhythmic eyeball oscillations that have a slow drift phase, followed by a fast corrective phase. This distinctive form of involuntary eye movement is termed a jerk nystagmus (see Video 20). Nystagmus results from dysfunction of the vestibular system and disruption to its important role in coordinating the position of the eyes relative to the position and movement of the head. Therefore, a jerk nystagmus is often observed concurrently with other clinical signs of vestibular dysfunction, such as a head tilt or ataxia of all limbs.

The characteristics of a jerk nystagmus may be useful to guide the neuroanatomic localisation. However, they are not definitive and should always be used in combination with other consistent neurological deficits.

- Direction of the fast 'jerk' phase
  The fast phase of a nystagmus represents the attempt by the body to correct for the slow drift phase that results from the underlying pathology. The fast phase is most commonly directed away from the side of the lesion, and a tip to remembering this is that it can be thought of as 'running away from the problem'!
  A nystagmus can be horizontal, vertical, or torsional (rotatory). A true vertical nystagmus may suggest the presence of a lesion affecting the central rather than peripheral vestibular system. However, lesions affecting the peripheral vestibular system can result in a diagonal nystagmus that is almost vertical and difficult to distinguish from a true vertical nystagmus, particularly in an animal with a head tilt and loss of balance. Disorders of the central vestibular system can also result in horizontal and torsional nystagmus, therefore whilst the presence of a true vertical nystagmus is supportive of a central lesion, its absence does not exclude disease of the central vestibular system. It has also been suggested that a lesion affecting the central vestibular system is more

likely if the fast phase of the nystagmus changes in direction when the head is placed into different positions (e.g. in dorsal recumbency or following head elevation). Further discussion of the approach to vestibular disease can be found in Chapter 6.

- Rate of nystagmus (beat frequency)
  It has been suggested that acute disorders affecting the peripheral vestibular system may result in a more rapid nystagmus compared to those affecting the central vestibular system, with a beat frequency >66 beats per minute being more suggestive of a peripheral lesion (Troxel et al. 2005).

- Positional nystagmus
  By adjusting the position of the head, a nystagmus can sometimes be induced in animals that do not have a spontaneous nystagmus when the head is in its normal position. This may be observed in animals with central vestibular disease or in those that are compensating for more chronic peripheral vestibular dysfunction. The easiest way to assess for positional nystagmus is by elevating the head so that it points towards the ceiling, or by placing the animal in dorsal recumbency with the neck extended if it will allow. Positional nystagmus is often observed in cats, which appear to be able to compensate more rapidly for vestibular dysfunction compared to dogs (see Video 25). Recognition of a positional nystagmus in an animal that otherwise appears normal is useful for determining the neuroanatomic localisation as it is a distinctive sign of vestibular dysfunction.

In animals that do not have a resting strabismus (see above), a ventral strabismus may also be observed when elevating the head to assess for positional nystagmus. This positional strabismus is not related to pathology affecting the cranial nerves innervating the extraocular muscles but is consistent with a lesion to the vestibular system on the same side as the affected eye. It results from an inability of the vestibular system to detect the change in head position and appropriately alter the eyeball position to point in the direction of the head. Disorders affecting the cranial nerves innervating the extra-ocular muscles (III, IV, VI) will result in a static strabismus that is present in all head positions, and not only when the head position is changed.

Other forms of spontaneous eye movement. In addition to disorders affecting the vestibular control of eye movement, other forms of involuntary eye movement are rarely observed secondary to disorders affecting the control of saccadic eye movements. Saccadic eye movements occur in the normal way to rapidly shift the direction of gaze from one object of interest to another when the head is in a static position. Disorders affecting their control result in involuntary, rapid eye movements that lack the initial drift phase characteristic of a nystagmus. These involuntary eye movements are called saccadic oscillations. Saccadic oscillations are rarely reported in small animals, but recognition of these unusual eye movements may help to guide a specific neuroanatomic localisation.

- *Convergence–retraction pulses.* This form of abnormal, spontaneous eye movement is characterised by rhythmic convergence and retraction of both eyeballs into the sockets and has been reported in dogs with lesions in the dorsal midbrain (Crawford et al. 2016).
- *Opsoclonus.* This distinctive form of spontaneous eye movement is characterised by rapid, multi-directional eye movements without a drift phase (see Video 26). The recognition of opsoclonus may suggest a cerebellar neuroanatomic localisation. Opsoclonus has been reported in a dog with neuronal ceroid lipofuscinosis and in dogs and a cat with idiopathic generalised tremor syndrome (Ives et al. 2018).

Vestibulo-ocular reflex testing. Movement of the head from side-to-side, or up-and-down, should result in coordinated, conjugate eyeball movements that realign the direction of gaze with that of head position. This is called the vestibulo-ocular reflex. The eyeballs initially appear to remain in a fixed position as the head is moved, but this actually represents a slow eyeball movement in an equal and opposite direction to head movement. This ensures that the gaze can remain fixed and stable on an object of interest in spite of small head movements during normal activity. As the head is moved further from the midline, there follows a fast corrective eye movement in the direction of head movement that realigns the head and eyeball position.

These movements are initiated and coordinated by the vestibular system, which includes parts of the cerebellum. Therefore, in addition to resulting in abnormal spontaneous eye movements, disorders of the vestibular system can also interfere with the normal vestibulo-ocular reflex. This may be clinically apparent with a vestibular lesion as an absent, incomplete, or slow corrective eye movement when the head is moved towards the side of the lesion (see Video 2a). Disorders affecting the vestibular system equally on both sides (e.g. bilateral otitis media/interna) may result in an absent vestibulo-ocular reflex when moving the head in any direction. Animals with bilateral vestibular dysfunction will not have a head tilt but may show wide head excursions, a crouched posture, ataxia of all limbs, and drifting to both sides when walking (Figure 3.10 and Video 27).

Lesions affecting the brainstem that involve the vestibular nuclei in the medulla oblongata can result in a poor vestibulo-ocular reflex when moving the head from side-to-side. This clinical sign will also be accompanied by other indications of severe brainstem dysfunction, such as a reduced level of mentation (stupor or coma), tetraparesis, and other cranial nerve deficits (e.g. poor gag reflex, miosis, or anisocoria). An absent or incomplete vestibulo-ocular reflex may be observed in association with brainstem compression secondary to increased intracranial pressure and herniation of brain parenchyma under the tentorium cerebelli or through the foramen magnum. The vestibulo-ocular reflex therefore forms an important part of the serial assessment of animals with

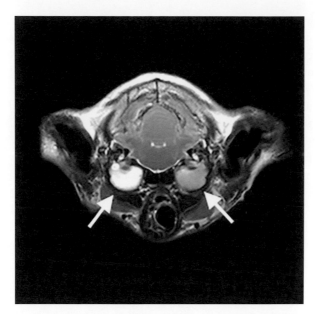

Figure 3.10 A transverse T2-weighted MRI at the level of the tympanic bullae in a 20-year-old, female neutered, domestic shorthair cat with a 4-week history of a crouched posture and progressive loss of balance. Neurological examination revealed ataxia of all limbs, drifting to both sides when walking, wide head excursions, an absent vestibulo-ocular reflex, and a mild right head tilt. Proprioception was normal in all limbs and withdrawal reflexes were strong in all limbs. The neuroanatomic localisation was bilateral peripheral vestibular system. Note the hyperintense material filling both tympanic bullae (arrows). The tympanic bullae should normally be gas-filled and appear black on MRI. Bilateral bacterial otitis media/interna was diagnosed following myringotomy; this was medically managed in the first instance in light of the cat's advanced age.

suspected elevated intracranial pressure (e.g. following head trauma) to allow early identification of a deteriorating clinical status and rapid intervention. The neurological assessment and monitoring of animals following head trauma is discussed further in Chapter 7.

Pupillary light reflex and dazzle reflex. The PLR and dazzle reflex can be assessed at the same time but may not significantly influence your neuroanatomic localisation in an animal that appears to be visual and does not have any pupil abnormalities (e.g. anisocoria). Therefore, if there is no history to suggest visual deficits, if the menace responses are intact, and if the pupils appear symmetrical and an appropriate size for the light levels and emotional state of the animal, it may not be necessary to perform these tests.

The PLR and dazzle reflex both rely upon a strong light source to allow accurate assessment. The most common reason for a subjectively poor PLR is use of a light that is not bright enough, particularly when trying to overcome increased sympathetic tone in a stressed patient.

- *Dazzle reflex*

  This is a subcortical reflex that tests the integrity of the visual pathways to the level of the midbrain, together with the facial nerve. It involves observing for a narrowing of the palpebral fissure in response to a bright light source.

- *Pupillary light reflex*

  As previously discussed, active pupil constriction is mediated by the parasympathetic component of the oculomotor nerve and is dependent on the environmental light levels. This information is transmitted via the optic nerve to the parasympathetic nucleus of the oculomotor nerve in the midbrain. Decussation of this information at both the level of the optic chiasm and between the pre-tectal nucleus and the oculomotor nuclei, means that light entering one eye will result in constriction of both pupils (Figure 3.11). Constriction of the pupil receiving the light is termed the 'direct PLR' and constriction of the contralateral pupil is termed the 'consensual PLR'.

This concept explains why blindness in one eye will often result in little appreciable anisocoria, that is until the visual eye is covered and there is passive dilation of the blind pupil. If light is shone into the blind eye there will be no change in the size of either pupil (no direct or consensual PLR). However, if light is shone into the visual eye then this will result in constriction of both pupils (intact direct and consensual PLRs).

If there is no anisocoria observed, then assessing for a normal direct PLR in each eye is all that is required. An indication that the PLR is likely to be normal can also be acquired by simply closing both eyes when in a bright environment,

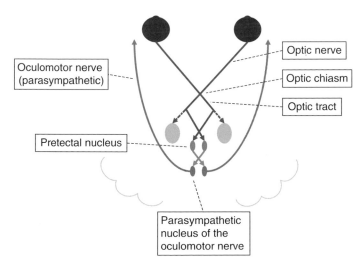

Figure 3.11 The pupillary light reflex. Light directed into either eye will stimulate the parasympathetic nuclei of the oculomotor nerves which will, in turn, result in reflex constriction of the pupils of both eyes.

followed by opening each eye in turn to observe for appropriate pupil constriction. Observing for a consensual PLR is primarily useful if there is anisocoria present:

Unilateral miosis. If this is the result of loss of sympathetic innervation to the affected eye (as part of a Horner syndrome), then the affected pupil will constrict further in response to light shone into either eye (assuming that the optic and oculomotor nerves are not affected).

Unilateral mydriasis. The most common neurological cause for unilateral mydriasis is a lesion affecting the parasympathetic component of the oculomotor nerve, resulting in an inability to constrict the pupil. Assuming that the optic nerve is unaffected, vision will still be present in this eye and the menace response will be intact. The affected pupil will not constrict when light is shone into it (absent direct PLR), but there will still be active constriction of the contralateral pupil (intact consensual PLR). Light shone into the unaffected eye will result in a direct PLR in this eye, but no change in the size of the mydriatic pupil (absent consensual PLR).

b. Mouth and jaws

Jaw tone. Jaw tone can be assessed by appreciating the resistance to opening of the mouth. This reflects the function of the motor component of the trigeminal nerve (mandibular branch). Bilateral loss of function is required before a reduced jaw tone is clinically apparent, as there is sufficient strength from the masticatory muscles on one side to result in normal jaw function.

Tongue symmetry and tone. This can be assessed when the mouth is open (see 'Hands-Off' Assessment).

Gag reflex (see Video 3a). If the animal is amenable, then the gag reflex can be assessed by gently placing one or two fingers to the back of the throat and feeling for reflexive contraction of the pharyngeal muscles around your fingers. Animals with a poor gag reflex will show little reluctance to this examination and the pharynx will not contract as expected around your fingers. Care should be taken so that you are not inadvertently bitten when performing this examination. This is particularly important as the results may add little to your neuroanatomic localisation if there is no history to suggest dysphagia or difficulty swallowing. Therefore, appropriate case selection is advised before performing the gag reflex. Individual variation in the interpretation of this test also needs to be considered, both in terms of the examiner and the patient. The gag reflex may appear subjectively poor in docile, large breed dogs such as Labrador Retrievers that do not appear to have a genuine neurological deficit.

Palpation of the masticatory muscles. The temporalis and masseter muscles should be assessed for atrophy or swelling (Figure 3.12). See Chapter 6 for further discussion regarding the different causes of masticatory muscle atrophy and the approach to these cases.

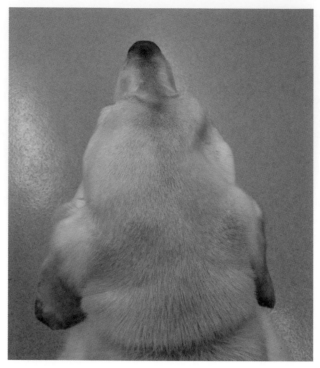

Figure 3.12 Marked, unilateral (right-sided) masticatory muscle atrophy in a 10-year-old Labrador Retriever with a peripheral nerve sheath tumour affecting the mandibular branch of the right trigeminal nerve. Note the prominent zygomatic arch and contours of the skull on the affected side compared to the normal left side.

c. Nose

Nasal septum nociception (see Video 4a). The end of a pair of closed haemostats can be used to gently apply a mild noxious stimulus to the inside of the nostril on each side of the nasal septum. This stimulus should elicit a conscious response of irritation, indicated by withdrawal or shaking of the head to avoid the stimulation. As for the menace response, this test screens both cranial nerve and cerebrocortical functions: the ipsilateral trigeminal nerve (sensory–ophthalmic branch) and the contralateral sensory cortex. If the ipsilateral palpebral reflex is intact then it can be assumed that the trigeminal (sensory) component of this test is functional. Therefore, a deficient response to stimulation on one side of the nasal septum compared to the other would be more consistent with a lesion involving the *contralateral* forebrain (see Video 5a). This would be further supported by the presence of other compatible neurological deficits, such as an absent menace response or proprioceptive deficits on the same side as the abnormal nasal nociception.

2. Limb palpation

The limbs should be examined in turn for focal or generalised muscle atrophy, for the general impression of limb muscle tone, and for any swellings or foci of discomfort. This is most easily performed in each limb with the animal standing and immediately prior to performing the proprioceptive tests described below. Further examination can then be performed, if required, at the time of withdrawal reflex testing.

- Focal atrophy of individual muscles is most consistent with denervation atrophy secondary to a lesion affecting the motor fibres in the peripheral nerve that innervates the affected muscle (e.g. suprascapular nerve for the supraspinatus and infraspinatus muscles – see Figure 3.13).
- Generalised atrophy of the muscles in a single limb could result from chronic disuse of that limb, a lesion affecting multiple nerve roots, or a lesion affecting the individual peripheral nerves innervating the affected muscles (e.g. brachial plexus lesion).
- Generalised atrophy of the muscles of all limbs could be consistent with a generalised neuromuscular disorder (primary myopathy or generalised motor polyneuropathy); however, cachexia related to a systemic disease process should always be considered (malnutrition, malabsorption, maldigestion, protein-losing conditions, heart failure, neoplasia).
- Reduced muscle tone in one or more limbs is clinically apparent as a reduced resistance to flexion and extension of the limb, and a general impression of flaccidity and increased joint mobility when the limb is moved. This is most often noticeable in the carpi and hocks.

3. Assessment of postural reactions (proprioceptive testing)

Proprioception can be defined as the perception of the relative position and movement of different parts of the body at any point in time. This information is important for adopting a normal posture and for planning and coordinating movements. Receptors called 'proprioceptors' are associated with the muscles and joints of the body and provide information about the current state of play (e.g. joint position, muscle stretch). This information is transmitted to the level of the spinal cord in peripheral sensory nerves. Large, myelinated axons within the spinal cord transmit this information up to the regions of the brain concerned with coordination and proprioception (forebrain and cerebellum). Dysfunction of the receptors, the pathways transmitting this information, or the areas of the brain involved with processing proprioceptive information can therefore result in abnormal postures and gaits. The vestibular system and its control of equilibrium and balance is also intimately involved in proprioception. This is termed 'special proprioception' and is grouped together with the other special senses of hearing, smell, taste, and vision.

Proprioceptive testing is a sensitive way to increase suspicion for an underlying neurological disorder and a proprioceptive deficit would not be expected for a primary orthopaedic condition. However, as normal proprioception relies upon the integrity of multiple neuroanatomic structures and long pathways from the limbs to the brain, identification of a proprioceptive deficit is poorly specific for a particular neuroanatomic localisation. A lesion anywhere between the limb being tested and the brain can result in a proprioceptive deficit on examination. Therefore, whilst identification of abnormal proprioception supports the presence of a neurological lesion, other tests that screen more specific regions of the nervous system are required to narrow down the neuroanatomic localisation.

Proprioception is a sensory modality; however, testing for proprioception also relies upon normal motor function to perform the corrective movements that we use to define a normal test result. Therefore, these tests will naturally be absent in a paralysed dog or cat even if the sense of proprioception is completely unaffected by the lesion responsible. Proprioceptive testing is unrewarding in these cases and does not need to be performed in limbs that are truly paralysed. Proprioceptive testing is extremely useful in animals with some degree of voluntary motor function (i.e. paresis) and it is vital that the animal's

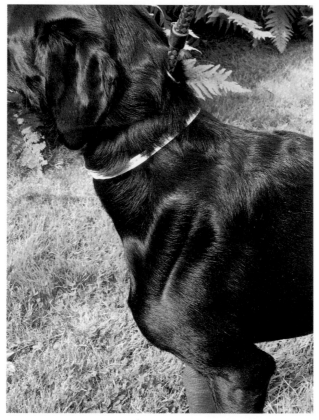

Figure 3.13 Marked, focal atrophy of the left supraspinatus and infraspinatus muscles in a dog following traumatic damage to the left suprascapular nerve. Note the prominent spine of the underlying scapula in this case.

weight is adequately supported when performing these tests. This is so that any attempt to initiate a corrective movement is observed, even if the movement is weak or incomplete. If the weight is not supported then an animal with neuro-muscular weakness, for example, in which the proprioception may in fact be normal, will collapse through the limb being tested; this will give the impression of absent proprioception. It is the attempt to correct for a change in limb or joint position that tells you whether an animal knows where the limbs are in space (i.e. has normal proprioception) and not the strength of the corrective movement itself.

There are several different tests, known as postural reactions, that can be performed to assess an animal's proprioception, but it is important to appreciate that performing all of these tests is not required in the majority of cases. Paw replacement is often the most useful first test and is easy to perform in most dogs.

a. Paw replacement
The animal being examined should be standing as squarely as possible, with their weight evenly distributed across all limbs (see Video 6a). A tabletop can be used for small dogs and cats, but larger dogs will feel more relaxed when examined on the floor. With the animal facing away from you, place your hand under the sternum to support some of the animal's weight. As previously discussed, providing this support is important to ensure that the animal does not collapse through the limb if it is weak, or that the animal does not shift their weight away from the limb during testing. This can result in the false impression that replacement of the paw is delayed. One front paw should be gently lifted and turned over so that the dorsal skin surface is in contact with the ground. The paw should be rapidly replaced into its normal position in a clean and coordinated manner. If you are unable to place the dorsal aspect of the paw onto the ground without the animal starting to replace it, then this test can be assumed as normal. The pelvic limbs can be assessed in an identical manner by supporting the weight under the abdomen during testing.

A delayed or absent paw replacement should be considered abnormal (Figure 3.14). However, considerations should also include:

- Reluctance to replace the paw secondary to limb or joint pain rather than a true proprioceptive deficit
- An inability to perform the replacing movement secondary to severe motor dysfunction (e.g. paralysis) rather than a lack of knowledge of abnormal paw position.
- Uneven weight bearing (i.e. shifting of weight away from the limb being tested).
- Severe systemic illness resulting in lethargy, generalised weakness, and a subjectively delayed paw replacement.

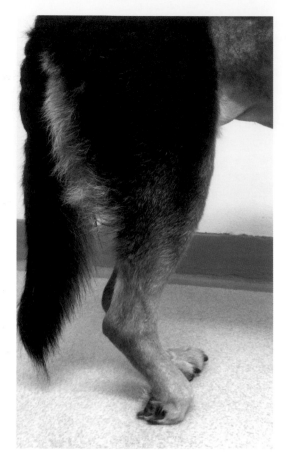

Figure 3.14 Absent paw replacement in the right pelvic limb of a dog with a spinal cord lesion affecting the T3–L3 spinal cord segments on the right side.

If paw replacement testing is convincingly abnormal, then other tests of proprioception may not be required to further refine your neuroanatomic localisation. If paw replacement testing is equivocal, then further proprioceptive testing should be performed. Hopping is the most useful test to perform next, particularly in cats for which paw replacement can be difficult to interpret and may appear normal unless a severe neurological deficit is present.

b. Hopping

Hopping requires more complex movements and coordination when compared to paw replacement. It therefore represents a complementary test and may reveal subtle proprioceptive deficits that are not apparent using paw replacement alone. Hopping can be performed on a tabletop for small dogs and cats, but it can be easier to interpret when the limb being examined is viewed from above and the animal is on the ground for testing.

Thoracic limbs. With the animal facing away from you, the thoracic limb on one side can be gently lifted away from the ground by holding the humerus immediately proximal to the elbow (see Video 7a). Your other arm should be placed under the abdomen just in front of the pelvic limbs so that the pelvic limbs can be lifted a small distance above the ground. This means that the animal is now bearing weight on a single thoracic limb. It is very important to take the majority of the animal's weight at this stage and not force the dog or cat to take its full weight on only a single limb. If the animal has neuromuscular weakness or is reluctant to bear weight on the limb due to pain, then it may collapse through the limb, which could be misinterpreted as a true proprioceptive deficit.

The body of the dog or cat should now be moved in a slow and steady manner towards the side of the limb being tested. This will move the shoulder of the tested limb lateral to the paw that is in contact with the ground. The normal response is for the animal to compensate for this change in body position by performing a small, coordinated hop that is initiated the moment you lose sight of the paw under the shoulder. This hop should result in the paw coming to rest on the ground immediately underneath the shoulder again. Several consecutive hops can be assessed on one side before assessment of the other limb in an identical manner. Repeated cycles of testing should be performed in each limb to gain an overall impression as to whether hopping is normal and symmetrical. Observing the limb being tested from above makes it easier to appreciate a subtle delay in the initiation of the hop when you start to lose sight of the paw. With practice, this test can be performed very quickly and with minimal stress to the patient.

Pelvic limbs. The easiest way to test hopping in the pelvic limbs is to stand at the side of the animal with their head facing either to your left or to your right. If the head is facing to your left, then the animal's right pelvic limb can be tested first by passing your left hand under the sternum to lift the thoracic limbs away from the ground. Your right arm can then be used to lift the left pelvic limb away from the ground, as this limb is closest to you. As for hopping the thoracic limbs, it is important that the animal's weight is adequately supported during testing. The animal's body can then be moved away from you so that you start to lose sight of the right hind paw as the hip moves laterally. At this stage, the animal should hop to replace the paw immediately under the new position of the hip. The initiation of the hop in the pelvic limbs is often slightly slower than for the thoracic limbs but it should still be a brisk and coordinated movement. The left pelvic limb can then be tested in an identical manner but with the animal facing to your right.

See Video 8a for an example of abnormal paw replacement and hopping in the pelvic limbs. In addition to a delay in the initiation of the hop, other abnormalities that can be appreciated when performing hopping include:

- Wide and inappropriate replacement of the paw to a new position that is further lateral than that of the hip or shoulder joint. This is often accompanied by a delay in the initiation of the hop and is consistent with abnormal proprioception.
- Excessive flexion of the limb during hopping and/or excessive force used to replace the paw on the ground. This inappropriate rate, range, and force of movement is termed 'dysmetria' and can be seen in association with disorders affecting the cerebellum. However, certain breeds such as pugs may also show apparent dysmetria when hopping as a normal breed variation.

c. Hemi-walking

Hopping can be difficult to perform and interpret in large or heavy dogs. If this is the case, then the thoracic and pelvic limbs on the same side can be assessed at the same time using hemi-walking. This is performed in a similar manner to pelvic limb hopping but instead of lifting both thoracic limbs away from the ground, only the thoracic and pelvic limbs on the side closest to you are lifted up. The animal's body is then moved away from you to assess the 'hopping' of the thoracic and pelvic limbs on the opposite side. The animal can then be moved to face in the other direction to test the contralateral limbs.

d. Wheelbarrow testing

This test can be useful to accentuate any subtle proprioceptive deficits that are suspected following gait assessment, paw replacement, and hopping. With the animal facing away from you, place your arms under the abdomen and lift both pelvic limbs a small distance above the ground. The dog or cat is then encouraged to walk forwards using only their thoracic limbs for weight support. Elevating the head using one hand placed under the muzzle can also help to accentuate any abnormal limb movements or positioning. Possible abnormalities that may be observed on wheelbarrow testing include:

- Scuffing of the thoracic limbs or erratic limb placement suggestive of a proprioceptive deficit in the affected limb(s).
- Excessive flexion of the limbs during protraction (hypermetria) in animals with cerebellar dysfunction.
- Animals with lower motor neuron paresis of the thoracic limbs (e.g. generalised neuromuscular disease or a C6–T2 spinal cord lesion) may struggle to perform wheelbarrow testing. This is clinically apparent as buckling of the affected limb(s) under the animal's weight, sometimes together with a low head carriage and performing a 'forward roll' in those with generalised neuromuscular weakness.

e. Extensor postural thrust

This test is most useful in cats or small dogs to further evaluate the pelvic limb proprioception. Place both hands around the thorax, just caudal to the shoulders, and hold the animal upright so that it is elevated from the ground. The animal is then lowered towards the ground and encouraged to walk backwards. The normal response should be for the dog or cat to extend the pelvic limbs in anticipation of them reaching the ground, followed by even and coordinated backward steps.

Animals with lower motor neuron weakness of the pelvic limbs (e.g. generalised neuromuscular disease or an L4–S1 spinal cord lesion) will show poor extension of the pelvic limb joints (stifles and/or hocks) and may collapse when trying to perform the stepping movements. Proprioceptive deficits in the pelvic limbs are apparent as a delay in the onset and termination of the corrective stepping movements, resulting in long steps with erratic placement of the affected limb(s).

f. Other tests of proprioception

Other tests that can be used to assess proprioception include the paper slide test and tactile placing. These tests need not be performed if a convincing proprioceptive deficit has already been identified using paw replacement or hopping.

Paper slide test. With the animal standing squarely and distributing weight evenly across all limbs, a piece of paper is placed under the paw of the limb being tested. This piece of paper is then pulled slowly in a lateral direction and the normal response is for the animal to briskly correct the position of the limb so that it lies underneath the body (e.g. under the shoulder for the thoracic limb, or under the hip for the pelvic limb). A proprioceptive deficit is suggested if there is a delay in the replacement of the paw back to its normal position. This test assesses proprioception in a similar way to hopping but in reverse, with the limb being moved lateral to the body rather than the body being moved lateral to the limb. It can therefore be useful for large or giant breed dogs, or for nervous animals, in which hopping may be difficult to perform and interpret.

Tactile placing. This test of proprioception can be useful in cats or small dogs, particularly within the confines a small consultation room (see Video 9a). The animal is held with one hand under the abdomen or thorax, and the other hand gently covering the eyes so that the dog or cat cannot see the examination table in front of them (see Video 10a). The thoracic and pelvic limbs are then tested in turn by moving the animal towards the edge of the table so that the dorsal aspects of the paws being tested contact the table edge. Contact with the table edge should induce a coordinated stepping movement so that the paws are placed onto the table. If there is a proprioceptive deficit, then there will be a delay in the initiation of the stepping action and the dorsal aspect of the paw will drag along the table edge before a corrective movement is observed. The results of this test should be confirmed using other tests of proprioception (e.g. hopping or paw replacement). Tactile placing can appear abnormal in animals that are nervous as they may be tense and hold their limbs in an extended position. It is also prudent to perform this test when holding the animal on each side of your body (e.g. alternating between using your right and left arm to cover the eyes), as the limb closest to your body can sometimes appear to show an abnormal response. This should only be interpreted as abnormal if repeatable with the animal held on both sides of your body.

4. Spinal reflex testing

Gait evaluation and proprioceptive testing are most useful to confirm the presence of a neurological problem and to determine which limbs are affected. However, they are non-specific in terms of localising the site of the lesion responsible. This is because numerous neuroanatomical structures, including components of the brain, spinal cord, and peripheral nervous system, are required for normal proprioception and to generate a normal gait. Other tests are therefore required, which assess the integrity of more limited regions of the nervous system, to determine a specific neuroanatomical localisation. This includes assessment of the local spinal reflexes in all limbs.

Similar to the cranial nerve examination, spinal reflex testing involves application of a tactile stimulus to a region of the body and the observation of an appropriate motor reaction to this stimulus. In doing so, these tests screen the function of three main components.

1. The peripheral sensory nerves that detect and transmit the sensory information to the level of the spinal cord.
2. The peripheral motor nerves that innervate the muscles responsible for the reflex movement.
3. The region of the spinal cord that contains both the cell bodies of the peripheral motor neurons involved in the reflex and the interneurons that connect the sensory component to these cell bodies.

A spinal reflex will be abnormal if there is dysfunction of one or more of these three components and spinal reflexes can therefore be affected by lesions involving the spinal cord or peripheral nervous system. It is important to remember that these local spinal reflexes do not require input from the brain or spinal cord UMNs to be normal. They will therefore be intact as long as the peripheral nerves and spinal cord segments required for reflex activity are functional, irrespective of brain or spinal cord lesions at distant sites. For example, the spinal reflexes in the pelvic limbs will appear normal even if the spinal cord is severed at a site cranial to the L3 spinal cord segment. This concept underlies the importance of separating the interpretation of spinal reflex testing and assessment for nociception ('deep pain sensation') in the limb being tested. Otherwise, confusion may arise regarding both the lesion localisation and the severity of the clinical signs. If the peripheral sensory nerve responsible for detecting a tactile or noxious stimulus is damaged, then both the flexor withdrawal reflex and nociception may be absent in the limb being tested. However, the flexor withdrawal reflex may be reduced or absent in a dog with a generalised peripheral motor polyneuropathy whilst nociception will remain normal as the sensory nervous system and spinal cord are not affected in these cases. In contrast, a severe thoracolumbar spinal cord lesion may result in loss of nociception in the pelvic limbs but the pelvic limb withdrawal reflexes will remain normal as the spinal cord segments responsible for the reflex are spared (L4–S1 spinal cord segments).

Spinal reflex testing is therefore most useful for:

- localising the site of a spinal cord lesion by screening the function of specific regions of the spinal cord
- assessing the integrity of the peripheral nerves required for reflex function.

a. Flexor withdrawal reflex

The flexor withdrawal reflex is the most useful spinal reflex to perform in the majority of cases (see Video 11a). It is particularly useful for refining the neuroanatomic localisation in an animal with a suspected spinal cord lesion. It should be assessed in both the thoracic and pelvic limbs and can initially be performed in a standing animal at the same time as proprioceptive testing (see Videos 12a and 13a). If there is any suspicion that the reflex is abnormal, then this should be confirmed by repeating the test with the patient in lateral recumbency.

The interdigital skin of the limb being tested is held between your thumb and forefinger, with the limb in extension. A gradually increasing pressure is then applied, which should induce flexion of the limb to pull it away from the stimulus; all of the joints in the limb being tested should flex at this time (shoulder, elbow, carpus, and digits for the thoracic limb, and the hip, stifle, hock, and digits for the pelvic limb). The animal should still be able to withdraw the limb even if you apply mild resistance to flexion by keeping hold of the interdigital skin between your fingertips. If there is no response to fingertip pressure, then fingernails can be used to apply a stronger stimulus. If no attempt is subsequently made to withdraw the limb, then artery forceps can be used to apply gentle pressure to the interdigital skin or nail bed of one digit. This pressure should be increased very gradually to avoid local trauma to the digit. If the animal does not withdraw the limb but demonstrates apparent discomfort at any time during testing (e.g. vocalisation, distress, trying to bite, or move away), then it can be assumed that the motor component of the reflex is abnormal and increasing pressure should not be applied.

The most important considerations when performing this test are:

- the strength of limb withdrawal
- whether all joints are adequately flexed at the time of withdrawal.

There is significant individual variation regarding the force required to elicit a withdrawal reflex between different animals. Therefore, an apparent delay in the onset of withdrawal or the fact that more force was required to elicit the reflex compared to another animal is not significant. The most important thing is whether the animal is able to perform normal limb flexion at any point during testing.

Other important factors to consider are:

- Is there a mechanical resistance to joint flexion that could influence interpretation of the test (e.g. marked osteoarthritis and reduced range of joint motion)?
- Is there a focus of limb pain that may make an animal reluctant (rather than unable) to withdrawal the limb?

Do not make this mistake: A strong withdrawal reflex does not mean that the animal is consciously aware of the stimulus being applied to the distal limb, only that the peripheral nerves and local spinal cord segments required for the reflex are functional. This is therefore *not* the same as having intact 'deep pain perception' (nociception) (see Video 15).

Thoracic limb withdrawal reflex. This test screens the integrity of the C6–T2 spinal cord segments, C6–T2 dorsal and ventral nerve roots, and the peripheral nerves that innervate the flexors of the shoulder (axillary nerve), elbow (musculocutaneous nerve), carpus, and digits (median and ulnar nerves). The sensory nerves responsible for detecting the stimulus reside within the radial nerve (dorsal aspect of the paw) and median and ulnar nerves (palmar aspect of the paw) if the second or third digits are stimulated (see Video 12a).

This test is most useful to refine the neuroanatomic localisation in an animal with tetraparesis/tetraplegia and a suspected spinal cord lesion between the C1 and T2 spinal cord segments. Strong thoracic limb withdrawal reflexes would be consistent with a lesion affecting the C1–C5 spinal cord segments, whereas weak thoracic limb withdrawal reflexes would imply a lesion involving the C6–T2 segments (or peripheral nerves).

Pelvic limb withdrawal reflex. This test primarily screens the integrity of the L6–S1 spinal cord segments, L6–S1 nerves roots, and the sciatic nerve that innervates the flexors of the stifle, hock, and digits. The hip flexors are innervated by the femoral nerve (L4–L6 spinal cord segments and nerve roots) and the lumbar spinal nerves. The sensory nerve responsible for detecting the stimulus depends on which digit is used to perform the test, with this being the sciatic nerve if the stimulus is applied to the fifth (lateral) digit and the femoral nerve for the first (medial) digit (see Video 13a).

This test is most useful for refining the neuroanatomic localisation in an animal with paraparesis/paraplegia and a suspected spinal cord lesion between the

T3 and S1 spinal cord segments. Strong pelvic limb withdrawal reflexes would be consistent with a lesion affecting the T3–L3 spinal cord segments, whereas weak pelvic limb withdrawal reflexes would imply a lesion involving the L4–S1 segments/nerve roots (or sciatic nerves) (see Video 14a).

A diffuse or multifocal spinal cord lesion affecting both the C6–T2 and L4–S1 spinal cord segments would be required to affect the withdrawal reflexes in both the thoracic and pelvic limbs concurrently. Such conditions are rare, and the scenario of reduced/absent withdrawal reflexes in all limbs is more commonly observed in association with generalised neuromuscular disorders that affect the peripheral nerves required for reflex function away from the spinal cord.

b. Patellar reflex

The patellar reflex is the most commonly performed tendon reflex in veterinary medicine, and familiarity with the same reflex in human medicine means that owners often find it entertaining to see it performed in their pet! However, this test may be of little use for refining the neuroanatomic localisation in many cases and there are several considerations to bear in mind when interpreting the results. The patellar reflex is most useful in animals that have an abnormal pelvic limb gait, show apparent pelvic limb weakness, or show poor stifle extension when standing.

The patellar reflex is most easily assessed with the animal in lateral recumbency and the limb being tested held partially flexed (see Video 15a). It may also be tested when the animal is standing, by holding the femur just proximal to the stifle and allowing the distal limb to hang beneath (see Video 16a). However, the limb should always be relaxed at the time of testing as increased extensor tone in the limb can complicate interpretation of a subjectively weak reflex. The patellar tendon that runs between the patella and the tibial tuberosity is struck briskly using a tendon hammer to elicit a reflex extension of the stifle. The handle of a pair of scissors or forceps can also be used to apply the blunt stimulus to the patellar tendon.

Striking the patellar tendon results in stretching of small, specialised myofibres called muscle spindles that lie within the quadriceps muscle. This results in firing of nerve endings associated with the muscle spindles, and this information is relayed to the spinal cord via sensory nerve fibres within the femoral nerve. These sensory axons connect directly (monosynaptically) to the cell bodies of motor nerve fibres that reside within the ventral grey matter of the L4–L6 spinal cord segments. These motor axons leave the spinal cord in the L4, L5, and L6 ventral nerve roots and form the motor component of the femoral nerve which innervates the quadriceps muscle responsible for stifle extension.

Important considerations when performing the patellar reflex are:

- The reflex may appear reduced/absent in animals with pre-existing stifle disease (e.g. cruciate ligament rupture, osteoarthritis).
- The reflex may appear reduced/absent if there is increased muscle tone in the limb being tested. This can often be the case for nervous animals or those that are intolerant of being held in lateral recumbency.
- The reflex will also appear absent if the patellar tendon is not struck cleanly, or if the patella or tibial tuberosity are inadvertently struck instead.
- The patellar reflex may appear reduced/absent in older dogs as an incidental finding. Interpretation of the reflex in this subset of animals therefore needs careful consideration. If an animal has a normal pelvic limb gait and is able to stand with a normal stifle posture, then femoral nerve function (motor) can be assumed to be adequate. A reduced/absent patellar reflex in these cases is unlikely to be significant and should not be used to guide the neuroanatomic localisation unless there are other neurological deficits consistent with abnormal sensory nerve function (e.g. reduction of other tendon reflexes, poor flexor withdrawal reflexes, proprioceptive deficits).

Top tip: If the animal is in lateral recumbency, the patellar reflex may appear reduced in either the recumbent or uppermost limb; if this is the case, then the reflex should be repeated with the animal in the opposite recumbency. If the patellar reflex is normal in one recumbency, then this does not need to be confirmed in the other recumbency.

A subjectively exaggerated patellar reflex could reflect:

- A spinal cord lesion rostral to the L4 spinal cord segment resulting in loss of UMN inhibition on reflex function. This can be apparent as clonus of the patellar reflex in which there is repetitive extension of the stifle in response to a single stimulus.
- Sciatic nerve dysfunction resulting in loss of tone in the antagonist stifle flexor muscles that would normally provide resistance to stifle extension. This is termed 'pseudo-hyperreflexia'.
- The patellar reflex may also appear exaggerated in a stressed or excited dog, therefore a subjectively 'strong' reflex should always be interpreted with caution. Given the degree of natural variation between animals it is more reliable to simply think of this reflex as being either normal or reduced/absent.

c. Other limb reflexes

In addition to the patellar reflex, other tests of reflex function include the extensor carpi radialis, biceps brachii, triceps, cranial tibial, and gastrocnemius reflexes.

These tests aim to assess the integrity of the specific spinal cord segments, their associated nerve roots, and the peripheral nerves involved in each reflex.

- *Extensor carpi radialis*: C7–T2 spinal cord segments and nerve roots; radial nerve (see Video 17a).
- *Biceps brachii*: C6–C8 spinal cord segments and nerve roots; musculocutaneous nerve.
- *Triceps*: C7–T1 spinal cord segments and nerve roots; radial nerve.
- *Tibialis cranialis*: L6–S1 spinal cord segments and nerve roots; peroneal nerve (see Video 18a).
- *Gastrocnemius*: L7–S1 spinal cord segments and nerve roots; tibial nerve.

The authors rarely perform these tests in practice as they are less reliable than the patellar reflex and their interpretation is complicated by the fact that they may be absent in the normal animal. Recent studies have also questioned the clinical utility of the cranial tibial and extensor carpi radialis reflexes as they can still be elicited in cats after anaesthetic blockade of the brachial and lumbosacral plexi (Tudury et al. 2017). This suggests that these reflexes are not strictly myotactic, as they appear independent of the reflex arc and are more likely to represent local muscle contraction in response to percussion of the muscle belly itself.

d. Perineal reflex, anal tone, tail tone, and bladder function

Perineal reflex and anal tone. The perineal reflex can be performed at the same time as assessment of anal tone and tail tone (see Video 19a). These tests are used to screen the integrity of the first sacral (S1) to fifth caudal (Cd5) spinal cord segments, the S1–Cd5 nerve roots, the pudendal nerves for anal sphincter tone, and the caudal nerves for tail tone and movement. The S1–S3 and Cd1–Cd5 spinal cord segments reside within the spinal canal of most dogs in the region of the L5 and L6 vertebrae, respectively. Their associated nerve roots then course caudally as part of the cauda equina to exit the spinal canal via their respective foramina. Pathology affecting the L5 and L6 vertebrae or their associated intervertebral discs may therefore affect these adjacent spinal cord segments, resulting in poor tail or anal tone. The termination of the spinal cord in cats is located more caudally within the spinal canal, typically at the level of the L7 to sacral vertebrae.

To assess the perineal reflex, artery forceps are used to gently pinch the skin either side of the anus. This should elicit a reflex contraction of the anal sphincter and flexion of the tail. Reduced or absent anal tone, indicating a lesion involving the S1–S3 spinal cord segments/nerve roots or the pudendal nerve, will be apparent as a relaxed anal sphincter that does not constrict around your finger when digital rectal examination is performed. There will also be little or no resistance to gentle opening of the anus using the ends of a pair of artery forceps.

Tail carriage. A low tail carriage can be the result of both neurological and non-neurological conditions.

- A flaccid tail that lacks voluntary movement and hangs limp would be most consistent with a lesion affecting the Cd1–Cd5 spinal cord segments, nerve roots, or caudal nerves. It is important to note that the flaccid tail may passively swing from side to side when the animal is walking, which may be mistaken for a voluntary tail wag.
- A spinal cord lesion involving the descending UMN tracts between the first cervical (C1) and seventh lumbar (L7) spinal cord segments may result in a low tail carriage and reduced voluntary tail function if the messages informing the tail to move are interrupted (e.g. an absent tail wag when greeting the owner). However, the muscle tone in the tail should be normal and reflex flexion should still be observed on perineal reflex testing.
- A low tail carriage with normal tail tone can be seen in nervous animals, or secondary to discomfort in the region of the tail base (e.g. lumbosacral disease, caudal disc extrusion, cat bite abscess).
- Reduced tone in the distal tail concurrent with firm, painful swelling of the tail base that is held rigidly extended can be seen in dogs with acute caudal myopathy (often colloquially called 'limber tail' or 'swimmer's tail'). This condition is more commonly seen in working dogs, with swimming being a risk factor. Recent research has suggested a possible genetic predisposition in Labrador Retrievers (Pugh et al. 2016). This condition is likely to reflect a form of compartment syndrome in which excessive use or trauma to the tail muscles results in swelling and an increase in pressure within muscles that are constrained by a tight fascia. This increased pressure can result in ischaemia of the caudal muscles and nerves.

Bladder function and palpation. If there is a history of urinary incontinence (either urine leakage or an inability to pass urine), then assessment of bladder size, tone, and ease of expression can help to guide the neuroanatomic localisation if a neurological lesion is responsible. However, non-neurological causes of urinary incontinence should always be considered first, as these are likely to be more common in general practice compared to neurological lesions, particularly in the absence of other neurological deficits such as paraparesis, paraplegia, or poor tail or anal tone. Non-neurological conditions to consider in these cases include urolithiasis and urethral obstruction (particularly in male cats), feline lower urinary tract disease, bacterial cystitis, bladder or urethral neoplasia, and urethral sphincter mechanism incompetence in spayed female dogs.

The detrusor muscle of the bladder and the urethral sphincters are primarily innervated by the autonomic nervous system (sympathetic and parasympathetic components). Contraction of the detrusor muscle for urination is mediated by the parasympathetic nervous system via the pelvic nerve, which has cell bodies in the S1–S3 spinal cord segments. Contraction of the striated muscle of the external urethral sphincter is mediated by the pudendal nerve, which also has cell bodies in the S1–S3 spinal cord segments (Figure 3.15). Therefore, a lesion that damages the S1–S3 spinal cord segments/nerve roots, or the pelvic and pudendal nerves themselves, can result in a flaccid bladder that is easy to express. Incomplete urine voiding will occur as the animal is unable to contract the detrusor muscle, and urine leakage may occur secondary to loss of tone in the external urethral sphincter. This is often termed a 'lower motor neuron' bladder and is frequently accompanied by poor tail and anal tone and/or a weak perineal reflex.

There is also an internal urethral sphincter that is made up of smooth muscle and is innervated by sympathetic nerve fibres in the hypogastric nerve. This nerve originates from cell bodies in the cranial lumbar spinal cord segments (L1–L4 in the dog) and can therefore be spared by lesions that affect the S1–S3 segments in the low lumbar/lumbosacral spine. Intact tone in the internal sphincter may therefore provide some resistance against bladder expression in animals with an otherwise flaccid 'lower motor neuron' bladder. The hypogastric nerve can be damaged, together with the pelvic and pudendal nerves, by lesions in the region of the pelvic plexus in the caudal abdomen (e.g. pelvic fracture, neoplasia). This will result in complete loss of internal and external urethral sphincter competence, and a leaking bladder that is very easy to express.

Voluntary control of urination is mediated by spinal cord UMNs that travel from the micturition centres in the brainstem to the cell bodies of the hypogastric, pelvic, and pudendal nerves that directly control bladder function (Figure 3.15). Spinal cord lesions between C1 and L7 may damage these UMN fibres, resulting in loss of the voluntary control of urination. In affected cases, the bladder will fill until the pressure inside it exceeds the tone of the urethral sphincters, and it starts to overflow. It is therefore very important to distinguish between voluntary urination and an overflowing 'upper motor neuron' bladder in animals with spinal cord lesions. This is to avoid the bladder becoming overstretched and non-functional. The pelvic nerves and pudendal nerves are unaffected in these cases, meaning that the bladder remains tonic and is often difficult to express against a contracted urethral sphincter. Loss of voluntary urination is usually observed with spinal cord lesions that are severe enough to result in

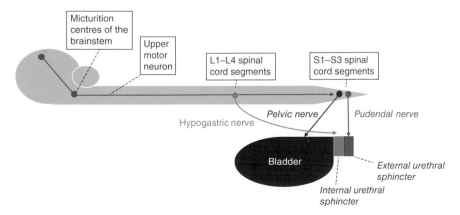

Figure 3.15 The innervation of the bladder.

paraplegia. It is therefore unusual (but not impossible) to see a loss of voluntary bladder function in animals that still have voluntary movement in their pelvic limbs (i.e. ambulatory or non-ambulatory paraparesis). Likewise, voluntary urination frequently returns at roughly the same time as pelvic limb movements in animals that are recovering from severe spinal cord injury. See Sections 6.10 'Paresis, Paralysis and Proprioceptive Ataxia' and 7.3 'Acute Spinal Cord Injury' in Chapters 6 and 7 respectively for further discussion regarding bladder management in animals with spinal cord lesions.

e. Cutaneous trunci reflex

The cutaneous trunci reflex is most useful when used to more accurately localise a suspected spinal cord lesion between the T3 and L3 spinal cord segments (see Video 20a). Assessment of this reflex in a dog or cat with a normal gait and normal proprioception in all limbs is not usually required. The term 'panniculus reflex' has been used for this test but is a misnomer as the word 'panniculus' refers to the layer of subcutaneous fat that is not involved in this reflex arc.

This test is performed by pinching the skin of the dorsum on either side of the vertebral spinous processes, which should elicit reflex contraction of the cutaneous trunci muscle on both flanks (Figure 3.16a). This is a bilateral reflex and pinching on one side of the dorsum should elicit contraction of the cutaneous trunci muscles on both sides. The cutaneous trunci reflex should be present in the majority of dogs from the level of the L5–L6 vertebrae. Testing should therefore start at this level and can be stopped if the reflex is present; further testing at more cranial levels is only required if no contraction of the cutaneous trunci is observed. Stimulation should be repeated sequentially at the level of each spinous process, moving forwards until contraction is observed.

If the cutaneous trunci reflex can only be elicited at a level more cranial than the L5–L6 vertebrae, then this would be consistent with a spinal cord lesion that is blocking the ascending sensory information travelling to the cell bodies of the lower motor neurons that innervate the cutaneous trunci muscle (Figure 3.16b). These cell bodies reside in the C8 and T1 spinal cord segments, with their associated axons forming the lateral thoracic nerve. A spinal cord lesion that interrupts the cutaneous trunci reflex may lie up to four vertebrae cranial to the level of reflex loss but is most commonly around two vertebrae cranial to the level of interruption (Gutierrez-Quintana et al. 2012). For example, if the cutaneous trunci reflex is absent caudal to the level of the L2 spinous process then this would be most consistent with a spinal cord lesion in the vicinity of the T13 vertebra (e.g. T13–L1 disc extrusion).

A bilateral lesion involving the C8–T1 spinal cord segments, C8–T1 nerve roots, or lateral thoracic nerves would result in an absent cutaneous trunci reflex at all levels of stimulation. However, it is important to note that this reflex may be difficult to elicit in some dogs and cats. An absent cutaneous trunci reflex at all levels of stimulation should therefore be interpreted with caution unless

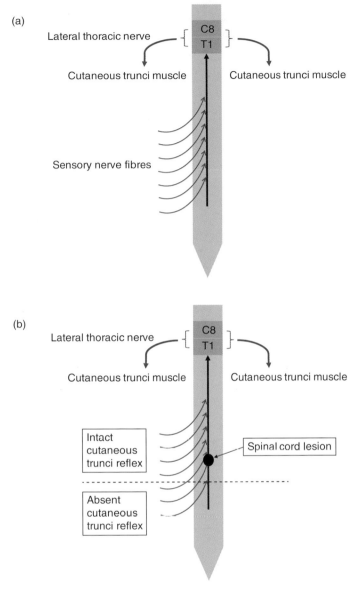

Figure 3.16 (a) The cutaneous trunci reflex. Stimulation of the skin overlying the dorsum results in reflex contraction of the cutaneous trunci muscle on both sides. (b) A spinal cord lesion that blocks the ascending sensory information from reaching the C8–T1 spinal cord segments will interrupt the cutaneous trunci reflex at a level roughly two vertebrae caudal to the level of the spinal cord lesion.

there are other neurological deficits consistent with a lesion affecting the C8–T1 spinal cord segments or nerve roots.

A unilateral lesion that involves the C8–T1 spinal cord segments, nerve roots, or lateral thoracic nerve will result in an ipsilateral loss of cutaneous trunci muscle contraction. This will be clinically apparent as contraction of the cutaneous trunci muscle on only one side (opposite to the side of the lesion) in response to stimulation of either side of the dorsum at any level. Other clinical signs that could be associated with a unilateral lesion affecting the C8–T1 spinal cord segments or nerve roots include lower motor neuron paresis of the ipsilateral thoracic limb, proprioceptive deficits in the ipsilateral pelvic limb, or Horner syndrome in the ipsilateral pupil.

5. Spinal palpation and neck manipulation

Tests that may be uncomfortable for the animal or that involve the application of a noxious stimulus should only be performed if the information is essential for determining the prognosis or to refine the neuroanatomic localisation (see Videos 21a and 22a). They should also be performed at the end of the examination so that the dog or cat remains cooperative.

Identification of a focus or foci of apparent discomfort when moving the neck or applying pressure to the vertebral column can greatly assist in supporting your lesion localisation. This can be performed by working from head to tail.

- Direct palpation of the cervical spine. This is most easily performed by applying pressure from laterally using your fingers on either side of the paraspinal muscles, working from the wings of the atlas to in front of the scapulae.
- Direct pressure applied to the transverse processes that protrude from the ventrolateral aspect of the C6 vertebra at the level of the thoracic inlet.
- Ventral flexion, dorsal extension, and lateral movement of the neck to the left and right sides. A normal dog or cat should allow the head to be moved so that the nose touches each flank. Resistance to such movement may imply discomfort, but mechanical restriction by a paraspinal mass should also be considered. Flexion of the neck in a young toy breed dog with suspected neck pain and/or neurological deficits in all limbs should be avoided due to the risk of exacerbating possible atlantoaxial instability.
- Direct palpation of the dorsal spinous processes from the first thoracic vertebra (T1) to the lumbosacral junction. Light pressure should be used initially, followed by cycles of palpation using increasing force to identify any foci of apparent discomfort.
- Lordosis testing of the lumbosacral junction can be performed by extending both hips and applying direct pressure to the lumbosacral region from dorsally using either your other hand or chin.
- Tail elevation may elicit discomfort in dogs with lumbosacral discomfort or tail pain.
- Digital rectal examination can be performed to assess for prostatic enlargement or discomfort, anal sac disease, intrapelvic mass lesions, or discomfort on direct pressure to the ventral aspect of the sacrum.

All innervated anatomical structures in the region of discomfort should be considered as a possible origin for any apparent pain that is elicited. This approach is particularly useful to guide further investigations if there are no other neurological deficits on examination (e.g. in an animal that presents with neck pain as the sole clinical finding). These anatomical structures include vertebrae, vertebral facet joints, paraspinal muscles, outer annulus fibrosus of the intervertebral disc, ligaments (e.g. dorsal longitudinal ligament), meninges, and nerve roots.

The spinal cord itself is comprised of many sensory nerve fibres but does not contain nociceptive nerve endings, therefore lesions affecting the spinal cord in isolation do not typically result in overt discomfort (e.g. intramedullary tumours). However, meningeal or nerve root involvement can result in severe pain, and parenchymal lesions that affect the processing of nociceptive information at the level of the dorsal horn may also result in apparent discomfort (e.g. syringomyelia).

6. Testing of pain perception (nociception)

Nociception is the response of the nervous system to a harmful or potentially harmful stimulus. This process involves the transmission of sensory information from the site of stimulation to the forebrain in order to determine the potential for harm. A conscious response to such stimulation therefore needs to be observed when testing for nociception, which could include vocalisation, turning to look at the site of stimulation, or attempting to bite. This is often termed 'deep pain perception' and involves applying firm pressure using a pair of artery forceps to the nail bed or digit of the limb being tested. Application of a noxious stimulus using artery forceps is of course not required if a conscious response to more gentle stimulation using your fingertips or fingernails is observed first.

This conscious response to stimulation is *not* the same as the reflex movement of a limb in response to the stimulus being applied, as described for the flexor withdrawal reflex (see Video 15). Reflex testing only screens the peripheral nerves and spinal cord segments involved in the reflex action and will remain present even if the spinal cord is transected away from the segments involved.

The presence of a conscious response to a noxious stimulus requires integrity of the axons within the spinal cord that transmit this information to the sensory cortex in the forebrain. These are small, unmyelinated axons that lie deep within the spinal cord on both sides, making them more resilient to injury compared to the more superficial, larger, myelinated proprioceptive and motor fibres. This is of clinical importance as it means that there is always an ordered loss of neurological function with increasing severity and extent of spinal cord injury:

- Loss of proprioception
- Loss of voluntary motor function (ranging from paresis to paralysis)
- Loss of nociception only when proprioception and voluntary motor function have both been lost (i.e. nociception will only be lost once the affected limb is paralysed).

The fact that a severe, transverse lesion to the spinal cord is required to stop the nociceptive messages being able to reach the brain, means that it is extremely useful for predicting lesion severity and likely prognosis in a paralysed animal. However, this also means that nociceptive testing is *only* required in animals with no appreciable voluntary movement in the limb(s) being tested. Performing this test in an animal that has voluntary movement or, even worse, that can still walk only adds unnecessary pain and distress. The interpretation of nociceptive testing can also be difficult in stressed or stoic animals, particularly in those that have another focus of pain or that have received recent analgesia, and this makes appropriate case selection even more important.

Testing for nociception in the thoracic and/or pelvic limbs in a tetraplegic animal is not inappropriate; however, it is unusual for a cervical spinal cord lesion to result in deep pain negative tetraplegia without also affecting the descending axons for respiration, resulting in death.

3.5 Summary of the Neurological Examination

As previously discussed, performing a complete neurological examination in every animal that presents to you with a possible neurological problem is always good practice. However, a more refined neurological examination can often be performed in the majority of patients and should take about 10 minutes to perform.

3.5.1 Observation
- Alertness and interaction with the environment ('mentation and behaviour').
- Posture of the head, limbs, joints, body, and tail.
- Gait: Is it normal? Which limbs are affected? What is the stride length in the affected limbs? Is limb placement predictable?
- Presence of any involuntary movements.
- Facial symmetry, voluntary blinking, eyeball position, jaw tone and position.

3.5.2 Hands-On Assessment
- *Cranial nerve examination*:
  - Eyes: palpebral reflexes, menace responses, observation for involuntary eye movements (spontaneous and positional), pupil size and symmetry.
  - Mouth and jaws: jaw tone, tongue symmetry, masticatory muscle bulk.
  - Nose: nasal septum nociception.
- *Limb palpation*: muscle atrophy, muscle tone.
- *Postural reactions*: paw replacement in all limbs, followed by hopping if paw replacement is normal or equivocal.
- *Spinal reflex testing*: withdrawal reflexes in all limbs, patellar reflexes if abnormal pelvic limb gait or posture.

- Perineal reflex and assessment of tail tone, anal tone, and bladder function.
- *Spinal palpation and neck manipulation*: for spinal hyperaesthesia.

The choice of additional tests will depend upon the presenting complaint, how tolerant the patient is of examination, and how confident you are of a neurological deficit(s) after performing the tests above. These tests could include the following:

- *Turning the patient into dorsal recumbency to look for positional nystagmus*. This is particularly useful to confirm vestibular dysfunction if there is a suspicion of intracranial disease, or if there are subtle signs of possible vestibular dysfunction (e.g. slight head tilt or drifting when walking) but no spontaneous nystagmus on cranial nerve examination.
- *Vestibulo-ocular reflex*. This test can be used to add support for a vestibular disorder but may offer little extra information if a head tilt, positional strabismus, or abnormal spontaneous nystagmus has already been identified. This test is most useful in animals with bilateral vestibular dysfunction or as part of a modified Glasgow Coma Scale (MGCS) to monitor trends in brainstem function.
- *Pupillary light reflex*. This test should be performed if anisocoria is present or if visual deficits are suspected in one or both eyes.
- *Gag reflex*. If it is safe to perform, this test is most useful in animals with a history of dysphagia, gagging, regurgitation, or difficulty swallowing. As for the vestibulo-ocular reflex, it is also useful to monitor trends in brainstem function.
- *Hemi-walking*. This test is only required if an animal is too large to perform hopping in individual limbs.
- *Wheelbarrow testing*. This test can be useful if there is a suspicion of neuromuscular weakness (e.g. generalised motor polyneuropathy). Animals with generalised weakness may find it difficult to support their head and can collapse on the thoracic limbs as if performing a forward roll. Elevating the head when performing wheelbarrow testing can also accentuate hypermetria in animals with cerebellar dysfunction.
- *Extensor postural thrust*. This test can be very useful in cats to assess for proprioceptive deficits in the pelvic limbs.
- *Tactile placing*. This is an additional test of proprioception that can be used to confirm or refute the findings of hopping or paw replacement if the results of these tests are equivocal.
- *Cutaneous trunci reflex*. This should be performed in all cases for which there is a suspicion of a spinal cord lesion between C6–L3 to further guide the neuroanatomic localisation.
- *Nociceptive testing*. This test should only be performed if there is no voluntary movement observed in one or more limbs (paralysis/plegia).

Bibliography

Crawford, A.H., Beltran, E., Lam, R., and Kenny, P.J. (2016). Convergence-retraction nystagmus associated with dorsal midbrain lesions in three dogs. *J. Vet. Intern. Med.* 30: 1229–1234.

Dewey, C.W. and da Costa, R.C. (2015). *Practical Guide to Canine and Feline Neurology*, 3e. Hoboken, NJ: Wiley Blackwell.

Gutierrez-Quintana, R., Edgar, J., Wessmann, A. et al. (2012). The cutaneous trunci reflex for localising and grading thoracolumbar spinal cord injuries in dogs. *J. Small Anim. Pract.* 53: 470–475.

Ives, E.J., MacKillop, E., and Olby, N.J. (2018). Saccadic oscillations in 4 dogs and 1 cat. *J. Vet. Intern. Med.* 32: 1392–1396.

Kent, M., Platt, S.R., and Schatzberg, S.J. (2010). The neurology of balance: function and dysfunction of the vestibular system in dogs and cats. *Vet. J.* 185: 247–258.

de Lahunta, A., Glass, E., and Kent, M. (2015). *Veterinary Neuroanatomy and Clinical Neurology*, 4e. St Louis, MO: Elsevier Saunders.

Lorenz, M.D., Coates, J., and Kent, M. (2011). *Handbook of Veterinary Neurology*, 5e. St Louis, MO: Elsevier Saunders.

Muguet-Chanoit, A.C., Olby, N.J., Babb, K.M. et al. (2011). The sensory field and repeatability of the cutaneous trunci muscle reflex of the dog. *Vet. Surg.* 40: 781–785.

Platt, S. and Olby, N. (2013). *BSAVA Manual of Canine and Feline Neurology*, 4e. Gloucester, UK: British Small Animal Veterinary Association.

Pugh, C.A., de C Bronsvoort, B.M., Handel, I.G. et al. (2016). Cumulative incidence and risk factors for limber tail in the Dogslife Labrador retriever cohort. *Vet. Rec.* 179: 275.

Quitt, P.R., Reese, S., Fischer, A. et al. (2019). Assessment of menace response in neurologically and ophthalmologically healthy cats. *J. Feline Med. Surg.* 21 (6): 537–543.

Sprague, J.M. (1953). Spinal border cells and their role in postural mechanism (Schiff–Sherrington phenomenon). *J. Neurophysiol.* 16: 464–474.

Troxel, M.T., Drobatz, K.J., and Vite, C.H. (2005). Signs of neurologic dysfunction in dogs with central versus peripheral vestibular disease. *J. Am. Vet Med. Assoc.* 227: 570–574.

Tudury, E.A., de Figueiredo, M.L., Fernandes, T.H. et al. (2017). Evaluation of cranial tibial and extensor carpi radialis reflexes before and after anesthetic blockade in cats. *J. Feline Med. Surg.* 19: 105–109.

Chapter 4 Lesion Localisation

Edward Ives

As discussed in Chapter 3, the neurological deficits identified on examination reflect the lesion location and *not* the underlying cause. This location is called the neuroanatomic localisation. It is essential that the neuroanatomic localisation is determined before you consider individual diseases and perform further tests. This is because some disorders will be more likely to affect certain regions of the nervous system and others less likely to do so. Conditions affecting different regions of the nervous system can also result in similar clinical signs. For example, an abnormal gait in all limbs could result from a lesion affecting the brain (e.g. cerebellar infarct), or the cervical spinal cord (e.g. intervertebral disc disease), or any part of the neuromuscular system (e.g. peripheral neuropathy, myasthenia gravis). If the neuroanatomic localisation is not considered before tests are performed, then the diagnostic approach is likely to become confused and expensive for the owner, with unnecessary tests being performed that are difficult to interpret.

The subjective nature of the neurological examination, together with the wide range of individual variation, means that it may be difficult to determine the significance of an individual examination finding. Therefore, after performing the full neurological examination it can be useful to classify your findings as follows:

- Tests that you feel confident were normal.
- Tests for which a clear neurological deficit was present (e.g. absent palpebral reflex, paraplegia, absent paw replacement).
- Equivocal findings (e.g. subjectively weak withdrawal reflex, poor patellar reflex, incomplete PLR in a stressed animal).

The tests for which a clear neurological deficit was present should then be used to determine the site of a *single* lesion that could explain all of these deficits. It can then be decided whether the equivocal findings:

a. support this localisation
b. are more likely to be insignificant or unrelated to the current problem
c. suggest a multifocal disease process.

A Practical Approach to Neurology for the Small Animal Practitioner, First Edition. Paul M. Freeman and Edward Ives.
© 2020 John Wiley & Sons Ltd. Published 2020 by John Wiley & Sons Ltd.
Companion Website: www.wiley.com/go/freeman/neurology

Many neurological tests involve the same test being performed on both sides of the body. This means that there is an internal control, and by comparing the results for the left and right sides, the potential significance of a subtle or equivocal finding may be determined. If there is clear asymmetry in the test results, then a subtle deficit is more likely to be significant than if your findings are similar for both the left and right sides.

As discussed in Chapter 3, if it is not possible to determine the site of single lesion to explain all of the neurological deficits, then a *multifocal* or *diffuse* neuroanatomic localisation should be considered.

It is always important to consider the clinical history and the owner's primary concerns when determining the neuroanatomic localisation. This ensures that unrelated, pre-existing neurological deficits are flagged up that could have otherwise complicated the interpretation of the current examination. These could include:

- a head tilt in an animal with a prior history of vestibular disease
- pelvic limb proprioceptive deficits in a dog that has had previous spinal surgery for intervertebral disc disease
- dysphonia, poor hock flexion on withdrawal reflex testing, or pelvic limb proprioceptive deficits in an old Labrador Retriever with a degenerative polyneuropathy.

4.1   Principles of Lesion Localisation

The nervous system can be broadly divided into two parts (Figure 4.1).

- *Central nervous system*: the brain and spinal cord.
- *Peripheral nervous system*: peripheral sensory nerves, peripheral motor nerves, the skeletal muscles responsible for movement, and the neuromuscular junction between the motor axons and skeletal muscles. It is important to remember that the cell bodies of the peripheral motor nerves reside within the central nervous system (ventral horn of the spinal cord grey matter), with the axons leaving the spinal cord in the ventral nerve roots before forming the individual, named, peripheral nerves (e.g. femoral nerve, radial nerve).

The first step in every case should be to decide whether the lesion responsible for the presenting clinical signs is most likely to be affecting the:

- *brain*
- *spinal cord*
- *neuromuscular system*.

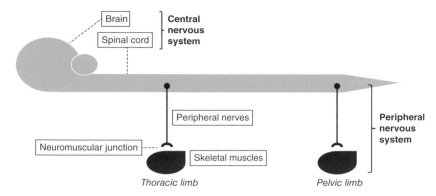

Figure 4.1 The anatomic division of the nervous system into central and peripheral components.

This will ensure that a large category of neurologic disease is not overlooked and aims to make the localisation process more approachable by limiting the initial choice to one of three broad regions.

In some instances, particularly for neuromuscular disorders, it may be difficult to refine the neuroanatomic localisation further based upon the neurological examination alone. However, the final goal of the neuroanatomic localisation should be to localise the lesion to one of the following 10 possibilities (Figure 4.2).

- Brain (intracranial)
  - forebrain
  - brainstem
  - cerebellum
- Spinal cord
  - C1–C5 spinal cord segments
  - C6–T2 spinal cord segments
  - T3–L3 spinal cord segments
  - L4–caudal (Cd) spinal cord segments

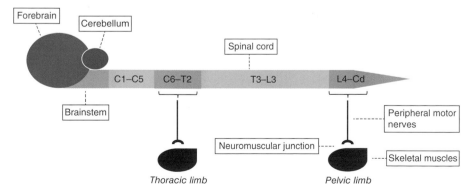

Figure 4.2 The nervous system divided into the regions that are used for lesion localisation.

- Neuromuscular system
  - peripheral neuropathy
  - neuromuscular junction disorder (junctionopathy)
  - myopathy

Any lateralisation of neurological deficits, if present, should also be considered to determine your final neuroanatomic localisation (e.g. left forebrain, right brainstem, or diffuse cerebellum if there is no lateralisation and the clinical signs are symmetric). This localisation can then be used to formulate a list of differential diagnoses, before planning further investigations.

4.1.1 Cranial Nerve Deficits

The neuroanatomic localisation for animals presenting with single (or multiple) cranial nerve deficits should also be mentioned, as where they fall within the 10 subcategories listed above is sometimes unclear. A cranial nerve deficit may result from damage to either the neuronal cell bodies that lie within the brainstem nuclei, or to the peripheral, axonal component of the cranial nerve. The neuroanatomic localisation relating to dysfunction at the level of the neuronal cell bodies would be brain (brainstem). In this scenario, other neurological deficits will usually be observed that would support this lesion location, such as tetraparesis or hemiparesis, ataxia of all limbs, other cranial nerve deficits, and an altered level of mentation. Dysfunction of the peripheral component of the cranial nerve outside the central nervous system is a common cause of cranial nerve dysfunction, and usually presents as an isolated deficit in the absence of other clinical signs (e.g. idiopathic facial paralysis, trigeminal neuropathy). The neuroanatomic localisation in these cases falls best within the neuromuscular (peripheral nerve) category, even if there are no other deficits found to support a generalised neuromuscular disorder affecting the rest of the body. Junctionopathies and myopathies may also result in clinical signs of cranial nerve dysfunction, including facial weakness, dysphagia, and megaoesophagus. The deficits in these cases usually reflect bilateral dysfunction. This should raise the index of suspicion for a neuromuscular localisation unless there are other neurological deficits to support an extensive/bilateral brainstem lesion.

A logical approach to the neuroanatomic localisation should start by considering if any of the presenting clinical signs or neurological deficits are consistent with a disease affecting the brain. If an intracranial lesion localisation appears unlikely, then a spinal cord lesion or neuromuscular disorder should be considered next.

4.2 Intracranial Lesions

The brain is an extremely complex neuroanatomical structure that processes sensory information from within and outside the body, before initiating and coordinating appropriate motor responses via the spinal cord and peripheral nervous system. Functions of the brain that can be screened by the neurological examination include:

- *level of alertness*
- *behaviour and interaction with the environment*
- *conscious response to noxious stimuli*
- *cranial nerve functions, including vision and vestibular function (balance)*
- *proprioception*
- *initiation and coordination of movements.*

Different regions of the brain are responsible for different functions and the brain can be divided into three broad regions when considering the neuroanatomic localisation: the forebrain, brainstem, and cerebellum. Classical clinical signs that would add support for a lesion involving these regions are discussed next.

1. Forebrain

- A history of epileptic seizures.
- Behavioural abnormalities (e.g. loss of house training, restlessness, pacing, altered interaction with the owner or other dogs).
- Change in the level of mentation (depression to stupor).
- Circling, most commonly towards the side of a forebrain lesion (see Video 22).
- Proprioceptive deficits affecting the thoracic and pelvic limbs on the opposite side to a lateralised forebrain lesion (Box 4.1).
- Visual deficits (e.g. an absent menace response in the eye on the opposite side to a lateralised forebrain lesion, see Video 28). A forebrain lesion that affects the central visual pathways at the level of the thalamus or visual cortex will result in blindness without affecting the pupillary light reflex.

Box 4.1

Top tip: The motor centres that are responsible for the initiation of movement in dogs and cats reside predominately within the brainstem. Therefore, whilst a forebrain lesion may result in reduced/absent paw replacement in the contralateral thoracic and pelvic limbs, the gait may appear subjectively normal if the animal is on an even surface as the brainstem motor centres are not affected.

---

2. Brainstem

The brainstem contains many important nuclei and neuronal pathways. Disease processes that affect these structures can result in profound neurological signs dependent on the extent of the lesion and the speed of onset. These structures include:

- *nuclei of cranial nerves III (oculomotor) to XII (hypoglossal)*
- *ascending reticular activating system (ARAS)*, responsible for level of wakefulness by diffuse stimulation of the cerebral cortex
- *central components of the vestibular system*
- *basal motor nuclei* responsible for the initiation and control of movement
- *respiratory and cardiac centres*
- *descending upper motor neuron tracts* destined to the travel down the spinal cord to initiate movement by stimulating the cell bodies of the peripheral motor nerves that innervate the skeletal muscles
- *ascending sensory and proprioceptive tracts* travelling from the periphery to the forebrain and cerebellum via the spinal cord.

A brainstem neuroanatomic localisation should be considered if one or more of the following neurological deficits is observed on examination.

- *Change in the level of mentation* (depression to coma).
- *Cranial nerve deficits (cranial nerves III–XII)*: see Box 4.2. Further discussion of individual cranial nerve deficits can be found in Chapter 6.
- *Vestibular syndrome* (e.g. head tilt, spontaneous nystagmus, ataxia of all limbs with drifting or rolling). Further discussion regarding the distinction between peripheral and central vestibular disorders can be found in Chapter 6.
- *Tetraparesis or ipsilateral hemiparesis.* Interruption to the descending upper motor neuron tracts will result in a long stride length in the affected limbs (delay in the onset and termination of the stride).
- *General proprioceptive ataxia of all limbs or the ipsilateral thoracic and pelvic limbs for a lateralised brainstem lesion.*
- *Proprioceptive deficits in all limbs or in the ipsilateral thoracic and pelvic limbs for a lateralised lesion.*

Seizures, loss of learned behaviours and visual deficits would not be expected for a lesion that is isolated to the brainstem. Therefore, a forebrain lesion or a

---

Box 4.2 Bilateral Cranial Nerve Dysfunction

Cranial nerve deficits that affect the same nerve on both sides (e.g. bilateral facial paralysis, or a dropped jaw as a result of bilateral loss of trigeminal [motor] nerve function) are more likely to reflect a disorder affecting these nerves outside the brainstem. This is particularly likely if the level of mentation is unaffected. A lesion that is extensive enough to result in dysfunction of the cranial nerve nuclei on both sides of the brainstem would also be expected to affect adjacent nuclei and pathways. This would result in a change to the level of mentation (stupor/coma), tetraparesis, proprioceptive deficits in all limbs, or even death secondary to interruption of the descending cardiorespiratory pathways.

multifocal disease process should be considered if these are observed or reported in the clinical history.

A lesion that involves the upper cervical spinal cord will also affect the ascending proprioceptive pathways and the descending upper motor neuron tracts to and from the brain. This means that it can sometimes be difficult to distinguish a brainstem lesion from a lesion affecting the cervical spinal cord. The concurrent presence of an altered level of mentation, vestibular syndrome, or ipsilateral cranial nerve deficits would be most consistent with a brainstem lesion in these cases.

3. Cerebellum

The cerebellum plays a vital role in coordinating the rate, range, and force of movements. This also includes learned responses, such as the coordination of blinking in response to objects approaching the eyes (menace response). The initiation of these movements originates in the forebrain and brainstem and does not involve the cerebellum. Therefore, a lesion that is isolated to the cerebellum may result in marked ataxia (see Video 18) and proprioceptive deficits (hopping in particular), but it will not result in appreciable upper or lower motor neuron paresis ('weakness'). In contrast to lesions that affect the ARAS in the brainstem or that diffusely affect the forebrain, cerebellar lesions also do not influence the level of mentation and animals will remain alert and responsive.

The cerebellum contains regions that are intimately associated with the control of balance and forms part of the central vestibular system. These regions exert a tonic inhibitory influence on the vestibular nuclei in the brainstem. Unilateral cerebellar lesions may reduce this inhibitory influence on one side, resulting in uneven output from the vestibular nuclei on each side of the brainstem and clinical signs of a head tilt or nystagmus. A disease process that affects the peripheral vestibular system or the brainstem vestibular nuclei will reduce the output from the ipsilateral vestibular nuclei, resulting in a head tilt towards the side of the lesion. In contrast, a unilateral cerebellar lesion will result in an increased output from the ipsilateral vestibular nuclei due to the loss of inhibition. This results in a 'paradoxical vestibular syndrome' in which the direction of the head tilt is away from the side of the lesion (see Video 19). Other regions of the cerebellum are usually also affected in these cases, resulting in additional neurological deficits that assist in the recognition of a cerebellar neuroanatomic localisation:

- *ipsilateral proprioceptive deficits* (particularly hopping)
- *ipsilateral hypermetria* (excessive flexion of the thoracic and pelvic limbs during protraction)
- *head and neck tremors* that are exacerbated by intention to perform movements
- *reduced/absent menace response in the ipsilateral eye*, without loss of visual tracking.

In summary, a cerebellar neuroanatomic localisation should be considered if a combination of the following neurological deficits is observed on examination:

- *ataxia of all limbs without apparent paresis* – normal stride length but inappropriate rate, range, and force of movement (see Video 18)
- *hypermetria* (excessive limb flexion during protraction) affecting all limbs or the ipsilateral thoracic and pelvic limbs for a lateralised lesion
- *head and neck tremors* – most noticeable with intention to perform a movement (e.g. lowering the head to a food or water bowl) (see Video 11)
- *central vestibular syndrome*, with a head tilt either towards or away from the side of the lesion
- *absent menace response(s) with normal vision*.

4.3 Spinal Cord Lesions

The spinal cord contains the descending upper motor neuron pathways that connect the motor centres in the brain to the cell bodies of the peripheral motor nerves that innervate the skeletal muscles of the limbs and trunk (Figure 4.3). These peripheral motor nerves, termed 'lower motor neurons', have cell bodies that reside within the ventral grey matter of the spinal cord. The spinal cord is also comprised of ascending sensory and proprioceptive pathways that transmit information from the peripheral sensory nerves to the cerebellum and sensory cortex of the forebrain. Other than rare, degenerative disease processes that may selectively affect certain tracts, a structural lesion to the spinal cord will indiscriminately affect the function of both the ascending (sensory) and descending (motor) pathways. Lesions affecting the ventral grey matter in certain regions of

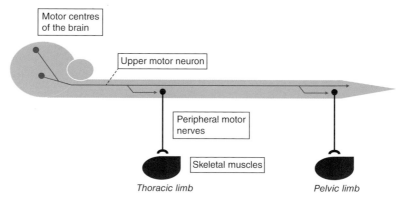

Figure 4.3 The upper motor neurons descend the spinal cord and connect the motor centres in the brain to the cell bodies of the peripheral motor nerves that innervate the skeletal muscles of the body and limbs.

the spinal cord can also damage the cell bodies of the lower motor neurons innervating the limb muscles. Disease processes that affect the spinal cord are termed 'myelopathies' and will result in a spectrum of clinical signs dependent on the location, severity, and extent of the lesion.

- *An inability to initiate movement or support weight in one or more limbs* – this is termed 'paresis' and results from damage to the spinal cord upper motor neuron tracts and/or the cell bodies of the lower motor neurons in the ventral grey matter.
- *Proprioceptive ataxia in one or more limbs ('incoordination').*
- *Proprioceptive deficits in one or more limbs.*
- *Reduced nociception caudal to the level of an extensive spinal cord lesion* – this will only be observed once all voluntary motor function is lost (i.e. in cases with paralysis/plegia).
- *Apparent discomfort on spinal palpation if adjacent innervated structures are affected* (e.g. meninges, nerve roots, vertebrae, muscles, ligaments, intervertebral facet joints, outer annulus fibrosus).

As previously discussed, whilst lesions affecting the brain can also result in an abnormal gait, ataxia, and proprioceptive deficits, there are some important factors to consider.

a. Animals presenting with a single, focal spinal cord lesion should not have any cranial nerve deficits. The main exception to this rule is Horner syndrome secondary to a spinal cord lesion affecting the C1–T3 spinal cord segments (see Chapter 6).
b. Animals with spinal cord lesions may appear 'dull' secondary to pain or distress at being recumbent; however, their level of mentation should be alert and appropriate. The presence of seizure activity, visual deficits, behaviour change, or an abnormal level of mentation should alert you to the presence of a multi-focal or diffuse disease process if the lesion otherwise localises to the spinal cord.
c. An intracranial lesion will only affect the gait and/or proprioception in all limbs, or in the thoracic limbs *and* pelvic limbs on one side if there is a lateralised lesion. Therefore, a lesion residing outside the brain should be suspected if only a single limb is affected, or if the pelvic limbs are affected without thoracic limb involvement.

The spinal cord can be divided into individual segments, each with an associated pair of peripheral sensory and motor nerves (one on each side). In the dog and cat, there are 8 cervical spinal cord segments, 13 thoracic segments, 7 lumbar segments, 3 sacral segments, and a variable number of caudal segments related to tail innervation.

The aim of the neuroanatomic localisation in an animal with a suspected spinal cord disorder is to localise the lesion to one of four broad regions (see Figure 4.2):

- C1–C5 spinal cord segments
- C6–T2 spinal cord segments
- T3–L3 spinal cord segments
- L4–Cd spinal cord segments.

These regions are chosen as we have a limited number of examinations that can be used to screen the function of specific spinal cord segments. The basis of these tests is that the cell bodies of the lower motor neurons to the thoracic limbs reside within the C6–T2 spinal cord segments, and those for the pelvic limbs and tail reside within the L4–Cd spinal cord segments. Therefore, tests which assess the muscle strength in the thoracic and pelvic limbs will screen both the integrity of the peripheral nerves innervating the muscles being tested, together with the spinal cord segments involved in the reflex activity (Figure 4.4). These tests are called segmental spinal reflexes and are further discussed in Chapter 3.

Having first excluded an intracranial neuroanatomic localisation, the first question to consider when assessing the gait and proprioception of an animal with a suspected spinal cord lesion is: 'How many limbs are affected?' Answering this question will assist in deciding which spinal cord segments are most likely to be affected.

- *C1–T2 spinal cord segments*: all limbs are affected, or the thoracic *and* pelvic limbs on one side are affected.
- *T3–Cd spinal cord segments*: only the pelvic limbs +/− tail are affected, or only one pelvic limb is affected.

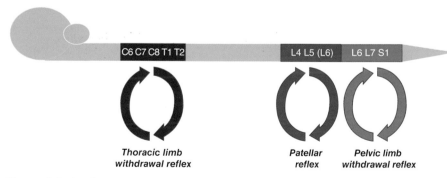

C6 C7 C8 T1 T2	L4 L5 (L6)	L6 L7 S1

Thoracic limb
withdrawal reflex   *Patellar*   *Pelvic limb*
reflex   *withdrawal reflex*

Figure 4.4 The thoracic limb withdrawal reflex tests the integrity of the C6–T2 spinal cord segments/ventral nerve roots and the peripheral motor and sensory nerves of the thoracic limb. The patellar reflex tests the integrity of the L4–L6 spinal cord segments/ventral nerve roots and the femoral nerve. The pelvic limb withdrawal reflex tests the integrity of the L6–S1 spinal cord segments/ventral nerve roots and the sciatic nerve. These reflexes do not require input or involvement of any other parts of the nervous system to be normal; they can therefore be intact even if the spinal cord is severed at a distant site.

The lesion can then be localised further, based on observation of the gait and posture, and on the use of neurological tests that screen certain regions of the nervous system. As discussed in Chapter 1, if the gait is abnormal in one or more limbs but the proprioception appears normal then non-neurological disease should always be considered (e.g. orthopaedic disease, reduced vascular perfusion).

1. All limbs are affected

If there are no neurological deficits to suggest an intracranial lesion, then the neuroanatomic localisation is most likely to involve one of following three regions (Figure 4.5):

- C1–C5 spinal cord segments
- C6–T2 spinal cord segments
- generalised neuromuscular disease.

Assessment of the thoracic limb withdrawal reflexes and thoracic limb muscle tone can now be performed to screen the integrity of the C6–T2 spinal cord segments, which contain the cell bodies of the lower motor neurons to the thoracic limbs. These lower motor neurons are responsible for extensor muscle tone to support the weight against gravity, and for flexor muscle strength that we can test using the withdrawal reflex. The thoracic limb withdrawal reflexes and muscle tone should be normal for a lesion affecting the C1–C5 spinal cord segments, as the lower motor neuron cell bodies will be unaffected. The gait associated with a C1–C5 lesion will also be long-strided in all limbs, with a characteristic 'over-reaching' of the thoracic limbs at the end of protraction, as there is a delay in onset and termination of the swing phase of the stride secondary to interruption of the upper motor neuron messages from the motor centres in the brainstem (see Video 29). In contrast, a lesion affecting the C6–T2 spinal cord segments would result in:

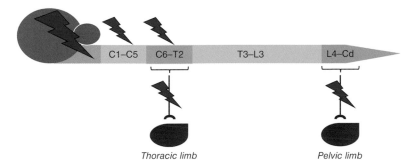

Figure 4.5 The potential locations for a neurological lesion ('lightning bolt' symbol) that could result in an abnormal gait in all limbs.

- reduced/absent thoracic limb withdrawal reflexes
- reduced muscle tone (flaccidity) in the thoracic limb muscles
- neurogenic atrophy of the affected thoracic limb muscles
- an inability to support weight against gravity for the thoracic limbs.

The inability to support weight on the thoracic limbs will result in a short-strided thoracic limb gait +/− collapse through the thoracic limbs when hopping is performed. This short-strided thoracic limb gait will contrast with the long-strided, ataxic pelvic limb gait that results from disruption of the upper motor neuron signals running down to the pelvic limbs via the C6–T2 spinal cord. This discrepancy between the thoracic and pelvic limb stride lengths for a C6–T2 spinal cord lesion is termed a 'two-engine' gait (see Video 30).

Assessment of the withdrawal reflexes will always be associated with a degree of subjectivity, and there can be a wide range of natural variation between individuals of different species, breeds, and temperaments. Therefore, it is not unreasonable to have a final neuroanatomic localisation of C1–T2 spinal cord segments if the tests above appear equivocal. This broader localisation can still be used to plan further investigations, such as diagnostic imaging, and remains far superior to deciding on further tests without a neurolocalisation at all.

The pelvic limb withdrawal reflexes and the patellar reflexes only involve the L4–S1 spinal cord segments, femoral nerve, and sciatic nerve. They will therefore be normal if there is a focal spinal cord lesion between the C1–T2 spinal cord segments. The muscle tone in the pelvic limbs will also be normal. A generalised neuromuscular disorder resulting in weakness of all limbs should be suspected if the withdrawal reflexes are weak in the thoracic *and* pelvic limbs. Unless there is a history of significant trauma, this would be more likely than the presence of a multifocal or diffuse spinal cord lesion that is concurrently affecting the C6–T2 and L4–Cd spinal cord segments (see below for further discussion of neuromuscular disease).

2. The thoracic and pelvic limbs on only one side are affected ('hemiparesis')

If there are no neurological deficits to suggest an intracranial lesion, then the neuroanatomic localisation is most likely to be:

- lateralised (ipsilateral) C1–C5 spinal cord segments
- lateralised (ipsilateral) C6–T2 spinal cord segments.

In exactly the same manner as for all limbs being affected, assessment of the thoracic limb withdrawal reflexes and thoracic limb muscle tone should be performed to further localise the lesion. These tests should be normal for a C1–C5 spinal cord lesion and reduced/absent if the lesion is affecting the lower motor neuron cell bodies in the C6–T2 segments. In contrast to the situation when all limbs are affected, a generalised neuromuscular disorder would be highly unlikely to only affect one side of the body whilst sparing the limbs on the other side.

3. The thoracic limbs appear normal but both pelvic limbs are affected ('paraparesis')

If the voluntary motor function, gait, and proprioception appear normal in the thoracic limbs, then we can reasonably assume that both the brain and the spinal cord down to the level of the T2 spinal cord segment are functioning normally. The neuroanatomic localisation in this situation is most likely to involve one of the following three regions (Figure 4.6):

- T3–L3 spinal cord segments
- L4–Cd spinal cord segments/nerve roots
- femoral nerves and/or sciatic nerves (bilateral).

The following neurological tests should be performed to distinguish between these scenarios:

- the patellar reflexes, testing the L4–L6 spinal cord segments and femoral nerves
- the pelvic limb withdrawal reflexes, testing the L6–S1 spinal cord segments and sciatic nerves
- the perineal reflex, anal tone, and tail tone, screening the S1–Cd spinal cord segments
- the pelvic limb flexor and extensor muscle tone, reflecting the integrity of lower motor neuron cell bodies in the L4–S1 spinal cord segments, the femoral nerves and the sciatic nerves.

All of these tests should be normal for a lesion affecting the T3–L3 spinal cord segments but may be reduced/absent for a lesion affecting the L4–Cd spinal cord segments. Lesions that affect the L4–Cd spinal cord segments may also result in weakness of the extensor muscles in the affected limbs. This will be clinically

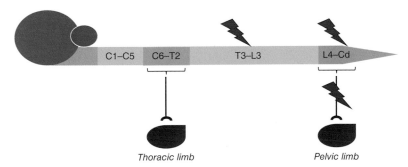

Figure 4.6 The potential locations for a neurological lesion ('lightning bolt' symbol) that could result in an abnormal gait in the pelvic limbs only (i.e. normal thoracic limbs).

apparent as an inability to support the weight against gravity and poor joint extension (e.g. dropped hock for a sciatic nerve lesion). The animal may also appear 'lame' as they rapidly shift weight away from the affected limb(s) to avoid collapse. This can mimic shifting weight away from a painful limb or limb weakness secondary to vascular compromise. Therefore, aortic thromboembolism, orthopaedic, and neurologic conditions should all be considered in animals with a short-strided or 'lame' gait in the pelvic limbs. This is in contrast to the gait typically observed for lesions affecting the T3–L3 spinal cord segments. In these cases, there is good tone in the pelvic limbs together with a long-strided, ataxic gait secondary to interference with the ascending proprioceptive tracts and descending upper motor neurons to the pelvic limbs (see Video 16).

It can be difficult to distinguish a lesion that is affecting the L4–Cd spinal cord segments at the level of the spinal canal, from the less common scenario of a bilateral lesion involving the femoral and/or sciatic nerves outside the vertebral column. The latter may be observed in trauma cases or in the early stages of a generalised neuromuscular condition, before clinical involvement of the thoracic limbs is observed. However, the tail function and perineal reflex will frequently be normal in cases with bilateral femoral and/or sciatic nerve involvement, as the sacral and caudal spinal cord segments and nerves are unaffected. This is in contrast to lesions at the level of the spinal canal, which typically also affect the sacral/caudal spinal cord segments or nerve roots in addition to the causing paraparesis (e.g. intervertebral disc disease, neoplasia).

It may be possible to further refine the location of a T3–L3 spinal cord lesion by using the cutaneous trunci reflex or by identification of a focus of spinal pain (see Chapters 3 and 6).

4. A single pelvic limb is affected ('monoparesis')

If only a single pelvic limb is affected, then non-neurological disease should always be considered as a cause of lameness that is mimicking a true monoparesis. Common underlying causes for this presentation include hip dysplasia, cruciate ligament disease, and patellar luxation. If non-neurological disease is excluded on the basis of the clinical history and good physical and orthopaedic examinations, then this situation can be approached in a similar manner to when both pelvic limbs are affected. A convincing proprioceptive deficit in the affected limb compared to the normal contralateral limb would also add support for an underlying neurologic cause:

- lateralised (ipsilateral) T3–L3 spinal cord segments
- lateralised (ipsilateral) L4–S1 spinal cord segments
- ipsilateral femoral and/or sciatic nerve lesion in the affected limb.

The most useful examinations that can be used to distinguish between these options would be:

- the patellar reflex testing the L4–L6 spinal cord segments and femoral nerve
- the pelvic limb withdrawal reflex testing the L6–S1 spinal cord segments and sciatic nerve
- the pelvic limb flexor and extensor muscle tone, reflecting the integrity of lower motor neuron cell bodies in the L4–S1 spinal cord segments, the femoral nerve, and the sciatic nerve.

These tests should be normal for a lesion residing within the T3–L3 spinal cord segments and may be reduced/absent in the case of a lateralised lesion affecting the L4–S1 spinal cord segments, L4–S1 nerve roots, femoral nerve, or sciatic nerve. A lesion affecting the L4–L6 spinal cord segments, L4–L6 nerve roots, or femoral nerve will affect the patellar reflex. A lesion affecting the L6–S1 spinal cord segments, L6–S1 nerve roots, or sciatic nerve will affect the withdrawal reflex. The perineal reflex, anal tone, and tail tone may be affected if the sacral and caudal spinal cord segments or nerve roots are also affected.

5. A single thoracic limb is affected ('monoparesis')

As for when a single pelvic limb is affected, non-neurological disease should always be considered as a cause for lameness rather than true paresis (e.g. orthopaedic disease affecting the shoulder or elbow, paw injury, nail bed infection). If local disease affecting the limb itself is excluded, then an intracranial or primary spinal cord localisation is highly unlikely in these cases. If this were the case, then the tracts to the ipsilateral pelvic limb should also be affected as they pass via the site of injury, resulting in hemiparesis. The most likely neuroanatomic localisation for thoracic limb monoparesis is therefore the ipsilateral peripheral nerve(s) to the affected thoracic limb.

6. Both thoracic limbs are affected but the pelvic limbs appear normal

Whilst uncommon, if both thoracic limbs are affected (e.g. proprioceptive deficits and weak withdrawal reflexes in both thoracic limbs) but the pelvic limbs appear normal, then the following rare clinical presentations could be considered:

- isolated damage to the peripheral nerves innervating both thoracic limbs (e.g. traumatic avulsion of the nerve roots to both brachial plexi, bilateral brachial plexus neuritis, bilateral nerve infiltration by lymphoma)
- a spinal cord lesion that damages the grey matter of the C6–T2 spinal cord segments with relative sparing of the surrounding white matter tracts to and from the pelvic limbs, termed a 'central cord syndrome' (e.g. traumatic spinal cord injury, intramedullary spinal neoplasia, spinal cord ischaemia).

See Boxes 4.3–4.6 for a summary of the most common clinical signs observed secondary to spinal cord lesions affecting the C1–C5, C6–T2, T3–L3, and L4–Cd spinal cord segments.

Box 4.3 C1–C5 Spinal Cord Segments

- Tetraparesis/tetraplegia or ipsilateral hemiparesis/hemiplegia: interruption to the descending upper motor neuron tracts resulting in a long stride length (delay in the onset and termination of the stride) (see Video 29).
- Proprioceptive ataxia in all limbs, or in the ipsilateral thoracic and pelvic limbs for a lateralised lesion.
- Proprioceptive deficits in all limbs, or in the ipsilateral thoracic and pelvic limbs.
- Normal flexor withdrawal reflexes in all limbs.
- Normal patellar reflexes.
- Normal tail and anal tone, intact perineal reflex.
- Cutaneous trunci reflex present at the level of L5.
- Possible neck pain.
- Possible Horner syndrome.

Box 4.4 C6–T2 Spinal Cord Segments

- Tetraparesis/tetraplegia or ipsilateral hemiparesis/hemiplegia: damage to the descending upper motor neuron tracts to the pelvic limbs results in a long pelvic limb stride length (delay in the onset and termination of the stride), and damage to the cell bodies of the lower motor neurons innervating the thoracic limb skeletal muscles results in a short thoracic limb stride length (extensor muscle weakness and inability to support weight). This is termed a 'two engine gait' as the short thoracic limb gait appears faster than the long pelvic limb gait (see Video 30).
- Proprioceptive ataxia in all limbs: this is more noticeable in the pelvic limbs as the weakness of the thoracic limbs and short stride length masks underlying ataxia.
- Proprioceptive deficits in all limbs, or in the ipsilateral thoracic and pelvic limbs.
- Weak thoracic limb withdrawal reflexes.
- Reduced thoracic limb muscle tone.
- Denervation atrophy of thoracic limb muscles.
- Normal pelvic limb withdrawal reflexes.
- Normal patellar reflexes.
- Normal tail and anal tone, intact perineal reflex.
- Cutaneous trunci reflex may be absent if the C8–T1 spinal cord segments or C8–T1 nerve roots are affected.
- Possible neck pain.
- Possible Horner syndrome.

---

7. Potential pitfalls in the localisation of spinal cord lesions

Two interesting phenomena that may complicate the localisation of spinal cord lesions are discussed below. These should always be considered in animals that present with acute spinal cord injury.

Box 4.5 T3–L3 Spinal Cord Segments

- Normal thoracic limb voluntary motor function, proprioception, and withdrawal reflexes.
- Paraparesis/paraplegia, or ipsilateral pelvic limb monoparesis/monoplegia: interruption to descending upper motor neuron tracts resulting in a long stride length (delay in the onset and termination of the stride).
- Proprioceptive ataxia in the pelvic limbs.
- Proprioceptive deficits in the affected pelvic limb(s).
- Normal pelvic limb withdrawal reflexes.
- Normal patellar reflexes.
- Normal tail and anal tone, intact perineal reflex.
- Cutaneous trunci reflex may be interrupted approximately two vertebrae caudal to the level of a transverse spinal cord lesion.
- Possible thoracolumbar spinal discomfort.

Box 4.6 L4–Cd Spinal Cord Segments

- Normal thoracic limb voluntary motor function, proprioception, and withdrawal reflexes.
- Paraparesis/paraplegia, or ipsilateral pelvic limb monoparesis/monoplegia. Damage to the cell bodies of the lower motor neurons innervating the pelvic limb skeletal muscles resulting in a short pelvic limb stride length and poor joint extension (extensor muscle weakness and inability to support weight).
- Proprioceptive deficits in the affected pelvic limb(s).
- Weak pelvic limb withdrawal reflexes (L6–S1).
- Reduced/absent patellar reflexes (L4–L6).
- Reduced pelvic limb muscle tone (L4–S1).
- Reduced hock and/or stifle extension.
- Denervation atrophy of pelvic limb muscles.
- Reduced/absent tail and anal tone, reduced/absent perineal reflex (S1–Cd).
- Cutaneous trunci reflex present at the level of L5.
- Possible lumbosacral spinal discomfort.

---

a. Schiff–Sherrington posture

The distinctive Schiff–Sherrington posture (see Video 23) has already been discussed in Chapter 3 and is characterised by increased extensor muscle tone in the thoracic limbs following an acute lesion affecting the T3–L3 spinal cord segments. The increased extensor tone may restrict an animal's ability to rise into sternal recumbency, meaning that they often present in lateral recumbency. This can mimic a lesion affecting the C1–T2 spinal cord segments. However, unlike an animal with a C1–T2 lesion, those with Schiff–Sherrington posture will have normal thoracic limb voluntary movement and proprioception when assisted to stand. This posture is commonly associated with acute, severe lesions to the T3–L3 spinal cord segments, but it has no prognostic significance and should not be used to guide an owner as to the prognosis for a functional recovery.

b. Spinal shock phenomenon

This is a poorly understood phenomenon that is observed in both humans and animals following experimental or natural spinal cord injuries (Smith and Jeffery 2005). It is characterised by a counterintuitive loss of local spinal reflexes (e.g. reduced/absent withdrawal reflexes +/− patellar reflexes) following an acute, often severe, lesion affecting the spinal cord segments lying rostral to those involved in the reflex arcs being tested. This is most commonly observed as a loss of pelvic limb withdrawal reflexes following an acute lesion affecting the T3–L3 spinal cord segments. The patellar reflexes may be lost for between minutes and hours following spinal cord injury in domestic animals but have often returned to normal by the time of presentation. In the author's experience, the pelvic limb withdrawal reflexes may remain weak for up to 5–7 days following an acute T3–L3 lesion if spinal shock is present.

This syndrome is thought to represent an acute loss of upper motor neuron input to interneurons involved in the local reflexes being tested. This results in a transient loss of reflex function and reduced muscle tone in the affected limbs. As for Schiff–Sherrington posture, whilst spinal shock is often associated with severe neurological deficits (e.g. paraplegia) it has not been shown to have individual prognostic significance. Therefore, the primary clinical significance is the possibility for an incorrect neuroanatomic localisation. A lesion affecting the L4–Cd spinal cord segments would sensibly be your first thought in a dog or cat that presents with:

- normal forelimb voluntary motor function and proprioception
- non-ambulatory paraparesis or paraplegia
- reduced muscle tone in the pelvic limbs
- weak pelvic limb withdrawal reflexes.

However, a lesion affecting the T3–L3 spinal cord segments with associated spinal shock should always be considered in cases with the same clinical presentation but that also have:

- intact patellar reflexes
- a cutaneous trunci reflex that is interrupted at or rostral to the level of L2–L3
- focal spinal discomfort in the region of the T3–L3 vertebrae.

This differentiation is very important in terms of deciding where to focus further imaging (e.g. radiography or MRI) and how to interpret any changes observed on these images.

4.4   Neuromuscular Disease

Disorders that affect the peripheral nerves, skeletal muscles, or the neuromuscular junction are less commonly encountered in general practice compared to conditions involving the central nervous system (Figure 4.7). A lack of familiarity with these conditions, coupled with the fact that the clinical signs may mimic disorders affecting the brain or spinal cord, may lead to misdiagnosis. As a result, there may be an inappropriate choice of further investigations (e.g. spinal radiography or advanced imaging) that delays reaching a diagnosis and can be costly for an owner.

Disorders that affect the peripheral motor nerves, neuromuscular junction, or skeletal muscles will cause variable degrees of lower motor neuron weakness in the affected body parts, resulting in one or more of the following clinical signs (see Video 31).

- Poor extensor muscle tone (flaccidity) and an inability to support weight against gravity. If the animal has enough strength to stand and walk, this results in a stiff, short-strided gait in the affected limbs as the animal shifts its weight away from a weak limb to avoid collapse. Poor extension of the joints when standing/walking may also be observed (e.g. tarsi, stifles, elbows).
- Weakness of the flexor muscles resulting in reduced/absent withdrawal reflexes.
- Reduced/absent tendon reflexes (e.g. patellar reflex).
- Muscle atrophy. This atrophy could reflect damage to the peripheral motor nerves and denervation of the affected muscle(s), or be the result of primary

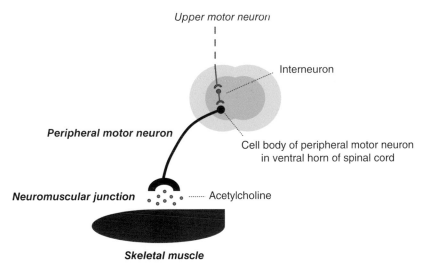

Figure 4.7 The motor arm of the peripheral nervous system comprises the peripheral motor nerves (with their cell bodies in the ventral horn of the spinal cord), the neuromuscular junction, and the skeletal muscles themselves. Disorders that affect any of these components are grouped under the broad term of 'neuromuscular disease'.

muscle damage in the case of generalised myopathies. Some animals with generalised neuromuscular disease may present with a primary clinical history of weight loss as a result of significant muscle atrophy.

- Exercise intolerance. Animals with disorders affecting the neuromuscular junction or skeletal muscles may present with exercise intolerance and/or exacerbation of their clinical signs during exercise. This results from an inability to meet the increased demand put on the muscles at the time of activity. This is in contrast to disorders affecting the brain, spinal cord, or peripheral motor nerves, for which the clinical signs are usually persistent and independent of exercise.

- The cranial nerves, masticatory muscles, and oesophageal muscles may be affected by neuromuscular disorders. These deficits are often bilateral and symmetric, and the most commonly affected nerves include the facial (VII) nerve resulting in facial paralysis, and the glossopharyngeal (IX) and/or vagus (X) nerves resulting in dysphagia, dysphonia, or megaoesophagus. The brain is not affected by neuromuscular disorders, therefore the mentation will remain alert and appropriate at all times. This is in contrast to animals with cranial nerve deficits secondary to a brainstem lesion. Animals with neuromuscular disease may also have other neurological deficits that would be incompatible with a brainstem neurolocalisation (e.g. weak withdrawal reflexes in all limbs).

The skeletal muscles and neuromuscular junction form part of the common motor pathway for movement and play no role in sensory functions such as proprioception or nociception. The same applies for the peripheral motor nerves. Therefore, unless a neuromuscular disorder affects the peripheral sensory nerves, which is uncommon for many of the disorders observed in general practice, the sensory function will be preserved. This means that in contrast to brain or spinal cord lesions, the proprioception remains normal for most neuromuscular cases. As long as there is sufficient motor function present for a small degree of limb movement, the animal will still attempt to initiate a corrective movement when performing proprioceptive testing, even if this movement is very 'weak' (see Video 31). For the same reason, if an animal with a neuromuscular disorder is able to walk then it will not be ataxic. The gait may appear stiff or short-strided secondary to generalised weakness, but limb placement should be predictable for each step. The relative sparing of sensory function in the majority of neuromuscular cases can be extremely useful to allow differentiation between these disorders from lesions affecting the brain or spinal cord that can also result in an abnormal gait in all limbs. Unless neuromuscular disease is considered, the proprioception in affected animals may appear 'confusingly' good given how weak the animal appears on examination.

A neuromuscular lesion localisation should therefore be considered in any animal presenting with an abnormal gait in all limbs. These animals will have a short-strided gait, may be exercise intolerant, and show generalised muscle atrophy, weak withdrawal reflexes in all limbs, and have possible cranial nerve deficits. However, the proprioception is often normal as long as the body weight is sufficiently supported during testing to avoid collapse (see Chapter 3). There will be no clinical signs to suggest an intracranial localisation (e.g. seizures, visual deficits, altered level of mentation), and the relative sparing of proprioception, absence of ataxia, and lower motor neuron weakness affecting all limbs would not be consistent with a focal spinal cord lesion. Further discussion regarding the diagnostic approach to neuromuscular disease can be found in Chapter 6.

Neuromuscular disorders are most commonly generalised conditions that concurrently affect all limbs. The appendicular muscles can be preferentially affected by some conditions (e.g. idiopathic polyradiculoneuritis), whilst others may also affect the cranial nerves and tail (e.g. botulism). In some instances, the pelvic limbs are initially affected before the disease progresses over days/weeks to involve the thoracic limbs. These cases can therefore be difficult to distinguish from a spinal cord lesion affecting the L4–S1 spinal cord segments before disease progression is observed. However, the presence of concurrent cranial nerve deficits (e.g. dysphonia, megaoesophagus, bilateral facial paresis), or exacerbation of the clinical signs by exercise, may help to increase suspicion for a neuromuscular disorder.

The clinical differentiation between peripheral neuropathies, junctionopathies, and myopathies may not be possible without performing further investigations. Therefore, a broader neuroanatomic localisation of 'neuromuscular disease' is a good starting point for planning these investigations. The following observations may be useful to refine your localisation but are not always reliable.

- Myopathies and junctionopathies only affect the motor component of the neuromuscular system, therefore proprioception will always be normal. It is unusual for these conditions to result in such severe weakness that an animal is unable to perform any corrective movement when proprioception is assessed.
- Peripheral neuropathies may also affect the peripheral sensory nerves, and the proprioception can therefore also be affected. However, the most common forms of peripheral neuropathy observed in general practice appear to predominately affect the motor nerves, with the proprioception being normal in these cases (e.g. idiopathic polyradiculoneuritis).
- Peripheral neuropathies more frequently progress to the point at which the animal is unable to walk compared to myopathies and junctionopathies. Exceptions to this include necrotising myopathies, fulminant myasthenia gravis, and botulism. In a similar manner, animals with absent withdrawal reflexes in all limbs and marked flaccidity of the trunk and limbs are more

likely to be affected by a generalised polyneuropathy than by a myopathy or junctionopathy, with botulism being the exception to this rule.

- Peripheral neuropathies usually present with persistent clinical signs that are less influenced by exercise or rest compared to myopathies and junctionopathies.

Chapter 5 will discuss how the neurological examination and final neuroanatomic localisation can be used, in conjunction with the clinical history, to formulate a meaningful list of differential diagnoses. It is always vital to consider the reported onset and progression of the clinical signs at this stage. Only then should further investigations be planned to rule in or out the most likely differential diagnoses.

Bibliography

Añor, S. (2014). Acute lower motor neuron tetraparesis. *Vet. Clin. North Am. Small Anim. Pract.* 44: 1201–1222.

Atkinson, P.P. and Atkinson, J.L. (1996). Spinal shock. *Mayo Clin. Proc.* 71: 384–389.

Berg, J. (1989). Problems in neurolocalisation. *Probl. Vet. Med.* 1: 358–365.

Brooks, N.P. (2017). Central cord syndrome. *Neurosurg. Clin N. Am.* 28: 41–47.

Dewey, C.W. and da Costa, R.C. (2015). *Practical Guide to Canine and Feline Neurology*, 3e. Hoboken, NJ: Wiley Blackwell.

Farrow, B.R., Murrell, W.G., Revington, M.L. et al. (1983). Type C botulism in young dogs. *Aust. Vet. J.* 60: 374–377.

Garosi, L., de Lahunta, A., Summers, B. et al. (2006). Bilateral hypertrophic neuritis of the brachial plexus in a cat: magnetic resonace imaging and pathological findings. *J. Feline Med. Surg.* 8: 63–68.

Glass, E.N. and Kent, M. (2002). The clinical examination for neuromuscular disease. *Vet. Clin. North Am. Small Anim. Pract.* 32: 1–29.

Henke, D., Vandevelde, M., Doherr, M.G. et al. (2013). Correlations between severity of clinical signs and histopathological changes in 60 dogs with spinal cord injury associated with acute thoracolumbar intervertebral disc disease. *Vet. J.* 198: 70–75.

de Lahunta, A., Glass, E., and Kent, M. (2015). *Veterinary Neuroanatomy and Clinical Neurology*, 4e. St Louis, MO: Elsevier Saunders.

Lorenz, M.D., Coates, J., and Kent, M. (2011). *Handbook of Veterinary Neurology*, 5e. St Louis, MO: Elsevier Saunders.

Parent, J. (2010). Clinical approach and lesion localization in patients with spinal diseases. *Vet. Clin. North Am. Small Anim. Pract.* 40: 733–753.

Platt, S. and Olby, N. (2013). *BSAVA Manual of Canine and Feline Neurology*, 4e. Gloucester, UK: British Small Animal Veterinary Association.

Smith, P.M. and Jeffery, N.D. (2005). Spinal shock – comparative aspects and clinical relevance. *J. Vet. Intern. Med.* 19: 788–793.

Sprague, J.M. (1953). Spinal border cells and their role in postural mechanism (Schiff–Sherrington phenomenon). *J. Neurophysiol.* 16: 464–474.

Thomas, W.B. (2010). Evaluation of veterinary patients with brain disease. *Vet. Clin. North Am. Small Anim. Pract.* 40: 1–19.

Thomsen, B., Garosi, L., Skerritt, G. et al. (2016). Neurological signs in 23 dogs with suspected rostral cerebellar ischaemic stroke. *Acta Vet. Scand.* 58: 40–48.

Chapter 5 Constructing the List of Differential Diagnoses

Edward Ives

The aim of this chapter is to bring together all of the information from the previous four chapters and to summarise how this can be used to construct a concise and appropriate list of differential diagnoses, upon which the most useful diagnostic investigations can be planned.

As discussed in the previous chapters, the primary goal of taking a complete clinical history and performing the general physical examination and a neurological examination is to answer two key questions:

1. *Does this animal have a lesion affecting its nervous system?*
2. *What is the location of that lesion?*

Only at this stage of the diagnostic process should specific categories of disease or individual disease processes be considered. This involves constructing a ranked list of conditions that could potentially result in a lesion in that location (from most likely to least likely). This is termed the 'list of differential diagnoses'. It is vital that other aspects of the clinical history and general physical examination findings are also considered at this stage in order to determine the most likely differential diagnoses (see Chapter 2). Dependent on the clinical history and neurological deficits, a list of three to five differential diagnoses can usually be chosen. This list can then be modified on the basis of focused further investigations, which aim to rule in or rule out your most likely diagnoses first.

Adopting this approach to every case is important. This is because diagnostic tests perform best when they are targeted to answering a specific clinical question – the limitations of the test are known and it is therefore easier to interpret the significance of a positive or negative test result. If you perform a test for a specific condition without first considering how common that condition is in the popula-

A Practical Approach to Neurology for the Small Animal Practitioner, First Edition. Paul M. Freeman and Edward Ives.
© 2020 John Wiley & Sons Ltd. Published 2020 by John Wiley & Sons Ltd.
Companion Website: www.wiley.com/go/freeman/neurology

tion of interest, or how likely it is to explain the clinical signs observed, then it is very difficult to know what to do if the test result is equivocal or 'positive'. This is particularly true for serum antibody testing, in which a high titre could represent active infection or incidental, historic exposure. Achieving an accurate diagnosis in the most efficient way possible means that treatment can be started promptly, more funds will be available for treatment, and the outcome is likely to be better.

Formulating the list of differential diagnoses relies upon the concept of clinical reasoning. This problem-orientated approach involves consideration of several aspects of the clinical history and presentation, together with how common certain diseases are in the population that the individual comes from. This will depend upon geographical location, travel history, and vaccination status. The most important aspects to consider when constructing the list of differential diagnoses are as follows:

1. *The signalment of the animal* (species, breed, age, and gender)
   As discussed in Chapter 2, some conditions are more common in (or specific to) a particular species or certain breed of dog or cat. Different disease processes will also be more common in animals of certain age groups, such as congenital anomalies in young animals or neoplastic disease in middle-aged and older animals. Gender is an important factor to consider for genetic disorders that may have different modes of inheritance (e.g. X-linked disorders in males) or in metastatic diseases from certain organs (e.g. prostatic adenocarcinoma in males, mammary gland adenocarcinoma in females).

2. *Signs of systemic disease from the clinical history and general physical examination*
   These clinical signs could include gastrointestinal disease (vomiting, regurgitation, diarrhoea), respiratory signs, pyrexia, or weight loss. Certain categories of disease will more commonly result in pyrexia or may affect other organ systems in addition to the nervous system. The index of suspicion for these categories will therefore be higher if systemic clinical signs are reported in the clinical history or are identified on the general physical examination. This is particularly relevant for infectious, neoplastic, and certain inflammatory conditions. The travel history and vaccination status of the affected animal are also important factors in deciding the relative likelihood of certain diseases to explain the presenting problem(s) (see Chapter 2).

3. *The reported onset and progression of the clinical signs*
   The speed of onset of clinical signs and how these signs progress over time may vary considerably dependent on the disease process responsible (Figure 5.1). This information is particularly useful to refine the list of differential diagnoses and makes disease onset and progression a vital part of clinical reasoning in veterinary neurology. For example, obstruction of blood flow to the brain or spinal cord will result in a sudden onset of clinical signs that may remain static or show a gradual improvement dependent on the collateral circulation and damage caused. In contrast, neoplastic and infectious dis-

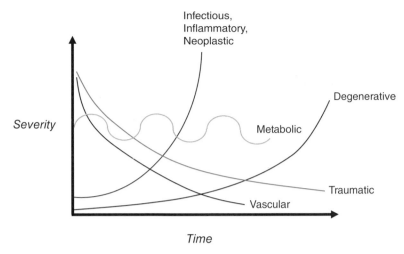

Figure 5.1 The speed of onset of clinical signs, and how these signs progress over time, may vary considerably, dependent on the disease process responsible.

orders would be expected to show a progressive clinical course unless treated and may have a more insidious onset. Further consideration of disease onset and progression in relation to different disease categories is discussed below. As discussed in Chapter 2, considering how the clinical course has, or has not, been influenced by previously administered medications, such as analgesics, antibiotics, or corticosteroids, can also help to refine the list of differential diagnoses.

4. *The neuroanatomic localisation, including lesion distribution and any lateralisation of neurological deficits*
   Certain disorders will only affect specific regions of the nervous system (e.g. myasthenia gravis for the neuromuscular junction, intervertebral disc disease for the spinal cord), whereas other conditions can affect any region (e.g. neoplasia, inflammation). Some disease processes are also more likely to present with focal, asymmetric clinical signs and lateralisation of neurological deficits compared to others (e.g. vascular disorders). Inflammatory and infectious conditions may result in multifocal clinical signs. The neurological deficits observed secondary to toxic or metabolic disorders tend to be diffuse and/or symmetric as there is even distribution of affected blood to all regions of the nervous system.

5. *The presence or absence of discomfort*
   Apparent discomfort may be reported in the clinical history, or be identified on examination, for many disease processes. It therefore represents a non-specific finding with many possible origins, including the meninges, nerve roots, peripheral nerves, vertebrae, muscles, joints, or ligaments. However, an absence of discomfort on examination may increase the index of suspicion for certain disorders, such as those involving the parenchyma of the brain or spinal cord that spare adjacent innervated structures (e.g. ischaemic lesions).

In summary, the five key areas that should be considered before formulating the list of differential diagnoses are:

1. *Signalment*
2. *Clinical history and presence/absence of non-neurologic signs*
3. *Onset and progression of clinical signs*
4. *Neuroanatomic localisation, including any lateralisation of deficits*
5. *Presence/absence of discomfort*

As an example, consider the most likely differential diagnosis for a 5-year-old, male, neutered Border Collie dog that is otherwise well and presents with a peracute onset of pelvic limb ataxia after running for a ball. There has been no progression of clinical signs over the last 48 hours, the lesion localises to the T3–L3 spinal cord segments, with the left pelvic limb being more affected than the right pelvic limb, and there is no apparent discomfort on spinal palpation. An ischaemic vascular event (e.g. fibrocartilaginous embolism) would be a common differential diagnosis to explain this peracute, non-progressive, non-painful, lateralised T3–L3 spinal cord lesion. This differential diagnosis would be highly unlikely if there had been progression of the clinical signs after the first 24 hours or if the dog appeared markedly painful on spinal palpation, even if the presentation was otherwise identical. Other differential diagnoses to consider in this case would include an acute non-compressive nucleus pulposus extrusion, an acute compressive nucleus pulposus extrusion, extrusion of a degenerate intervertebral disc, and possibly acute decompensation of underlying neoplasia.

5.1 Categories of Disease

In order to simplify the approach to formulating a list of differential diagnoses, broad categories of disease should be considered before individual conditions. This is similar to determining the neuroanatomic localisation, when three broad regions of the nervous system are initially considered (brain, spinal cord, or neuromuscular), before refining the localisation further. This ensures that an entire category of disease is not overlooked and that the most appropriate diagnostic investigations are chosen first. These broad categories of disease can be easily remembered using the mnemonic *VITAMIN D*:

- Vascular
- Inflammatory, Infectious
- Toxic, Traumatic
- Anomalous

- Metabolic
- Idiopathic
- Neoplastic, Nutritional
- Degenerative

These categories may be further subdivided before specific conditions are chosen as possible differential diagnoses (Box 5.1).

When formulating the list of differential diagnoses, each broad category of disease should be considered in turn and a specific category chosen if there is a consistent clinical picture for the individual case. This process is made easier by the fact that the different categories may typically affect animals of different ages, show a different onset and progression, affect different regions of the nervous system, or be more or less likely to result in discomfort on examination (Box 5.2). However, this should only be seen as a general guide and is unfortunately not a strict set of rules that every case will follow.

5.1.1 Vascular

Interruption of the normal blood supply to the nervous system is most commonly the result of vascular obstruction. This leads to ischaemia of the tissues within the territory of the affected vessel. The typical presentation for an ischaemic vascular event would be:

- acute onset (minutes to hours)
- static or improving clinical signs (over hours to weeks)
- focal neuroanatomic localisation
- lateralisation of neurological deficits is commonly observed, as a single vessel on one side of the brain or spinal cord is affected
- non-painful on spinal palpation or neck manipulation.

An animal of any species, age, or breed can theoretically be affected by ischaemic events, dependent on the nature of the occluding material. However, vessel obstruction by blood clots is more commonly observed in older animals and systemic diseases that predispose to clot formation may also result in non-neurologic clinical signs on examination (e.g. chronic renal disease, hyperadrenocorticism).

Haemorrhagic vascular events are a less common cause of neurological dysfunction when compared to ischaemia. They typically have an acute onset but may show progressive clinical signs if there is continued haemorrhage and an enlarging haematoma. Haemorrhage may also be associated with pain on examination as a result of mass effect, nerve root compression, or meningeal irritation. If there is a systemic disease process that has predisposed to vessel leakage or hypocoagulability, then haemorrhage may occur in multiple locations resulting in a multifocal neuroanatomic localisation.

Box 5.1 Subdivision of the categories of disease that are used to formulate a list of differential diagnoses

Vascular
- ischaemic/blood vessel obstruction (e.g. ischaemic stroke, fibrocartilaginous embolism)
- haemorrhagic/blood vessel rupture or leakage (e.g. coagulation disorder, *Angiostrongylus vasorum*)

Inflammatory
- sterile/non-infectious (e.g. meningoencephalitis of unknown origin)
- infectious: bacterial, viral, fungal, protozoal, rickettsial, algal

Traumatic
- external trauma (e.g. road traffic accident, kick, fall)
- internal trauma (e.g. acute non-compressive nucleus pulposus extrusion)

Toxic
- topical exposure (e.g. permethrin in cats)
- ingestion (e.g. metaldehyde)

Anomalous
- primary (e.g. hydrocephalus)
- secondary (e.g. vertebral malformation)

Metabolic
- excess (e.g. hepatic encephalopathy, uraemia, hypernatraemia)
- deficit (e.g. hypoglycaemia, hypocalcaemia, hyponatraemia)

Idiopathic

Neoplastic
- primary central nervous system neoplasia (e.g. glioma, meningioma)
- local extension (e.g. nasal adenocarcinoma invading the cranial vault)
- metastasis from a distant site (e.g. haemangiosarcoma)

Nutritional
- excess (e.g. vitamin A)
- deficiency (e.g. thiamine)

Degenerative
- primary degeneration of neurons (e.g. motor neuron disease)
- degeneration of structures that secondarily affect the nervous system (e.g. intervertebral disc disease)

> **Box 5.2** Here the different disease categories are divided according to their most common clinical presentation.
>
> **Onset**
> - Acute: vascular, inflammatory, infectious, traumatic, toxic, idiopathic, (neoplastic, nutritional)
> - Chronic: inflammatory, anomalous, metabolic, neoplastic, nutritional, degenerative
>
> **Clinical Course**
> - Static: vascular, traumatic, (anomalous), idiopathic
> - Improving: vascular, traumatic, toxic, idiopathic
> - Waxing-waning: inflammatory, metabolic
> - Progressive: inflammatory, infectious, anomalous, metabolic, neoplastic, nutritional, degenerative
>
> **Lesion Distribution**
> - Focal: vascular, traumatic, anomalous, idiopathic, neoplastic, degenerative
> - Multi-focal: inflammatory, infectious, (traumatic), (neoplastic)
> - Diffuse and symmetrical: toxic, metabolic, nutritional, degenerative
>
> **Apparent Discomfort**
> - Non-painful: vascular, toxic, anomalous, metabolic, idiopathic, degenerative
> - Painful: inflammatory, infectious, traumatic, neoplastic, degenerative

Typical presentation: Acute, non-progressive, non-painful, lateralised clinical signs.

5.1.2 Inflammatory/Infectious

Inflammatory or infectious diseases can have an acute or chronic onset but tend to be progressive over time without treatment. The severity of clinical signs associated with sterile inflammatory conditions, which are currently thought to represent autoimmune disorders, may also wax and wane over time.

Dependent on the specific disease process, inflammatory or infectious diseases can present with focal clinical signs (e.g. single abscess, granuloma, or discospondylitis) or produce lesions that are scattered throughout the nervous system, resulting in a multifocal lesion localisation.

In contrast to ischaemic events, inflammatory or infectious disease can result in foci of pain on examination and may also present with concurrent pyrexia, dependent on the disease process. However, inflammatory disorders should never be excluded on the basis of an absence of pyrexia or pain on examination.

Typical presentation: Acute or subacute, progressive, focal or multi-focal, possible discomfort on examination.

5.1.3 Traumatic

Traumatic events that result in neurological dysfunction will have an acute onset and are usually accompanied by a consistent clinical history or other examination findings suggestive of trauma. The severity of clinical signs may progress over 1–3 days secondary to oedema formation and expansion of the primary injury into the adjacent parenchyma. This process is termed secondary injury. The clinical signs will then remain static or show gradual improvement, dependent on the nature and severity of the injury. A traumatic event that results in instability of the vertebral column would be an exception to this rule, as progressive clinical signs may be observed secondary to recurrent spinal cord injury at the site of instability.

Traumatic events may affect a single region of the nervous system, resulting in a focal neuroanatomic localisation. However, the presence of multiple sites of injury should always be considered, particularly following blunt force trauma such as road traffic accidents. Pain is a common feature of trauma cases, secondary to direct neuronal injury (e.g. nerve roots) and/or damage to adjacent soft tissues and bones.

Typical presentation: Acute, non-progressive, painful, consistent clinical history.

5.1.4 Toxic

External toxins typically result in an acute onset of neurological signs following ingestion or topical administration, usually within minutes to hours of exposure. There may be a high suspicion of toxin exposure from the clinical history; young animals are often affected, given their inquisitive nature. If there is no further exposure to the toxin and the initial dose is not fatal, then the clinical signs should improve over time as the levels of toxin within the body and nervous system decline. As for metabolic disorders, toxicity most commonly results in symmetric neurological deficits as the toxin is distributed diffusely via the bloodstream.

Typical presentation: Acute, diffuse/symmetric clinical signs, non-painful, consistent clinical history.

5.1.5 Anomalous

As discussed in Chapter 2, anomalous disorders include congenital or developmental anatomic abnormalities. Congenital anomalies are present from birth and should always be considered in young, growing animals. However, an anomaly should never be excluded in middle-aged or older animals as decompensation may occasionally occur in later life. The clinical signs will typically be chronic in onset unless the anomaly predisposes to acute instability (e.g. atlantoaxial subluxation). These clinical signs can remain static, or they may show gradual progression if there is lesion expansion and secondary effects on the adjacent neuronal tissue (e.g. hydrocephalus, intradural spinal arachnoid diverticulum).

Typical presentation: Highly variable (see above).

5.1.6 Metabolic

Metabolic disorders can have an acute onset but may also present with a waxing-waning or episodic clinical history due to fluctuation in the levels of electrolytes, nutrients, or internal toxins. The index of suspicion for certain metabolic disorders may be higher in animals of certain ages or breeds (e.g. portosystemic shunting and hepatic encephalopathy in a young Yorkshire Terrier with poor growth). Non-neurologic signs may also be reported in the clinical history, such as gastrointestinal signs or polyuria/polydipsia.

Both toxic and metabolic disorders occur secondary to an excess or deficit of certain substances within the bloodstream. This blood is distributed to the entire nervous system and most commonly results in diffuse, symmetric neurological deficits reflecting involvement of the brain or neuromuscular system. A focal spinal cord neuroanatomic localisation would be unlikely to result from a metabolic or toxic disease process. It is also uncommon for metabolic disorders to present with apparent discomfort on examination.

Typical presentation: Concurrent non-neurological signs, diffuse/symmetric deficits, non-painful.

5.1.7 Idiopathic

An idiopathic disorder should only be suspected if there is a known condition (for which the underlying cause is currently unknown) that could result in the specific neurological signs displayed in an individual animal. A good example would be idiopathic facial paralysis in a dog that has had an extensive work up to exclude other possible causes for facial paralysis. The term should not be used as a 'diagnostic dustbin' simply because a definitive diagnosis has not been reached or when a reported idiopathic condition does not exist that would explain the presenting neurological signs.

The onset, progression, and lesion distribution for idiopathic disorders are specific to each condition. However, they frequently result in an acute onset of non-progressive or improving clinical signs. This most commonly reflects involvement of the peripheral nervous system, particularly individual cranial nerves, but an important exception is idiopathic epilepsy. It is uncommon for idiopathic disorders to present with a history of discomfort or pain on examination.

Typical presentation: Variable dependent on condition but typically acute, non-painful, and non-progressive.

5.1.8 Neoplastic

Neoplasia is typically associated with focal mass lesions that enlarge over time. Therefore, it would appear reasonable to assume that the associated clinical signs should have a chronic onset and be progressive in nature. Whilst this may be the case, the clinical signs associated with spinal neoplasia can have an acute onset secondary to pathological fracture, sudden haemorrhage, or vascular decompensation as the mass reaches a critical size. An acute onset of seizure activity is also a common presenting sign for intracranial neoplasia.

The index of suspicion for a neoplastic process should be higher in older animals, but certain forms of neoplasia may also be seen in young to middle-aged dogs (e.g. medulloblastoma, glioma) and cats (e.g. lymphoma). A focal neuroanatomic localisation is most common for neoplastic disorders; however, multi-focal or diffuse lesions can be seen for metastatic disease or in association with round cell neoplasms such as lymphoma or histiocytic sarcoma. Invasion of surrounding tissues and/or meningeal stretching or nerve root compression often result in pain on examination. However, an absence of discomfort should not be used to exclude a neoplastic process. Non-neurologic signs may be reported in the clinical history and abnormalities identified on general physical examination in cases with systemic involvement or metastatic neoplasia.

Typical presentation: Acute or chronic, progressive, middle-aged or older animals.

5.1.9 Nutritional

Nutritional disorders are rare in domestic species but may be observed in animals fed on an imbalanced, home-cooked diet or if there has been a manufacturing fault for commercial diets. The clinical signs can have an acute or chronic onset, dependent on the nutritional excess or deficiency, and are often progressive over time until treated. As for metabolic and toxic disorders, the lesion distribution is most commonly multifocal or diffuse unless there is susceptibility of certain regions of the nervous system to a particular nutritional deficiency (e.g. thiamine).

Typical presentation: Progressive, multi-focal or diffuse, non-painful, concurrent non-neurologic signs.

5.1.10 Degenerative

Disorders resulting from primary neuronal degeneration typically present with a chronic onset of progressive clinical signs. Certain disorders may be seen in specific breeds, with different ages at onset dependent on the individual condition. Degenerative disease should always be considered in a young animal that presents with chronic, progressive neurological signs, particularly if there is no apparent discomfort on examination. However, other degenerative conditions may not present until later in life and they should therefore still be considered in older animals (e.g. degenerative myelopathy, laryngeal paralysis-polyneuropathy, certain cerebellar abiotrophies). Different disorders may preferentially affect neurons in different regions of the nervous system, particularly the cerebellum, and the clinical signs tend to have a symmetric distribution as neurons on both sides are equally affected. If a degenerative disorder is suspected, then a literature search should be performed to look for reported conditions in the same breed that could explain the clinical history and examination findings.

Degeneration of anatomical structures that lie in close association with the nervous system, such as the intervertebral discs or articular facet joints, can result in neurological signs secondary to compression and neuronal injury. Whether this category should be classified as degenerative or fall within a sub-category of internal trauma is arguable (see Box 5.1). These disorders can have an acute onset (e.g. intervertebral disc extrusion) or a more chronic, progressive course, dependent on the pathology and nature of the injury. Clinical signs are typically progressive over time and discomfort may be present on examination secondary to meningeal or nerve root compression.

Typical presentation: Chronic, progressive, non-painful (the primary exception being degenerative intervertebral disc disease – see above).

5.2 Summary

The construction of a meaningful list of differential diagnoses for any given neurological problem relies upon a systematic and logical approach, with consideration of the following factors:

- *Signalment*
- *The clinical history – onset and progression of the clinical signs, owner-perceived discomfort, response to previous medications, concurrent non-neurologic signs*
- *The neuroanatomic localisation – lesion location, distribution, and symmetry*
- *Presence/absence of apparent pain on examination*

In the following chapter, we will discuss how to use this approach when managing the most common neurological presentations in general practice.

Bibliography

Armasu, M., Packer, R.M., Cook, S. et al. (2014). An exploratory study using a statistical approach as a platform for clinical reasoning in canine epilepsy. *Vet. J.* 202: 292–296.

Cardy, T.J., De Decker, S., Kenny, P.J., and Volk, H.A. (2015). Clinical reasoning in canine spinal disease: what combination of clinical information is useful? *Vet. Rec.* 177: 171.

da Costa, R.C. and Moore, S.A. (2010). Differential diagnosis of spinal diseases. *Vet. Clin. North Am. Small Anim. Pract.* 40: 755–763.

Dewey, C.W. and da Costa, R.C. (2015). *Practical Guide to Canine and Feline Neurology*, 3e. Hoboken, NJ: Wiley Blackwell.

de Lahunta, A., Glass, E., and Kent, M. (2015). *Veterinary Neuroanatomy and Clinical Neurology*, 4e. St Louis, MO: Elsevier Saunders.

Platt, S. and Olby, N. (2013). *BSAVA Manual of Canine and Feline Neurology*, 4e. Gloucester, UK: British Small Animal Veterinary Association.

Stanciu, G.D., Packer, R.M.A., Pakozdy, A. et al. (2017). Clinical reasoning in feline epilepsy: what combination of clinical information is useful? *Vet. J.* 225: 9–12.

Chapter 6 A Practical Approach to Common Presentations in General Practice

Edward Ives and Paul M. Freeman

The previous five chapters have summarised the initial approach to any case with suspected neurological disease, including how to determine if there is likely to be a lesion affecting the nervous system, where that lesion is located, and how to formulate a list of appropriate differential diagnoses. The next step is to decide whether urgent referral is indicated, or whether diagnostic tests can initially be performed in general practice. For those cases in which referral is not an option, the decision regarding which tests should be performed is particularly important. The aim of this chapter is to provide a logical approach to the diagnosis and treatment of the most common neurological presentations in general practice. The reader is referred to the many excellent 'disease-orientated' texts for more in-depth discussion regarding the pathophysiology, diagnosis, and treatment of the individual diseases mentioned. The neurologic syndromes discussed in this chapter are as follows:

- epileptic seizures
- movement disorders
- altered mentation
- blindness
- abnormalities of pupil size
- cranial nerve dysfunction
- vestibular syndrome
- cerebellar dysfunction
- neck and/or spinal pain

A Practical Approach to Neurology for the Small Animal Practitioner, First Edition. Paul M. Freeman and Edward Ives.
© 2020 John Wiley & Sons Ltd. Published 2020 by John Wiley & Sons Ltd.
Companion Website: www.wiley.com/go/freeman/neurology

- paresis, paralysis, and proprioceptive ataxia
- monoparesis and lameness
- neuromuscular weakness.

6.1 Epileptic Seizures

Edward Ives

The term 'seizure' can refer to any sudden attack or paroxysmal event. It is therefore a non-specific term but one that is frequently used to describe a seizure of neurological origin, or an 'epileptic seizure'. Owners may also use other non-specific terms for epileptic seizures, such as a 'fit' or 'convulsion'.

Epileptic seizures represent one of most common neurological presentations in small animal general practice. A logical and systematic approach is essential to achieve an accurate diagnosis and to plan the most appropriate treatment. Client communication is also vital, as expectations may differ greatly, management is frequently lifelong, and factors such as the requirement for daily medications and regular monitoring all depend upon good owner compliance.

6.1.1 What Is an Epileptic Seizure?

An epileptic seizure is not a disease entity itself but represents a clinical sign resulting from excessive and often hypersynchronous neuronal activity in the cerebral cortex (Berendt et al. 2015). This is most commonly apparent as transient, involuntary motor activity affecting a part or parts of the body, together with an altered level of mentation. Neurons are excitable cells that are constantly held in check, with the normal activity of neural networks reflecting a balance between excitatory and inhibitory connections between neurons. Each neuron has a threshold for excitation dependent on the environment surrounding it. This environment includes neighbouring neurons, supporting cells (e.g. astrocytes), neurotransmitter levels, electrolyte levels, and oxygen levels. Alterations to this environment, such as genetically determined factors, inflammation, oedema, or adjacent mass lesions, can result in a decrease in the neuronal threshold of activation that is sufficient to result in a seizure. Put simply, epileptic seizures are the result of either excessive excitation (via neurotransmitters such as glutamate) or inadequate inhibition (via neurotransmitters such as gamma-aminobutyric acid [GABA] or glycine). The initial seizure focus may involve only a small number of unstable neurons. However, this can induce surrounding neurons to discharge, resulting in seizure activity that affects a local region of the cerebral cortex, or that propagates to involve both cerebral hemispheres. The specific manifestation of a seizure will depend upon the area(s) of brain affected. For this reason, any unusual, involuntary phenomena that are episodic and recurrent should be investigated as possible epileptic seizures.

The term *'epilepsy'* is used to describe recurrent seizure activity (i.e. the occurrence of more than one confirmed or highly suspected epileptic seizure, irrespective of the underlying cause). Epilepsy is therefore a clinical sign and should not be confused with the condition 'idiopathic epilepsy', which is a specific diagnosis of exclusion.

6.1.2 Seizure Classification
1. Classification by clinical presentation
a. Focal seizures

Focal seizures occur when the excessive, hypersynchronous neuronal activity remains localised to a specific region of the cerebral cortex. This typically results in lateralised clinical signs, such as rhythmic contraction of the facial muscles on one side of the face or flexion of a single limb (see Video 2 and 32). These signs should be contralateral to the side of the seizure focus and are often accompanied by autonomic signs such as salivation. Structural brain lesions may present as focal seizures if they stimulate excessive neuronal activity in surrounding cerebral tissue (e.g. a neoplastic mass). However, focal seizures are also recognised in dogs for which no identified cause of the seizures can be found. These dogs will have a diagnosis of idiopathic epilepsy or 'epilepsy of unknown cause'. A study of 404 dogs with seizures of intracranial origin reported that the seizure pattern (focal versus generalised versus mixed) could not be used to differentiate dogs with asymmetric structural lesions ($n = 135$) from those with symmetric structural lesions ($n = 11$) or epilepsy of unknown cause ($n = 258$) (Armaşu et al. 2014).

Focal seizures may secondarily generalise to involve both cerebral hemispheres if the abnormal neuronal activity propagates across the midline. Generalisation of focal seizures is frequently observed in certain breeds of dog with idiopathic epilepsy (IE), such the Belgium Shepherd Dog.

b. Generalised seizures

Generalised seizures are the most common form of epileptic seizure observed in general practice. They are a manifestation of excessive neuronal activity that is affecting both cerebral hemispheres. This results in a loss of consciousness, bilaterally symmetric involuntary motor activity, rhythmic jaw movements, and recumbency (see Video 1). Generalised seizures are frequently accompanied by autonomic signs such as mydriasis, urination, defecation, and hypersalivation.

Generalised seizures frequently follow a set pattern, with each event having a similar appearance in an individual animal. This stereotypical nature is likely to reflect the same seizure focus being responsible for each recurrent seizure event. A generalised epileptic seizure can be divided into four main parts.

1. *The prodrome*: the period of abnormal behaviour that may be observed hours to days before a seizure occurs (e.g. restlessness, seeking the owner).

2. *The aura*: the sensory signs that occur seconds or minutes before a seizure. In humans, this may involve an unusual metallic taste or visual hallucinations. A genuine aura may therefore be difficult to appreciate in veterinary patients. However, the owners of dogs with recurrent seizures will often recognise when their pet is about to have a seizure as the dog may appear agitated, and either hide away or seek their owner immediately prior to the event.

3. *The ictus*: this is the seizure event itself. The majority of generalised epileptic seizures are self-limiting, with a duration between 30 seconds and 3 minutes.

4. *The post-ictal phase*: this is the period of abnormal behaviour that follows a seizure. This may last for several hours, up to several days, and typical signs include disorientation, ataxia, proprioceptive deficits, blindness, pacing, and polyphagia. If an animal is examined shortly after a seizure, then the potential influence of post-ictal signs on the findings and interpretation of your neurological examination should always be considered. For this reason, it is prudent to repeat the examination after a few hours, or the following day, to ensure that any neurological deficits are interpreted correctly.

Acute repetitive seizures, also termed 'cluster seizures', refers to when two or more individual seizures occur over a 24-hour period, with a complete recovery between events.

Status epilepticus is the term used to describe a seizure that is not self-limiting. It is specifically used if a single seizure is greater than 5 minutes in length, or if two or more seizures occur over a 30-minute period without a complete recovery between them. The emergency management of status epilepticus and acute repetitive seizures is discussed in Chapter 7.

Box 6.1.1 Reflex Seizures

Epileptic seizures are classified as 'reflexive' if they are triggered by certain stimuli. Reflex epilepsy is widely reported in humans but rarely described in veterinary medicine. It has been reported in dogs with stimulus-specific seizures, such as in response to certain sounds (e.g. lawnmower engine, doorbell ringing), exercise, car journeys, and visits to the vets or groomers (Forsgård et al. 2019; Shell et al. 2017). Some dogs may have multiple triggers for their seizures. A condition named 'audiogenic reflex seizures' has also been reported in older cats (median age 15 years) (Lowrie et al. 2016). These events are associated with high-pitched noises, such as crinkling of tin foil, chinking of glass, keys jangling, or metal spoon contact with a ceramic food bowl. Birman Cats appear over-represented and levetiracetam appears to provide good seizure control when compared to phenobarbitone (Lowrie et al. 2017).

2. Classification by underlying aetiology
See Figure 6.1.1 for a summary.

a. Extracranial disorders (reactive seizures)
Reactive seizures result from abnormal blood being pumped to a normal brain. This change in blood composition alters the neuronal environment in favour of excitation. Extracranial disorders usually present with generalised seizures +/– symmetric neurological deficits as there is equal delivery of abnormal blood to both cerebral hemispheres. Examples of extracranial causes of epileptic seizures include:

1. *Metabolic disorders* – hypoglycaemia, hepatic encephalopathy, uraemic encephalopathy, hypoxia, electrolyte abnormalities (e.g. hypocalcaemia, hypernatraemia, hyponatraemia)
2. *External toxin exposure* – lead, ethylene glycol, organophosphates, metaldehyde (found in slug pellets), chocolate, strychnine, illegal drugs, permethrin (in cats).

b. Intracranial disorders
If the blood being pumped to the brain is normal, then epileptic seizures may reflect a structural brain lesion that is detectable on diagnostic investigations, or may reflect a functional disorder that lowers the threshold for neuronal excitation.

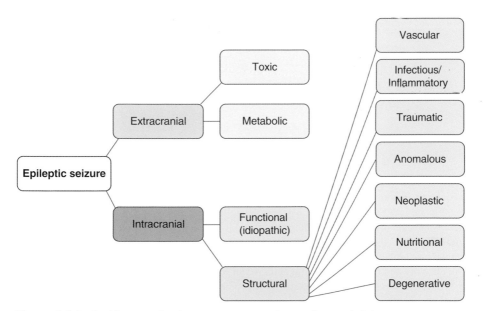

Figure 6.1.1 Classification of epileptic seizures according to their underlying cause.

i. Structural epilepsy

A structural brain lesion may sufficiently alter the neuronal environment to favour excessive neuronal excitation. Advanced imaging +/− cerebrospinal fluid (CSF) analysis is usually required for the diagnosis of these conditions.

- *Vascular* – cerebrovascular disease (haemorrhage or ischaemic stroke).
- *Infectious/inflammatory* – e.g. bacterial, viral, fungal or protozoal meningoencephalitis, meningoencephalitis of unknown origin (MUO).
- *Traumatic* – seizures may occur at the time of head trauma, or the onset can be delayed by weeks to months. Post-traumatic epilepsy has been reported to affect 6–10% of dogs following significant head trauma (see Chapter 7).
- *Anomalous* – e.g. hydrocephalus, porencephaly, meningoencephalocele.
- *Neoplastic* – primary (e.g. glioma, meningioma), metastatic, locally invasive (e.g. nasal adenocarcinoma) (Figure 6.1.2).
- *Degenerative* – e.g. neuronal ceroid lipofuscinosis (NCL), Alaskan Husky encephalopathy.

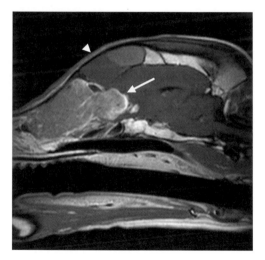

Figure 6.1.2 A parasagittal image (left side) from a brain MRI of a 12-year-old, male neutered Labrador Retriever with a clinical history of intermittent sneezing and eight generalised epileptic seizures over a 4-day period. Neurological examination revealed a depressed level of mentation, circling to left, and a left head turn. The neuroanatomic localisation was the left forebrain. The MRI demonstrated a large mass lesion occupying the caudal nasal cavity that had invaded through the cribriform plate, resulting in compression of the olfactory and frontal lobes of the brain (white arrow). Note also the accumulation of fluid in left frontal sinus secondary to obstruction of drainage by the nasal mass (arrow head). A nasal adenocarcinoma was suspected in this case, but histopathology was not performed to confirm the diagnosis.

ii. Idiopathic epilepsy ('epilepsy of unknown cause')

Idiopathic epilepsy (IE) is a functional intracranial disorder in which the lowered seizure threshold is likely to result from a combination of genetic, environmental, and developmental factors. A genetic component is supported by the fact that IE appears to be more common in certain breeds of dog, with evidence to suggest inheritance in breeds such as the Border Collie, Labradors Retriever, and German Shepherd Dog (Hülsmeyer et al. 2015).

Idiopathic epilepsy is the most common diagnosis for recurrent seizures in dogs, with a prevalence of 0.62% reported by a study of over 87 000 dogs from a UK general practice population (Kearsley-Fleet et al. 2013). It appears to be less common in cats, likely related to their more diverse genetic background. However, IE is increasingly recognised in this species and has been reported as the underlying cause of recurrent seizures in 20–60% of cats (Barnes Heller 2018; Pakozdy et al. 2013; Pakozdy et al. 2014; Stanciu et al. 2017; Wahle et al. 2014).

Idiopathic generalised epilepsy represents a group of epileptic disorders in humans, with specific subtypes that differ in relation to seizure type, age at onset, and whether a known genetic mutation is responsible. The term 'idiopathic epilepsy' is currently used in veterinary medicine as an umbrella-term to describe all seizure disorders for which an underlying cause cannot be identified. However, there are also likely to be specific subtypes of idiopathic epilepsy in different species and breeds of animal. This is supported by the fact that epilepsies of unknown cause may have a specific presentation in certain breeds of dog (e.g. juvenile myoclonic epilepsy in Rhodesian Ridgeback dogs [Wielaender et al. 2018]), and that the disease progression may differ dependent on the breed of dog; some breeds will typically show a relatively benign clinical course of IE (e.g. Finnish Spitz, Belgian Shepherd), whereas other breeds may present with a more severe phenotype and seizures that are difficult to control in spite of multiple medications (e.g. Italian Spinone, Australian Shepherd dog, Border Collie). Knowledge of these breed-specific differences is important when planning treatment and for managing owner expectations.

The onset of seizures in dogs with IE most commonly occurs between 6 months and 6 years of age. In spite of this, IE should never be excluded from the list of differential diagnoses in older dogs; between 13% and 45% of dogs with a seizure onset at >7 years old were diagnosed with IE in two studies (Ghormley et al. 2015; Schwartz et al. 2013). However, a study of over 400 dogs with recurrent seizures reported that the odds of an asymmetric structural brain lesion compared to IE increased by 1.6-fold for each additional year of age (Armaşu et al. 2014). Therefore, performing further investigations to exclude structural epilepsy is always advised in dogs with an onset of seizures at >6 years of age. A diagnosis of structural epilepsy is more likely in cats that are >7 years old at the time of seizure onset (Stanciu et al. 2017). However, the lower incidence of IE in cats compared to dogs means that further investigations should ideally be performed in all cats that present with a history of seizures (see Box 6.1.2).

The clinical course of IE can be extremely variable dependent on the individual. Many dogs will initially present with infrequent single seizures; however, some dogs may show cluster seizures or status epilepticus as their first presentation of IE. The occurrence of cluster seizures has been associated with a worse long-term prognosis in dogs with IE. This unpredictable clinical course should always be discussed with the owner at the time of diagnosis.

Dogs and cats with IE should have a normal neurological examination during the inter-ictal period. One study reported that dogs with an abnormal neurological examination were 16.5 times more likely to have an asymmetric structural brain lesion and 12.5 times more likely to have a symmetric structural brain lesion (e.g. hydrocephalus) compared to a diagnosis of IE (Armaşu et al. 2014). A structural brain lesion is also more likely in cats with an abnormal neurological examination (Stanciu et al. 2017). However, the possibility of pre-existing neurological deficits, post-ictal deficits, and the influence of recently administered antiepileptic medications on the neurological examination should also be considered. These deficits may mimic those associated with a structural brain lesion and the examination should be repeated if there is any uncertainty.

Idiopathic epilepsy is currently a diagnosis of exclusion, with no abnormalities being found on diagnostic investigations. Inter-ictal electroencephalography (EEG) does not appear to be a useful screening method to distinguish dogs with IE from those with structural epilepsy (Brauer et al. 2012). Recent guidelines for the diagnosis of IE in dogs have defined 3 tiers of diagnosis in practice.

Box 6.1.2 Epilepsy in Cats

The diagnostic approach to epileptic seizures in cats is broadly similar to that for dogs. However, there are some important considerations in this species which include:

- Third-degree AV block resulting in cerebral hypoxia is an important differential diagnosis for episodic, seizure-like episodes in cats.
- Idiopathic epilepsy is an increasingly recognised cause for recurrent seizures in cats, particularly in young cats with a normal inter-ictal neurological examination (Stanciu et al. 2017). However, structural epilepsy remains more common in cats than dogs and performing further investigations is always advised in this species.
- Phenobarbitone is currently the first-line treatment of choice for the majority of cats with recurrent seizures. Other treatment options include levetiracetam, imepitoin, and zonisamide (Bailey et al. 2008; Engel et al. 2017).
- Levetiracetam is reported to be the treatment of choice for audiogenic reflex seizures in older cats (Lowrie et al. 2017).
- Potassium bromide should not be used in cats as it has the potential to cause severe, potentially fatal, bronchial irritation.

Tier I
- Two or more unprovoked seizures at least 24 hours apart.
- Age at onset between 6 months and 6 years old.
- Normal inter-ictal physical and neurological examination.
- No abnormalities on haematology, serum biochemistry and urinalysis.

Tier II
- As for Tier I, together with negative findings on serum bile acid stimulation testing, magnetic resonance imaging (MRI) of the brain, and CSF analysis.

Tier III
- As for Tiers I and II, together with consistent EEG abnormalities.

6.1.3   Diagnostic Approach to Epileptic Seizures
The diagnostic approach to epileptic seizures should be logical and systematic so that the most appropriate investigations are performed in the first instance, and so that the management can be individualised to each case.

1. Establish if the events described are likely to represent epileptic seizures
This is vital before pursuing further investigations as owners may describe various forms of abnormal event as a 'seizure' (Box 6.1.3). The widespread popularity of smartphones has made access to videos of abnormal events much easier. This can be incredibly useful to further characterise an event, particularly if they are short, do not occur during veterinary visits, or if the clinical examination is normal between events. EEG during an episode can be used to confirm an

---

Box 6.1.3 Seizure Mimics

- Syncope or cardiorespiratory disease (e.g. third-degree AV block in cats)
- Vestibular syndrome
- Systemic disease resulting in weakness or collapse (e.g. hypoadrenocorticism)
- Narcolepsy/cataplexy (see Video 6)
- Pain (e.g. cervical disc disease resulting in pain and cervical muscle spasm, see Video 8)
- Stereotypical behaviours or obsessive compulsive behaviour disorders (e.g. tail chasing, fly catching)
- Rapid eye movement (REM) sleep disorders (see Video 9)
- Movement disorders (e.g. paroxysmal dyskinesia) (see Video 10, 33 and 37)
- Neuromuscular weakness (e.g. myasthenia gravis)
- Tetanus.

Box 6.1.4 When to Suspect an Epileptic Seizure

- Acute, often unexpected onset.
- Frequently occurring at times of rest, particularly when associated with idiopathic epilepsy. However, seizures associated with structural brain disease can occur at any time.
- A stereotypical pattern for each event in an individual cat or dog.
- Involuntary motor activity lasting <5 minutes. Unless representing status epilepticus, or if the owner has included the post-ictal period in the total duration of an event, generalised seizures most commonly last between 30 seconds and 3 minutes. A movement disorder should be considered if the abnormal motor activity lasts for more than 5–10 minutes, particularly if the animal has a normal level of mentation during the event.
- Increased muscle tone during the event, usually accompanied by rhythmic limb movements and facial muscle contractions (see Video 1).
- The presence of autonomic signs during the event (salivation, urination, defecation).
- A reduced level of mentation or a lack of response to the owner during the event.
- The presence of a distinct post-ictal phase (e.g. ataxia, disorientation, hyperactivity, polyphagia, visual deficits).

---

epileptic seizure. However, access to this equipment is currently limited in veterinary medicine and there are practical considerations regarding its use in dogs and cats, particularly for infrequent events. A positive response to an antiepileptic medication may suggest that previously observed events did represent epileptic seizures. However, a temporal association between starting a medication and a reduction in episode frequency does not always imply causation, and naturally regressive or waxing/waning disorders should also be considered. A general guide for when to suspect an epileptic seizure can be found in Box 6.1.4. Further discussion regarding the distinction between epileptic seizures and other paroxysmal events can be found in Chapter 1.

2. Formulate a list of differential diagnoses

As discussed in Chapter 5, a list of differential diagnoses should always be made *before* planning further tests. This list will depend upon the neuroanatomic localisation, the signalment of the animal, the clinical history, the disease onset, and the clinical progression.

Neuroanatomic localisation: an epileptic seizure is a manifestation of abnormal neuronal activity in the cerebral cortex, irrespective of whether the inciting cause is extracranial or intracranial in origin. Therefore, the neuroanatomic localisation for any animal with epileptic seizures is the forebrain. However, epileptic seizures may also be accompanied by other neurological deficits that could indicate a multi-focal or diffuse disease process.

Signalment: certain disorders are more common in animals of a particular age, breed, or sex. Therefore, the signalment can be used to rank the list of differential diagnoses (see Chapters 2 and 5).

- *Female animals* – decreased seizure threshold during oestrous in intact female dogs, metastatic mammary adenocarcinoma.
- *Young animals* (<1 year of age) – portosystemic shunt, hydrocephalus, hypoglycaemia, infectious diseases (e.g. canine distemper virus [CDV] encephalitis).
- *Middle-aged animals* (1–6 years of age) – idiopathic epilepsy (particularly in breeds with known heritability such as Border Collies and Labradors), meningoencephalitis of unknown origin (MUO).
- *Older animals* (>6 years of age) – intracranial neoplasia (particularly in brachycephalic breeds of dog), hypoglycaemia secondary to insulinoma, MUO, idiopathic epilepsy.

Clinical history: Important questions to ask when taking the clinical history should include:

- The age at the time of the first seizure.
- The seizure frequency and the presence or absence of cluster seizures.
- If there are any known or suspected trigger factors, such as seizures after eating in the case of a portosystemic shunt.
- The vaccination status and travel history of the affected animal.
- Concurrent medical conditions and any medications being administered.
- The diet and any known or suspected toxin exposure.
- A history of seizures in the parents or siblings would increase the index of suspicion for idiopathic epilepsy; a contagious disease or intoxication should also be considered if there is an acute onset of seizures in multiple animals at the same time.

The general clinical examination: a thorough general clinical examination is important to assess for signs of systemic disorders that could cause seizures (i.e. extracranial disease), mimic seizures, or that would affect the prognosis or risks associated with sedation/general anaesthesia.

The neurological examination: the neurological examination should ideally be performed in the inter-ictal period to avoid overlap of post-ictal deficits, such as ataxia, circling, vision loss, and proprioceptive deficits. Antiepileptic medications may also cause sedation and ataxia, which could influence the interpretation of the examination findings.

The inter-ictal neurological examination should be normal for all animals with IE but may also be normal for other diseases. These include waxing/waning metabolic conditions or intracranial neoplasia in 'silent' brain regions (e.g. the olfactory lobe) (Figure 6.1.3). Structural epilepsy should therefore never be

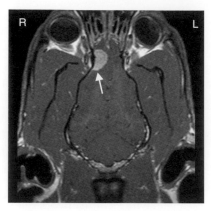

Figure 6.1.3 A T1-weighted MRI in the dorsal plane following the administration of intravenous contrast media in an 8-year-8-month-old, female neutered, German Shepherd Dog with a history of three generalised epileptic seizures over the last 6 weeks. There were no neurological deficits at the time of examination in the inter-ictal period, and haematology, serum biochemistry, and urinalysis were normal. Magnetic resonance imaging of the brain demonstrated a 1.5 × 1.5 × 1 cm, ovoid, broad-based, contrast-enhancing, extra-axial mass in the right olfactory lobe (white arrow). These imaging characteristics were most consistent with a meningioma as the cause of structural epilepsy in this case.

excluded on the basis of a normal neurological examination. A previous study of dogs with a normal inter-ictal neurological examination identified a cause for the observed seizures on brain MRI in 3% of dogs that were <6 years old and in 25% of dogs that were >6 years old (Smith et al. 2008). Very similar findings were reported for epileptic cats with a normal inter-ictal neurological examination; a detectable lesion was observed on MRI in 5% of cats between 1 and 6 years old and in 23% of cats >6 years old (Raimondi et al. 2017). Neurological deficits that would be consistent with an asymmetric structural brain lesion include a contralateral menace response deficit (see Video 28), contralateral proprioceptive deficits, reduced nasal septum nociception in the contralateral nostril, a head turn, circling (see Video 22), an altered level of mentation, and possibly neck pain.

3. Perform further investigations in general practice

The decision whether to perform further investigations in general practice, and when to perform them, will depend on many factors. These include the nature and frequency of the episodes, the inter-ictal examination findings, the list of differential diagnoses, the degree of owner concern, and the funds available for referral or further investigations.

If an animal has had a single episode that is suspected to represent an epileptic seizure, if it has fully recovered by the time of assessment, and it has a normal physical and neurological examination, then it is not unreasonable to monitor for further episodes. The owner should be encouraged to video any future events and should always be made aware that the option of performing further investigations is available at any time.

If an animal has had two or more isolated epileptic seizures, a cluster of seizures, or status epilepticus, then performing further investigations is advised (De Risio et al. 2015). In general practice, this should start by excluding extracranial disorders as referral for advanced imaging is generally required to diagnose intracranial disease. The specific investigations to perform will depend upon the signalment and list of differential diagnoses.

- *Haematology, serum biochemistry, and urinalysis* should be performed in all cases.
- *Blood pressure testing*, particularly in geriatric cats.
- *Bile acid stimulation testing +/– serum ammonia*, particularly if a portosystemic shunt is suspected.
- *Thyroid function testing* – total thyroid hormone (T4), free T4, thyroid stimulating hormone (TSH).
- *Fructosamine and insulin levels* if an insulinoma is suspected.
- *A coagulation profile* if a disorder of blood clotting is suspected (e.g. rodenticide ingestion or petechiae or ecchymoses on clinical examination).
- *Infectious disease testing* dependent on the species and relative risk of exposure – *Toxoplasma gondii* in cats and dogs, *Neospora caninum* or CDV in dogs, feline leukaemia virus (FeLV), feline immunodeficiency virus (FIV), and feline coronavirus in cats.
- *Urine metabolic screening* if an inborn error of metabolism is suspected (e.g. young animal with seizures and progressive neurological disease).
- *Toxicology* for known or suspected toxin exposure.
- *Thoracic radiography, abdominal ultrasonography,* or *thoracic and abdominal computed tomography (CT)* – if metastatic neoplasia or an extracranial cause of seizures is suspected, particularly if referral for further investigations is not possible.

It is not unreasonable to make a presumptive diagnosis of idiopathic epilepsy in general practice on the basis of the clinical history, signalment, a normal inter-ictal neurological examination, and normal blood/urine tests (Tier I classification). This diagnosis becomes extremely likely if the seizures remain infrequent and the neurological examination remains normal over a period of 6–12 months. However, the animal's owner should always be made aware that this is not a definitive diagnosis and the option of referral for further investigations should be discussed. This is particularly relevant if the seizures are difficult to control, or if the subsequent disease progression is incompatible with a diagnosis of idiopathic epilepsy (e.g. the appearance of inter-ictal neurological deficits).

4. Refer for further investigations

Referral to a veterinary neurologist should be offered to the owner of any animal that has had one or more suspected epileptic seizures. Further investigations may not necessarily be performed at this time, but the consultation gives the opportunity for further neurological assessment and an in-depth discussion regarding the causes and management of epilepsy.

If an extracranial cause for the events has been excluded, and if funds are available, then advanced imaging of the brain and CSF sampling may be advised. This is to achieve a diagnosis of either a structural brain lesion or idiopathic epilepsy (Tier II classification). MRI of the brain is the gold standard imaging modality in light of its superior soft tissue resolution compared to CT. A general guide as to when advanced imaging of the brain would be recommended is as follows:

- All cats with a history of epileptic seizures given the higher incidence of structural epilepsy in this species.
- Dogs with a seizure onset at <6 months or >6 years of age for which an extracranial cause has not been identified.
- Any animal with a history of cluster seizures or status epilepticus.
- Animals with inter-ictal neurological deficits that are consistent with a forebrain neuroanatomic localisation.
- Animals with a presumptive diagnosis of idiopathic epilepsy that appear refractory to antiepileptic drug (AED) therapy despite adequate serum drug levels.

6.1.4   Management of Epileptic Seizures

1. Owner communication

Good owner communication is vital throughout every step in the diagnosis and management of their pet's condition. This is to ensure that they are well-informed regarding the diagnosis, treatment options, and likely prognosis. The owner should also be made aware of the potential requirement for lifelong daily medication, regular monitoring of treatment, and the associated costs. This can be a big responsibility and one that may not be appropriate for all owners. It is always better to discuss these factors and to manage an owner's expectations prior to starting treatment, rather than have the owner feel misinformed at a later date.

Encouraging an owner to keep a record of their pet's seizures in the form of a seizure diary will assist in the monitoring of disease progression and the response to treatment. It may also help to keep the owner motivated, allow them to feel involved with the management of their pet's condition, and help to de-emotionalise the seizures for them at the time of an event. There are some recent smartphone applications that some owners may find useful for this purpose.

2. Goals of seizure management

The primary goal of seizure management is a reduction in the frequency and severity of seizures, with minimal adverse effects of treatment (Bhatti et al. 2015; Potschka et al. 2015). The overall quality of life for the animal should be prioritised, with the aim of reducing seizure-related morbidity and mortality. Whilst seizure freedom is the ideal management goal, this is rarely achieved in veterinary patients. Some studies have estimated that only 15–25% of epileptic dogs may become seizure-free on medication. A commonly used definition of a 'responder' is if a >50% reduction in seizure frequency is seen following the introduction of a medication or other intervention. Whether this is a satisfactory result for an individual animal (and owner) will obviously depend upon the seizure frequency before starting treatment. A reasonable goal to discuss with the owner of an animal with IE would be to achieve a single, short, self-limiting seizure every 3 months.

3. When to start treatment

The decision when to start treatment will depend upon:

- the underlying cause for the seizures
- seizure type and frequency
- the effects of the seizures on the owner
- the effects of the seizures on the animal's quality of life and its brain
- the adverse effects and costs of medication.

It has been suggested that long-term management of idiopathic epilepsy in dogs may be more successful if treatment is started early in the course of the disease, particularly in dogs with a high seizure density (i.e. a short time interval between seizures). However, several questionnaire studies have also documented that the adverse effects of medications have a large impact on owner-perceived quality of life for their pet (Chang et al. 2006). This is important, as dogs with epilepsy have an increased risk of premature death as a result of euthanasia, which is driven in part by a combination of economic burden and the emotional stress on the owner (Podell et al. 2016). Chronic behaviour changes are increasingly reported in dogs with recurrent seizures, including fear and anxiety-related behaviours (Packer and Volk 2015; Shihab et al. 2011; Watson et al. 2018; Winter et al. 2018). These can also contribute to owner-perceived poor quality of life for their pet and drive a decision to euthanasia. A general guide as to when to start medical management of epileptic seizures can be found in Box 6.1.5.

Box 6.1.5 When to Start Treatment

'No?'

- *A single, self-limiting seizure-like event and a normal neurological examination – monitor the animal closely for further events or abnormalities.*
- *Infrequent, short, self-limiting seizures in an animal with suspected idiopathic epilepsy (i.e. one seizure every 2–3 months).*
- *Seizures that are affecting an animal's quality of life less than the expected adverse effects of medications (e.g. infrequent, short, or focal seizures).*
- *Seizures following toxin exposure, after their initial management.*

'Yes?'

- *>2 seizures over a 6-month period, or an increasing frequency or severity of seizures.*
- *Cluster seizures or status epilepticus.*
- *An underlying progressive disease (i.e. structural epilepsy).*
- *Owner distress or a desire to treat when aware of the expected adverse effects of medications and responsibilities required.*
- *Severe post-ictal signs (e.g. aggression or blindness).*

---

4. How to manage epileptic seizures

a. Correct the underlying disease

This could include medical management or surgical attenuation of a portosystemic shunt, medical or surgical management of an insulinoma, radiotherapy or surgery for intracranial neoplasia, or medical management of meningoencephalitis. Antiepileptic medications are commonly used as an adjunctive treatment for these conditions until the underlying disease is deemed to have resolved. Long-term medical management is frequently required for conditions such as meningoencephalitis of unknown origin or intracranial neoplasia, for which a cure is not often possible.

b. Antiepileptic medications

Antiepileptic drugs (AEDs) are most commonly used for the long-term management of idiopathic epilepsy and in the palliative treatment of structural epilepsy. They exert their clinical effect by reducing neuronal excitability and increasing the threshold of neuronal excitation. There are three AEDs that are currently licensed in the United Kingdom (UK) for use in dogs: phenobarbitone, potassium bromide, and imepitoin. The choice of medication to use in an individual animal will depend upon multiple factors, including tolerability, efficacy, whether concurrent diseases are present (e.g. hepatic dysfunction, renal disease), and owner-related factors (e.g. financial, lifestyle). A flow diagram summarising a suggested approach to the management of idiopathic epilepsy in dogs using imepitoin, phenobarbitone, and/or potassium bromide can be found in Figure 6.1.4.

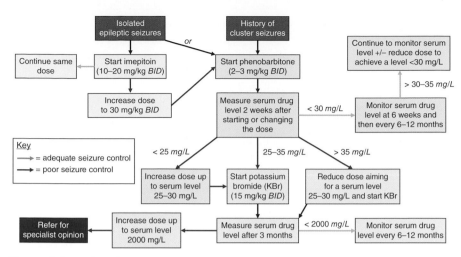

Figure 6.1.4 A flow diagram summarising a suggested approach to the management of idiopathic epilepsy in dogs using imepitoin, phenobarbitone, and/or potassium bromide.

Phenobarbitone

License: Phenobarbitone is licensed in the UK as a first-line medication for the management of epileptic seizures in dogs.

Mechanism of action: Poorly understood but likely works by enhancing the effects of the inhibitory neurotransmitter GABA, reducing the excitatory effects of glutamate, and decreasing calcium flow into neurons.

Clinical indications: First-line medication for dogs with generalised seizures, licensed treatment of choice for dogs with cluster seizures, first-line medication of choice in cats with epileptic seizures. Phenobarbitone is also useful in the emergency management of cluster seizures and status epilepticus (see Chapter 7).

Contraindications: Pre-existing hepatic dysfunction. If used, the hepatic parameters and drug serum levels should be carefully monitored.

Metabolism and excretion: Hepatic metabolism by microsomal enzymes, taking 7–14 days to reach a steady-state serum concentration (15–35 mg/l). Phenobarbitone auto-induces the hepatic cytochrome p450 system, resulting in a decreased half-life with chronic therapy. Gradually increasing oral doses are therefore often required over the life of an animal to maintain an adequate serum level.

Starting dose: 2–3 mg/kg per os twice daily in dogs and cats. Smaller dogs often require higher oral doses to achieve the same serum level when compared to larger dogs. Administration every 8 hours can be considered in dogs with inadequate seizure control on twice daily administration and a phenobarbitone elimination half-life of less than 20 hours (estimated by measuring peak and trough serum concentrations) (Stabile et al. 2017).

Serum level monitoring: 14 days after starting treatment or a change in the dose. Then at 6 weeks, 6 months, and every 6–12 months if the seizures are well-controlled.

The blood sample should be taken into a plain serum tube (not a serum gel tube) and can be taken at any time after the last dose in the majority of animals. However, it should ideally be taken at a similar time of day for each blood test to allow a fair comparison with previous levels. A trough serum drug concentration (i.e. one that is taken immediately before the next dose) can be considered in animals that show seizures close to when their next dose is due, or if a drug reaction is suspected.

The therapeutic range should be determined on an individual basis; toxicity may occur in some animals below the upper limit of the reference range, and some animals may be well controlled with a serum level below the lower limit (Bhatti et al. 2015, Podell et al. 2016).

- *Adequate seizure control at a serum level <25–30 mg/l.* No change in oral dose required (even if the serum level is below the lower limit of the 'therapeutic range', i.e. <15 mg/l).
- *Adequate seizure control but the serum level is >30 mg/l.* Continue to monitor the serum level and if it remains >30–35 mg/l then reduce the oral dose, aiming for seizure control at a level of <30 mg/l.
- *Inadequate seizure control and the serum level is <30 mg/l.* Increase the oral dose and recheck the serum level after 14 days, aiming for a level of 25–30 mg/l before considering other treatment options.
- *Inadequate seizure control with a serum level 25–35 mg/l.* Introduce potassium bromide (see below).

Adverse effects: Common adverse effects include polydipsia, polyuria, polyphagia, sedation, and ataxia. Significant sedation and ataxia will usually be self-limiting and markedly improve after the first 1–2 weeks. Less common adverse effects include superficial necrotising dermatitis, blood dyscrasias (e.g. anaemia, thrombocytopenia, or pancytopenia), and hepatotoxicity (Bersan et al. 2014; Charalambous et al. 2016). Hepatotoxicity may be seen as an idiosyncratic reaction that is independent of the oral dose. It can also be associated with chronic phenobarbitone therapy, but this is rare if the serum levels are kept below 35 mg/l.

Adverse effect monitoring: A complete blood cell count, biochemical profile, bile acid stimulation test at 3 months and then every 6–12 months.

Phenobarbitone induces alkaline phosphatase (ALP) in dogs and this parameter is frequently elevated as a 'normal' finding on serum biochemistry in treated dogs. Alanine aminotransferase (ALT) may also be mildly elevated in dogs, but the levels of both ALP and ALT should be monitored for further increases over time. Both aspartate aminotransferase (AST) and gamma glutamyltransferase (GGT) are useful for hepatic monitoring in dogs as their levels are not directly induced by phenobarbitone. Liver enzymes do not appear to be influenced by phenobarbitone use in cats at serum levels between 15 and 45 mg/l

(Finnerty et al. 2014). Phenobarbitone does not affect adrenocortical assessment (e.g. adrenocorticotropic hormone [ACTH] stimulation testing) but may alter the levels of total thyroid hormone (T4) and TSH, complicating the interpretation of thyroid function testing in dogs receiving phenobarbitone.

Potassium bromide

License: Potassium bromide (KBr) is licensed in the UK as an adjunctive medication in dogs with seizures that are refractory to phenobarbitone alone.

Mechanism of action: Incompletely understood but likely involves hyperpolarisation of the neuronal cell membrane and elevation of the seizure threshold as negatively charged bromide ions compete with chloride to enter via anion channels.

Clinical indications: Most commonly used as an add-on medication to phenobarbitone in dogs that continue to show a high seizure frequency in spite of an adequate phenobarbitone serum level (25–30 mg/l). KBr has been reported to be less effective when used as a monotherapy compared to phenobarbitone in dogs with idiopathic epilepsy (Boothe et al. 2012). Its use may also be associated with more severe adverse effects. However, KBr can be a useful first-line medication in dogs that cannot tolerate phenobarbitone (e.g. hepatic disease or previous idiosyncratic reaction).

Contraindications: Potassium bromide should not be used in cats due to the risk of potentially fatal eosinophilic bronchitis. Use with care in dogs with a history of pancreatitis. Serum levels should be monitored closely in dogs with renal disease.

Metabolism and excretion: Excreted unchanged via the kidneys, with a long serum half-life of 24–36 days. KBr takes 3–4 months to reach a steady state serum concentration (1000–2500 µg/ml in dogs) and the levels will fall slowly after a dose reduction.

The salt content of the diet should be kept constant in animals receiving KBr (Larsen et al. 2014; Shaw et al. 1996). Bromide and chloride compete for reabsorption by the kidneys, therefore a high dietary salt content (e.g. urinary diet) will result in reduced bromide reabsorption, increased renal excretion, and the potential for low KBr serum levels. Conversely, a low dietary salt content (e.g. cardiac diet) will result in increased bromide reabsorption, reduced renal excretion, and higher KBr serum levels. The use of loop diuretics (e.g. furosemide) can also increase KBr excretion, potentially resulting in loss of seizure control. Renal insufficiency may result in reduced renal excretion, an increase in the KBr serum level, and the potential for bromide intoxication if the dose is not appropriately adjusted.

Starting dose: 20–40 mg/kg/day per os. The long serum half-life means that KBr can be administered as a single daily dose; however, twice daily administration with food is recommended to reduce the incidence of gastrointestinal irritation.

Oral loading regimes have been described to achieve therapeutic serum levels more rapidly in dogs with frequent seizures (e.g. 125 mg/kg/day divided into four to six daily doses for 5 days). The use of loading doses may be associated with significant sedation, ataxia, and/or vomiting, therefore loading should only be performed if absolutely required and hospitalisation of the animal should be considered over the loading period. This is particularly recommended if rapid loading regimes are used (e.g. 625 mg/kg over 2 days divided into 8–12 separate doses).

Serum level monitoring: 3 months after starting treatment or a change in the dose, then every 6–12 months if the seizures are well controlled. The level can be checked after 1 month if a loading regime is used.

Adverse effects: The adverse effects of KBr are similar to those for phenobarbitone and include polydipsia, polyuria, polyphagia, sedation, and ataxia. Nausea, vomiting, irritability, restlessness, and erythematous dermatitis may also be observed (Baird-Heinz et al. 2012; Rossmeisl and Inzana 2009). Intravenous administration of sodium chloride (0.9%) can be used to increase renal excretion and reduce serum bromide levels more rapidly in the event of severe adverse effects or overdose.

Adverse effects monitoring: A complete blood cell count and serum biochemistry should be checked every 6–12 months in dogs on chronic therapy. KBr will artefactually elevate the chloride level on serum biochemistry as the laboratory machines cannot distinguish between chloride and bromide ions. Elevated serum canine pancreatic lipase immunoreactivity (cPLI) concentrations may also be observed in dogs receiving KBr; however, clinically significant pancreatitis is reported as a rare adverse reaction affecting less than 1 in 10 000 animals.

Imepitoin

License: Imepitoin is licensed in the UK for the reduction of the frequency of generalised seizures due to idiopathic epilepsy in dogs after evaluation of alternative treatment options. It has also recently been licensed for the reduction of anxiety and fear associated with noise phobia in dogs.

Mechanism of action: Imepitoin is a low affinity partial agonist at the benzodiazepine receptor and potentiates GABA-mediated inhibition, whilst also having a weak Ca-channel blocking effect.

Clinical indications: Imepitoin represents a first-line medication for dogs with isolated generalised seizures and highly suspected or confirmed idiopathic epilepsy (Rundfeldt et al. 2015; Tipold et al. 2015). The rapid onset of action, lack of serum monitoring requirements, and the possibility of milder adverse effects makes it an attractive option in these cases. However, its use is not recommended in dogs with a history of cluster seizures or status epilepticus. Dogs that are currently stable on an alternative AED should not be transitioned onto imepitoin unless there is evidence of poor efficacy or severe adverse effects associated with the other medication(s).

Imepitoin appears to be well tolerated in cats but its efficacy for seizure control remains unknown in this species (Engel et al. 2017).

Contraindications: Severe renal, hepatic, or cardiac disease.

Metabolism and excretion: Imepitoin reaches a maximum blood concentration 2 hours after oral dosing, followed by rapid blood clearance via the faecal route.

Starting dose: 10–30 mg/kg per os twice daily, with a constant timing of dosing in relation to food recommended (e.g. always with food, or always on an empty stomach).

There is currently limited data on the use of imepitoin in combination with other AEDs; however, it has been used in combination with phenobarbitone, potassium bromide, and levetiracetam without reported harmful clinical interactions (Neßler et al. 2017; Royaux et al. 2017). If seizure control is inadequate in dogs receiving 10–20 mg/kg of imepitoin twice daily, then the oral dose should be increased to 30 mg/kg twice daily (Bhatti et al. 2015). If seizure control remains inadequate, then phenobarbitone or potassium bromide can be added to the treatment regime. The addition of an adjunctive medication was reported to improve seizure control in 79% (phenobarbitone) and 69% (potassium bromide) of dogs with idiopathic epilepsy that was refractory to imepitoin monotherapy (Royaux et al. 2017). If the epilepsy is subsequently well controlled, then imepitoin withdrawal over 3 months can be considered (20 mg/kg twice daily for 1 month, 10 mg/kg twice daily for 1 month, 10 mg/kg once daily for 1 month). This did not result in an increase in monthly seizure frequency in one study, and also improved the adverse effects experienced by the dogs (Stee et al. 2017). Conversely, the addition of imepitoin may improve seizure control in dogs with idiopathic epilepsy that is resistant to treatment with phenobarbitone, with or without other adjunctive medications (Neßler et al. 2017). A lower starting dose of 5 mg/kg twice daily is recommended in these cases to reduce the incidence of adverse effects.

Serum level monitoring: No serum level monitoring is required as the blood levels correlate poorly with clinical effect.

Adverse effects: Potential adverse effects are similar to other AEDs but are generally mild and transient. These may include ataxia, polydipsia, polyuria, polyphagia, sedation, apathy, hyperactivity, vomiting, diarrhoea, anorexia, and hypersalivation. Aggression has been uncommonly reported and the use of imepitoin should therefore be carefully considered in dogs with a history of aggressive behaviour.

Adverse effects monitoring: Imepitoin does not induce hepatic enzyme elevation; however, a complete blood cell count and serum biochemistry is recommended every 6–12 months in any dog receiving daily, long-term medication.

c. Antiepileptic drug withdrawal

If an animal with idiopathic epilepsy becomes seizure-free on medication, then it can be difficult to know whether or when to attempt AED withdrawal. This can be considered if the animal has been in remission (seizure-free) for greater than 12 months. However, there will be an associated risk of seizure recurrence and it can be difficult to regain seizure freedom if AEDs are subsequently re-introduced. A small study reported seizure recurrence in 7 out of 11 dogs in which treatment had been stopped after a period of remission (Gesell et al. 2015). Only three of the seven dogs regained seizure freedom after resuming AED therapy. Seizure recurrence after cessation of treatment also appears to be common in cats that were previously in remission (Pakozdy et al. 2013). These considerations should therefore always be discussed with the owner before the decision is made to withdraw treatment.

d. Other antiepileptic medications

In recent years, there has been a trend in veterinary medicine towards the use of novel AEDs from human medicine, particularly in cases that are refractory to the veterinary licensed drugs discussed above. Examples of these medications include felbamate, zonisamide, gabapentin, and levetiracetam. The original branded formulations of these AEDs were often prohibitively expensive in the majority of veterinary cases. However, the increased availability of generic formulations means that their use is more feasible for many owners. It is important to consider that, at the time of writing, there are no veterinary-licensed versions of these medications. Their use is therefore off-label and the prescribing cascade should be adhered to at all times. Owners should always be made aware when any off-label medication is prescribed to their pet, an information sheet regarding the medication should be provided, and a disclaimer signed by the owner.

Potential advantages of these medications over phenobarbitone, potassium bromide, and imepitoin include a reduced incidence of adverse effects and the potential for a novel mechanism of action. This latter advantage may be useful for treating seizures that are refractory to drugs with other common mechanisms of action (e.g. GABA-mediated inhibition). However, the short half-life of several medications (e.g. levetiracetam) means that they ideally need to be administered three times a day to maintain adequate serum concentrations. This may not be feasible for some owners in terms of both lifestyle and cost.

Levetiracetam

License: No authorised veterinary formulation in the UK.

Mechanism of action: Levetiracetam is thought to exert its anti-seizure activity via binding to a synaptic vesicle glycoprotein called SV2-A and inhibiting the release of excitatory neurotransmitters.

Clinical indications: Levetiracetam is most commonly used as a third-line adjunctive medication in dogs that have poor seizure control in spite of adequate serum levels of phenobarbitone and potassium bromide (Volk et al. 2008). A randomised, placebo-controlled, crossover trial of levetiracetam for the treatment of idiopathic epilepsy in 34 dogs that were refractory to phenobarbitone and potassium bromide did not demonstrate a significant reduction in seizures compared to placebo (Muñana et al. 2012). However, this study had a low power and a number of dogs had levetiracetam plasma drug concentrations that were below the lower limit of the suggested therapeutic range.

The efficacy of levetiracetam as an off-label monotherapy in dogs is currently unknown. A small, single-blinded, randomised, phenobarbitone-controlled trial of levetiracetam as a monotherapy for dogs with newly diagnosed epilepsy did not report a significant difference in the monthly number of seizures before and after treatment for the levetiracetam group (Fredsø et al. 2016). Five of the six dogs in the phenobarbitone group showed a >50% reduction in seizures per month, whilst none of the dogs treated with levetiracetam fulfilled this definition of a responder. The use of levetiracetam as a monotherapy in dogs with idiopathic epilepsy is therefore not currently advised. However, the favourable adverse effect profile of levetiracetam means that its use has been suggested for dogs with structural brain disease to avoid the additional sedation and ataxia that may be associated with phenobarbitone administration (Kelly et al. 2017).

Levetiracetam has been used anecdotally as a pulse treatment to reduce the number of seizures per cluster in dogs with a tendency to experience cluster seizures (Packer et al. 2015). The suggested regime, in addition to the dog's daily maintenance medications, is to administer a single 60 mg/kg oral dose immediately following a seizure. The drug is then continued at a lower dose of 20–30 mg/kg per os three times a day until there have been no seizures for 48 hours. The administration of levetiracetam is then stopped until further seizures are observed.

Levetiracetam is well tolerated in cats (Bailey et al. 2008; Carnes et al. 2011), and appears particularly effective in the management of audiogenic reflex seizures (Lowrie et al. 2017). It has been suggested that the extended release formulation can be used once daily in cats if three times daily dosing of the standard, intermediate-release formulation is not practical or feasible (Barnes Heller et al. 2018).

The intravenous formulation of levetiracetam is expensive but can be useful in the management of acute cluster seizures and status epilepticus (Hardy et al. 2012) (see Chapter 7).

Contraindications: Severe renal disease.

Metabolism and excretion: Levetiracetam does not undergo hepatic metabolism and 70–90% is excreted unchanged in the urine.

Starting dose: 20–30 mg/kg per os every 8 hours (every 12 hours for the extended release formulation). Concurrent administration of phenobarbitone has been shown to increase levetiracetam clearance in epileptic dogs, meaning that increased oral doses of levetiracetam may be required in these cases (Muñana et al. 2015).

Serum level monitoring: Infrequently performed but can be measured in animals with a poor response to treatment or if toxicity is suspected.

Adverse effects: A serious adverse event has been reported following the rapid intravenous administration of undiluted levetiracetam; therefore, care should be taken during its preparation and administration (Biddick et al. 2018). Adverse effects associated with oral administration are generally mild and include sedation or ataxia.

Adverse effects monitoring: A complete blood cell count and serum biochemistry is recommended every 6–12 months in any dog receiving daily, long-term medication.

Zonisamide

License: No authorised veterinary formulation in the UK.

Mechanism of action: Numerous suggested mechanisms of action, including blockade of voltage-gated sodium and T-type calcium channels, facilitation of dopaminergic and serotonergic neurotransmission, enhancement of GABA activity in the brain, and inhibition of glutamate-mediated neuronal excitation.

Clinical indications: Zonisamide is primarily used as an adjunctive medication in dogs or cats with seizures that are refractory to licensed AEDs (phenobarbitone, imepitoin, and/or KBr).

Contraindications: Severe hepatic impairment and pregnancy.

Metabolism and excretion: Zonisamide is metabolised by the liver and primarily excreted by the kidneys. The elimination half-life is 15–17 hours in the dog. Zonisamide is metabolised by the same hepatic microsomal enzymes that metabolise phenobarbitone, therefore the elimination half-life is likely to be shorter in dogs that are receiving both medications.

Starting dose: 5 mg/kg per os twice daily (monotherapy in dogs and cats), 10 mg/kg per os twice daily (add-on therapy to phenobarbitone in dogs).

Serum level monitoring: Infrequently performed but can be measured in animals with a poor response to treatment or if toxicity is suspected.

Adverse effects: Adverse effects include sedation, ataxia, anorexia, and vomiting. Uncommon adverse effects include hepatotoxicity and renal tubular acidosis in dogs, and lymphadenopathy, hyperglobulinaemia, and cytopaenia in one feline case report (Collinet and Sammut 2017).

Adverse effects monitoring: A complete blood cell count and serum biochemistry is recommended after 1 month and then every 6–12 months if the animal is otherwise well and the seizures are well controlled. Blood tests should be performed immediately if the animal is unwell and there is a suspicion of an adverse reaction.

e. Non-pharmacological treatment options

Non-pharmacological treatment options for canine and feline epilepsy include dietary modification (Larsen et al. 2014; Law et al. 2015), and the implantation of deep brain electrodes or vagus nerve stimulators (Long et al. 2014; Martlé et al. 2016).

A randomised trial of a commercially available, ketogenic, medium-chain triglyceride (MCT) diet was performed in 21 dogs that were on chronic AED drug therapy for idiopathic epilepsy (Law et al. 2015). A reduction in seizure frequency was reported in the dogs receiving the trial diet compared to those receiving a standardised placebo diet. This study had low power but suggested a potential role for MCT diets in the management of dogs with idiopathic epilepsy.

The use of surgically implanted vagus nerve stimulators and deep brain electrodes has been reported for the management of drug-resistant epilepsy in certain human cases (Martlé et al. 2014). The high cost and complexity of implant placement currently limits the use of these implants in veterinary medicine. However, studies have demonstrated that their implantation appears to be safe and feasible in dogs, and the availability of these interventions may become more widespread in the future (Long et al. 2014, Martlé et al. 2016).

6.1.5 Refractory Epilepsy

Epilepsy is deemed to be refractory to treatment if an animal's quality of life is compromised by severe adverse effects of medication and/or frequent or severe seizures in spite of appropriate drug therapy (i.e. drug serum levels at the upper end of the therapeutic range). An estimated 25–30% of dogs with idiopathic epilepsy may be refractory to treatment and owners should always be warned of this possibility at the time of diagnosis. A history of cluster seizures appears to be a risk factor for refractory epilepsy.

The underlying basis of refractory epilepsy is likely to be multifactorial and will vary from case to case. Factors to consider should include:

* inadequate/inappropriate drug choice or dose
* poor owner compliance regarding administration of medications
* seizures related to changes in oestrogen and/or progesterone levels in entire female dogs
* a change in patient size or weight
* an incorrect diagnosis (e.g. idiopathic epilepsy in a dog with a non-epileptic movement disorder or intracranial neoplasia)
* natural progression of an underlying disease (e.g. meningoencephalitis, intracranial neoplasia)
* dietary changes
* newly developed systemic disease.

The approach to these cases should include a review of the diagnosis and previous investigations, measurement of serum drug levels if applicable (e.g. phenobarbitone and potassium bromide), the addition of adjunctive AEDs if appropriate, dietary modification, or referral for a specialist opinion.

6.1.6 Seizure Management in the Home Environment

A small supply of rectal diazepam can be dispensed to the owner of any animal that has a history of epileptic seizures. This can be administered *per rectum* at a dose of 1–2 mg/kg in the event of a seizure lasting for longer than 2–3 minutes. This ensures that medications are administered in the home environment before the potential onset of status epilepticus. Owners will also feel reassured and more in control of their pet's condition if they have this medication at home or in the car. As summarised above, levetiracetam can also be used as a pulse therapy in animals with a history of cluster seizures.

6.2 Movement Disorders

Edward Ives

Involuntary motor activity is a hallmark of epileptic seizures, but there are a number of other disorders that are also characterised by involuntary movement. These 'movement disorders' are also known as dyskinesias, derived from '*dys*' meaning abnormal, and '*kinesia*' meaning movement. Movement disorders are increasingly recognised in veterinary medicine and it is therefore important that a general practitioner is aware of their existence. This ensures that they are not mistaken for epileptic seizures and that the most appropriate tests and treatment are chosen in the first instance. As discussed in Chapter 1, there are certain characteristics of a movement disorder that can be useful to distinguish them from epileptic seizures.

- An alert level of mentation throughout an episode, even if the involuntary motor activity is affecting multiple limbs and/or both sides of the body (see Video 33). If both sides of the body were affected by epileptiform seizure activity, then this would imply involvement of both cerebral hemispheres and it is highly unlikely that the level of mentation would remain normal.
- An absence of autonomic signs (e.g. salivation, urination, defecation).
- An episode duration that may be longer than expected for epileptic seizure activity (e.g. >5–10 minutes).
- The absence of a post-ictal phase, despite a long episode duration.

There are still many unanswered questions regarding movement disorders in veterinary medicine, including the precise terminology that should be used to describe them, how they should be classified, and how they may relate to similar conditions in human medicine. Different forms of involuntary movement may also occur concurrently, further complicating a simple framework for classification. The aim of this section is to provide a basic summary of the different forms of involuntary movement that may be encountered in dogs and cats. It is hoped that this will allow the reader to more easily recognise a potential movement disorder if an animal presents with a history of constant or episodic abnormal motor activity. The reader is referred to the Bibliography section for more in-depth discussion regarding this complex subject in both human and veterinary medicine (Lowrie and Garosi 2016, 2017a,b; Urkasemsin and Olby 2015; Vanhaesebrouck et al. 2013).

Involuntary movements of the limbs, head, or body can be classified according to either their appearance (e.g. tremor, myoclonus) or their origin (e.g. muscle, peripheral nerve, or central nervous system [CNS]). The broad categories of involuntary movement that will be covered in this section are:

- tremors
- disorders of peripheral nerve hyperexcitability (fasciculations, myokymia, neuromyotonia, tetanus, and tetany)
- myoclonus
- paroxysmal dyskinesias.

6.2.1 Tremors

A tremor can be defined as an involuntary, rhythmic, oscillatory movement of a body part. These movements may vary in amplitude, but often have a specific frequency for each disorder. Resting tremors, as observed in Parkinsonian movement disorders in humans, have not been described in veterinary medicine. The pathologic tremors observed in animals are therefore 'action-related' and are termed 'kinetic tremors' if they affect body parts involved in active movements, or 'postural tremors' if they affect body parts involved in the maintenance of posture against gravity (Lowrie and Garosi 2016).

Examples of kinetic tremors reported in veterinary medicine include:

- *Intention tremors secondary to diffuse conditions affecting the cerebellum (e.g. degenerative disorders, inflammatory or infectious diseases)* – intention tremors predominately affect the head and are most noticeable during attempts to perform a purposeful movement, such as eating or drinking from a bowl (see Video 11). Further discussion regarding the approach to cerebellar disorders can be found in Section 6.8 'Cerebellar Dysfunction'.
- *Abnormalities of myelin production or development (hypomyelination or dysmyelination)* – affected dogs typically show clinical signs of generalised body tremors and ataxia when they first start to walk at 2–6 weeks of age. Any breed may theoretically be affected but commonly reported breeds include the Springer Spaniel, Samoyed, Chow Chow, Dalmatian, Weimaraner, and Bernese Mountain Dog. If myelin development is delayed, and not absent, then a spontaneous clinical improvement may be observed over the first year of life.

- *Idiopathic generalised tremor syndrome* (see Video 7) – this condition results in an acute onset of generalised body tremors that are exacerbated by excitement, stress, or exercise (Wagner et al. 1997). It predominately affects young (<2-year-old), small breed dogs and was previously known as 'little white shaker syndrome' given its frequent occurrence in small, white dogs such as Maltese Terriers. However, it may be observed in dogs of any breed and coat colour and has also been reported in cats (Mauler et al. 2014). It is assumed to represent an autoimmune inflammatory disorder, predominately affecting the cerebellum, with an unknown trigger. MRI of the brain is usually normal but CSF analysis may reveal an elevated protein and a mildly increased white blood cell count. Infectious disease testing should be negative. The response to immunosuppressive treatment using prednisolone is usually favourable (1 mg/kg twice daily, tapering over weeks/months to the lowest dose required to control the clinical signs).

Examples of postural tremors reported in veterinary medicine include:

- *Orthostatic tremor* – this condition most commonly affects young, giant breed dogs (e.g. Great Danes) and results in high frequency tremors that are triggered by standing and predominately affect the limbs (Garosi et al. 2005). These tremors may result in difficulty standing or lying down but disappear when the affected limbs are not bearing weight (see Video 13).
- *Benign, idiopathic postural tremor* – this condition affects the pelvic limbs of older dogs when they are standing (see Video 14). These tremors are not visible during movement and no treatment is advised. They may become more severe with increasing age.
- *Canine idiopathic head tremor syndrome* – this condition is characterised by episodes of involuntary side-to-side or up-and-down head tremors that start and stop spontaneously (see Videos 12 and 34). Affected animals are typically young at the time of the first episode and are otherwise normal between events. The condition can be observed in any breed, but English Bulldogs, Dobermans, and French Bulldogs appear over-represented (Guevar et al. 2014). Animals remain alert during the episodes, which can last for seconds, minutes, or hours. Stress has been reported as a potential trigger factor for some dogs. In contrast to typical epileptic seizures, animals with idiopathic head tremors can be distracted at the time of an episode and the episodes will often abate if the animal is given a toy or food. These episodes appear benign and do not usually require treatment. Over 50% of affected dogs are reported to show a spontaneous resolution over time and antiepileptic medications do not appear effective in controlling the episodes. Episodic head tremors have also been reported secondary to structural brain lesions (particularly those involving the thalamus) and advanced imaging of the head should be always

be considered in these cases, particularly in dogs that are older at the time of onset (e.g. >6 years old).

A tremor can be often recognised by its distinctive rhythmic, oscillatory nature. If a tremor is suspected in general practice, then a high suspicion for a specific disorder can often be made on the basis of the animal's signalment, the region of the body affected, and the onset of the tremors. A clinical approach to tremors in dogs should therefore include the following considerations:

- *The part of the body that is predominately affected* – head (intention tremors, idiopathic head tremors), limbs (orthostatic tremor, benign postural tremor), or whole-body tremors (hypomyelination, idiopathic generalised tremor syndrome).
- *The age of the animal* – hypomyelination in puppies, benign postural tremor in older dogs.
- *Whether the tremors are unpredictable and episodic* (e.g. idiopathic head tremors), *or only present at specific times* (e.g. when standing for orthostatic tremor, or when performing a purposeful movement for intention tremors).

6.2.2 Peripheral Nerve Hyperexcitability

Hyperexcitability of the peripheral motor nerves results in sustained or intermittent contraction of the skeletal muscles. The level of mentation remains normal, even if the entire body is affected, as the areas of brain responsible for wakefulness are not involved. In contrast to the characteristic rhythmic, oscillatory nature of a tremor, peripheral nerve hyperexcitability results in less regular involuntary muscle activity that has a variable frequency, may be sustained, and does not typically result in movement of the affected body part (Lowrie and Garosi 2017). Different phenotypic variants have been described, each with their own clinical and electrophysiological characteristics.

- *Fasciculations* – a flicker movement under the skin as a result of brief contraction of a small number of myofibres.
- *Myokymia* – rippling of the skin overlying a muscle that is affected by continuous muscle contractions at a rate of 5–150 Hz.
- *Neuromyotonia* – generalised muscle stiffness, with delayed relaxation, that persists during sleep or general anaesthesia and is seen as a consequence of high frequency (150–300 Hz) motor nerve activity. Myokymia and neuromyotonia are often observed concurrently as they generally represent a continuum of the same underlying pathology (Vanhaesebrouck et al. 2013).
- *Tetanus and tetany* – sustained muscle contraction without relaxation, predominately affecting the extensor muscles. The term 'tetanus' is most commonly

used to describe the increased extensor muscle tone seen following *Clostridium tetani* infection, whilst the term 'tetany' is most commonly used to describe the clinical signs resulting from hypocalcaemia.

The clinical signs associated with peripheral nerve hyperexcitability may be restricted to a single cranial nerve or appendicular muscle(s), or they can be generalised and affect the whole body.

Focal hyperexcitability may result from:

- local irritation to a peripheral nerve (e.g. following radiotherapy or compression by an adjacent vascular structure) (Rogatko et al. 2016)
- loss of central inhibition to peripheral nerve firing secondary to a focal brain or spinal cord lesion (Holland et al. 2010).

Generalised clinical signs can occur secondary to a number of different aetiologies:

- intoxications
- electrolyte disturbance (acute dehydration, hypocalcaemia)
- endocrine disorders (hypothyroidism, hypoadrenocorticism)
- neurodegenerative diseases
- hereditary or acquired disorders affecting the peripheral nerves and their associated ion channels; voltage-gated potassium channel dysfunction, disrupting repolarisation and termination of the action potential, is postulated to be the most frequent cause of generalised peripheral nerve hyperexcitability in humans (Gilliam et al. 2014; Vanhaesebrouck et al. 2013).

The most widely described syndrome of generalised peripheral nerve hyperexcitability in veterinary medicine is myokymia and/or neuromyotonia affecting young Jack Russell Terriers (onset <3 years old) (Bhatti et al. 2011; Vanhaesebrouck et al. 2010). These dogs are commonly also affected by the hereditary condition spinocerebellar ataxia (SCA), reported in 84% of Jack Russell Terriers with generalised myokymia and/or neuromyotonia in one study. Spinocerebellar ataxia results in characteristic clinical signs of cerebellar dysfunction, including hypermetria, truncal ataxia, head tremors, and reduced menace responses. The myokymia that may be observed in these dogs presents as rippling of the skin overlying affected muscles, and the neuromyotonia presents as transient episodes of severe generalised muscle stiffness which may be fatal. This disorder should therefore be highly suspected in a young Jack Russell Terrier that presents with this distinctive combination of cerebellar signs and abnormal muscle activity. Generalised myokymia and/or neuromyotonia has also been reported in two Yorkshire Terriers, one Dachshund, a crossbreed dog, a Border Collie and one adult cat, with concurrent SCA only reported in the Dachshund (Galano et al. 2005; Vanhaesebrouck et al. 2013).

If a disorder of peripheral nerve hyperexcitability is suspected from the clinical history or physical examination, then a previous history of radiotherapy for focal cases or toxin exposure in generalised cases should be excluded. Additional investigations should include haematology, serum biochemistry, and endocrine testing to exclude a metabolic disorder. Tetanus is usually a clinical diagnosis made on the basis of identification of a wound or anaerobic focus of infection, together with consistent clinical signs of focal or generalised increased extensor muscle tone. Further investigations are often limited in general practice as they rely upon complex electrophysiological testing, with or without advanced imaging. Contacting a specialist centre for advice or referral is therefore advised in these cases if possible.

6.2.3 Myoclonus

Myoclonus is the term used to describe a sudden, brief, involuntary, *shock-like* movement or 'jerk', which usually results in gross movement of the affected body part(s) (Lowrie and Garosi 2017). Whilst rhythmic myoclonic movements may appear similar to a tremor, tremors do not have an interval between movements and lack the 'shock-like' nature of a myoclonus. Disorders resulting from peripheral nerve hyperexcitability also lack this brief and sudden nature, and more commonly result in muscle rippling or sustained muscle contraction that does not move the affected body part. The classification of myoclonus is complex and remains controversial. A recent review on this subject in veterinary medicine attempted to classify myoclonus as either 'epileptic' or 'non-epileptic' based upon the association with concurrent epileptic seizures or degenerative encephalopathy (Lowrie and Garosi 2017).

1. Epileptic myoclonus

Myoclonic movements can be observed in association with several disorders that also result in generalised epileptic seizures and/or progressive intracranial signs.

a. Lafora disease

Lafora disease is a late-onset myoclonic epilepsy that is most widely recognised in the Miniature Wire-haired Dachshund, but has also been reported in Beagles, Basset Hounds, and several other breeds (Swain et al. 2017). The median age at the time of onset is 7 years old and dogs typically present with sudden jerking head and neck movements in response to visual or auditory stimuli (see Video 3). It is a progressive disease that may also be accompanied by intermittent generalised tonic-clonic seizures. A mutation in the EPM2B (NHLRC1) gene has been demonstrated in Miniature Wire-haired Dachshunds and a Beagle with this condition. A gene test to confirm the presence of this causative mutation is now commercially available.

b. Neuronal ceroid lipofuscinosis

NCL is one of a group of lysosomal storage disorders that can result in myoclonic seizures, in addition to other multifocal signs of neuronal degeneration such as blindness, behaviour change, and cerebellar dysfunction. Breed-specific gene testing is commercially available for many NCL subtypes.

c. Feline audiogenic reflex seizures

This recently described condition predominately affects older cats and is commonly associated with myoclonic seizures triggered by high-frequency sounds (see Section 6.1 'Epileptic Seizures') (Lowrie et al. 2016).

d. Myoclonic epilepsy of unknown origin in older dogs

Intermittent myoclonic movements, particularly affecting the head, may be observed in older dogs that otherwise appear normal. Cavalier King Charles Spaniels (CKCSs) are anecdotally over represented (see Video 35). Some dogs may show a gradual cognitive decline over months to years, but it remains uncertain as to whether this is related to the myoclonic episodes or is reflective of an unrelated, age-related canine cognitive dysfunction. Cardiac disease resulting in partial syncope, or structural epilepsy resulting in focal seizure activity, should always be considered in these cases.

2. Non-epileptic myoclonus

Constant, repetitive myoclonic movements of the limbs or facial muscles may be observed in dogs that have recovered from CDV encephalomyelitis (see Video 36). These movements can persist under general anaesthesia or during sleep. This condition is most commonly encountered in the United Kingdom as a static clinical sign in rescue dogs that have been imported from countries in which routine CDV vaccination is less common. Affected dogs do not show associated epileptic seizures, and an alternative cause for any reported seizure activity should always be investigated in these cases.

A condition called 'hemi-facial spasm' may also represent a form of non-epileptic myoclonic disorder. This condition is most commonly idiopathic and results in spontaneous, intermittent, and sudden contraction of the facial muscles on one side of the face. This is observed in the absence of facial paresis or paralysis, and the palpebral reflex is therefore intact between episodes of contraction. This is in contrast to cases of chronic facial nerve paralysis with denervation atrophy of the affected facial muscles. Referral for further assessment and advanced imaging of the head is advised in these cases to exclude an underlying structural cause for this unusual clinical sign.

6.2.4 Paroxysmal Dyskinesias

The paroxysmal dyskinesias are a large group of self-limiting, *episodic* movement disorders that, in light of their clinical presentation and episodic nature, are the most likely of all movement disorders to be mistaken for epileptic seizures (De Risio et al. 2015). Important differences between paroxysmal dyskinesias and an epileptic seizure include the absence of autonomic signs during an episode of dyskinesia, the maintenance of an alert mentation in spite of involuntary movements affecting multiple limbs, and the fact that episodes may last significantly longer than expected for an epileptic seizure (>5–10 minutes) (see Video 33). The onset and cessation of involuntary movements are frequently abrupt for dyskinesias, which also lack the post-ictal disorientation, ataxia, restlessness, or visual disturbance that typically follow epileptic seizures. The neurological examination should be normal between episodes, as for idiopathic epilepsy.

A paroxysmal dyskinesia should therefore be considered in any animal that is not responding as expected to treatment for epileptic seizures and the diagnosis reviewed at this time. Conversely, it is important to consider that movement disorders and epilepsy can potentially co-exist as separate conditions, without the requirement for a shared pathophysiology. This may rarely be observed in breeds with an apparent genetic predisposition for both idiopathic epilepsy and paroxysmal dyskinesia (e.g. Labrador Retrievers), or in dogs with a long-term dyskinesia that acquire a new structural cause for epilepsy in later life (e.g. intracranial neoplasia).

A number of different paroxysmal dyskinesias have been reported in veterinary medicine, with their names frequently including the breed of dog in which the condition was first recognised (Lowrie and Garosi 2017; Urkasemsin and Olby 2014). However, irrespective of the breed, a paroxysmal dyskinesia should be considered in any dog that presents for self-limiting episodes of involuntary muscle activity, without a loss of consciousness during the events.

Paroxysmal dyskinesias appear less common or poorly recognised in cats. Drug-induced dyskinesias have been rarely reported following the administration of phenobarbitone and propofol, underlying the importance of a complete clinical history in these cases.

The diagnosis of a paroxysmal dyskinesia is often made on the basis of the clinical history and the characteristics of an observed episode. With a few notable exceptions, further diagnostic testing is often unrewarding and expensive, being primarily aimed at excluding other potential causes. Differential diagnoses are similar to those listed for seizures in Section 6.1 'Epileptic Seizures'. In light of the low diagnostic yield of investigations such as MRI and CSF analysis, it is not unreasonable to make a presumptive diagnosis of a paroxysmal dyskinesia if there is a consistent clinical history, a known disorder in that particular breed, a normal neurological examination between episodes, and blood tests have excluded a metabolic or endocrine cause for involuntary motor activity. However, referral to a veterinary neurologist for further assessment and discussion regarding the suspected diagnosis should always be offered to the owners of these dogs.

A short summary of the most common paroxysmal dyskinesias that may be encountered in general practice is given below. The reader is referred to the

Bibliography for more in-depth discussion regarding the numerous paroxysmal dyskinesias that are increasingly reported in veterinary medicine.

1. Paroxysmal gluten-sensitive dyskinesia in the Border Terrier

This condition has been formerly referred to as 'Spike's disease' and 'canine epileptoid cramping syndrome'. It can affect Border Terriers of any age (from 6 weeks to over 7 years old) but the majority of dogs have their first episode before 3 years of age. The episodes typically present as stiffness, difficulty walking, apparent ataxia, tremors, abnormal muscle tone, and contraction of the muscles of the neck or limbs (see Video 4). These episodes most frequently affect all four limbs and last for between 5 and 30 minutes; however, they may last for several hours in some cases. Gastrointestinal signs, such as vomiting, diarrhoea, and borborygmi, may also be observed in around 50% of dogs, either in close association with an episode or between episodes (Black et al. 2014).

A recent study demonstrated anti-canine gliadin IgG and anti-canine transglutaminase-2-IgA antibodies in affected Border Terriers (Lowrie et al. 2015). It was therefore concluded that this disorder represents a manifestation of gluten sensitivity in the breed. This hypothesis was supported by a clinical improvement and reduction in serum antibody levels after institution of a strict gluten-free diet. Testing for anti-canine gliadin IgG and anti-canine transglutaminase-2-IgA antibodies is therefore recommended in Border Terriers that present with episodic clinical signs consistent with a dyskinesia. However, careful interpretation of these results is required. Antibody testing appears highly specific for this condition, but false positive results can be seen in dogs with other clinical manifestations of gluten sensitivity, such as gastrointestinal disease or dermatological signs (Lowrie et al. 2016). These tests also lack sensitivity, as in a study of 45 Border Terriers with presumed paroxysmal dyskinesia 16% of dogs had anti-canine gliadin IgG levels within the control range and 9% had levels of anti-canine transglutaminase-2-IgA antibodies within the control range (Lowrie et al. 2018). Differential diagnoses for this condition should include other causes of intermittent discomfort or reluctance to walk, with or without gastrointestinal signs, such as spinal pain, pancreatitis, gastro-oesophageal reflux, or hypoadrenocorticism.

2. Episodic hypertonicity syndrome in Cavalier King Charles Spaniels

This condition has also been termed 'episodic falling syndrome' (Herrtage and Palmer 1983). Clinical signs are usually first observed between 3 months and 4 years of age. Episodes are typically triggered by excitement, stress, or exercise and are characterised by increased muscle tone in the pelvic and/or thoracic limbs. This results in a crouched posture, difficulty walking, falling over, or lifting of the thoracic limbs above the level of the head. These clinical signs abate at times of rest and affected individuals appear otherwise normal. A mutation of the brevican gene (BCAN) has been identified as the cause of this condition in the Cavalier King Charles Spaniel (Gill et al. 2012). This gene encodes a proteoglycan complex that is required for normal axonal conduction and synaptic stability. The commercial availability of a gene test for this condition simplifies the diagnosis in suspected cases, with further testing for alternative diagnoses recommended if the results are negative. The use of acetazolamide and clonazepam has been reported as treatment for this condition, particularly if episodes are adversely affecting the quality of life in an individual dog.

3. 'Scottie cramp' in Scottish Terriers

'Scottie cramp' is a form of paroxysmal dyskinesia that affects young Scottish Terriers, with the majority of dogs showing their first episode at less than 1 year of age (Urkasemsin and Olby 2015). Female dogs were over-represented in one study. Episodes are triggered by excitement, stress, or exercise and typically last for between 5 and 20 minutes. Clinical signs vary in severity between individual dogs, and range from skipping, bunny-hopping, and kicking of the pelvic limbs during exercise, to progressive lowering of the neck, arching of the spine, and increasing spasticity of the limbs until the dog is unable to walk or falls over. The frequency and duration of these episodes may spontaneously decrease over time, with or without reduced exposure to known trigger factors. Fluoxetine has been used to treat more severely affected cases with some reported success (Geiger and Klopp 2009). Patellar luxation and hip dysplasia are important differential diagnoses in any young dog that presents with a skipping pelvic limb gait or bunny hopping. A thorough orthopaedic examination should therefore always be performed in these cases. A similar, milder form of exercise-induced dyskinesia may be responsible for the intermittent pelvic limb 'skipping' observed in some other small breed dogs in which orthopaedic examination is normal (e.g. Jack Russell Terriers).

4. Paroxysmal nonkinesigenic dyskinesia in Labrador Retrievers and Jack Russell Terriers

Affected dogs are typically young at the time of the first episode, with a reported median age at onset of 2 years old for Labrador Retrievers and 4 years old for Jack Russell Terriers (Lowrie and Garosi 2016). In some cases, the episodes may not be observed until 8–10 years of age, potentially related to acquired conditions acting as secondary trigger factors. The episodes of dyskinesia are characterised by an acute onset of involuntary limb movements in the absence of mentation change, autonomic signs, post-ictal signs, or inter-ictal abnormalities (see Video 37). These episodes are self-limiting and typically last for 2–10 minutes. They are most commonly observed in the home environment and may be triggered by excitement, sudden movements, or being startled (Labrador Retrievers), or by extremes of temperature (Jack Russell Terriers). The results of extensive diagnostic investigations are unremarkable in these dogs. The natural history of this condition appears to be regressive, with 75% of dogs showing improvement and 32% entering spontaneous remission over a median follow-up of 7.5 years in one study (39% of Labradors and 22% of Jack Russell Terriers). Dogs showing clusters of episodes appear less likely to achieve remission (Lowrie and Garosi 2016).

Similar forms of paroxysmal dyskinesia have been reported in other breeds of dog (e.g. Chinook Dogs) and it is likely that many breeds are affected by these under-recognised disorders (Packer et al. 2010; Urkasemsin and Olby 2014).

6.3 Altered Mentation

Paul M. Freeman

Changes in mentation are common with neurological disease, and in some situations may be the only abnormality seen. Any animal presenting with a history of altered mentation immediately provides both a diagnostic and managemental challenge, and a careful, methodical, and logical approach is required to ensure a successful outcome.

6.3.1 Definitions and Terminology

There are a plethora of terms associated with the field of mentation and behaviour, and this alone can lead to confusion and potential complications, particularly when conversations between colleagues are required for in-house or external referral of patients. The term *mentation* may be used to describe the animal's level of consciousness as well as the appropriateness of its behaviour. Some neurologists prefer the terms 'consciousness' and 'behaviour' rather than mentation per se, and some like to divide mentation into the *level* of mentation (consciousness) and the *quality* of mentation (behaviour).

For the purposes of this text, we will consider that the term mentation describes both the level of *consciousness* and the *behaviour* of the animal. We will look at consciousness and behaviour in turn, although in many situations both may be affected, and an abnormality of mentation may be considered to include either or both of these.

1. Consciousness (level of mentation)

There are also many terms used to describe an animal's state of consciousness. In general terms, what we are talking about is the animal's awareness of its surroundings and its responsiveness to external stimuli. An animal with a normal level of consciousness may be described as being *alert* and the acronym BAR, standing for 'bright, alert, and responsive', is the first entry in many consultation notes. This is very reasonable, and in fact may be considered a part of the neurological examination as well as the physical examination; an alert animal with a normal level of consciousness should be bright and responsive to normal external stimuli such as sounds, visual stimuli, touch, smell, people, and other animals in the vicinity.

An animal that is able to walk, has generally normal reflexes and voluntary movement, but which exhibits reduced responsiveness to external stimuli, may be described as *obtunded*. Obtundation implies a reduced awareness or willingness to respond to stimuli, although some response is still seen. The state of obtundation may describe a wide range of reduced consciousness, from an animal that is just a bit 'quiet', through to an animal which prefers to lie in a corner sleeping. The latter is still considered obtunded if it can be woken by noise or touch. The term 'depressed' may be applied to animals in this state, but is best avoided since its use has connotations of certain behavioural changes in humans which may not strictly apply to an obtunded animal.

An animal whose level of mentation is so severely depressed that they are only rousable with a noxious stimulus may be described as *stuporous*. Stupor describes a very severely reduced level of mentation, where the animal does not respond to touch, visual stimulation, or sound stimulation. However, the application of a painful stimulus will rouse the animal at least for a short time.

Finally, animals may enter the state of *coma*, where their mentation is so reduced that they are not rousable even with a noxious stimulus. Coma implies severe pathology, often intracranial, and immediately demands a high level of monitoring and urgent investigation. Comatose animals may show altered cardiorespiratory parameters associated with brain lesions and/or raised intracranial pressure (ICP), increasing the level of care required in the hospital environment.

2. Behaviour (quality of mentation)

Behaviour may simply be classified as normal or abnormal for any individual animal in their current situation. This may be difficult to determine, since an animal's behaviour may be affected by stress and anxiety, and reference to the owner and careful history taking may help the clinician to decide whether any observed apparent behavioural abnormality is genuine or normal for the individual.

Behaviour consists of an animal's normal performance of day-to-day functions, and abnormalities may include changes in temperament, changes in sleeping or eating pattern, excessive chewing or grooming, abnormal levels of anxiety (especially in novel situations), excessive vocalisation, abnormal autonomic activity (including sexual activity), and compulsive pacing, amongst other things. Obsessive compulsive behavioural activities can be episodic, such as 'fly catching' and tail chasing, and may also be described as part of an altered, abnormal behaviour.

Whenever a behavioural abnormality is encountered as part of the presenting complaint, an attempt must be made to establish whether the particular change(s) in question are part of a true neurological syndrome, or whether they may be more correctly considered a purely 'behavioural' abnormality. For the purposes of this text, we are concerned only with genuine neurological disease, and not with primary behavioural disease. However, it is often difficult to be sure whether an observed or reported abnormality of behaviour could have an underlying neurological cause. Once again careful history taking may give clues regarding the development of a behavioural problem, and perhaps the reasons why it has developed, and in many situations the advice of a properly trained animal behaviourist can be helpful.

Episodic behavioural abnormalities, especially obsessive or compulsive behaviours such as 'fly catching' (see Video 5), can in some instances be a manifestation of a focal seizure disorder. A simple test that can be applied to determine whether a behaviour pattern is more likely to be behavioural or potentially neurological in origin, is whether the behaviour can be interrupted in any way once started. Focal seizure activity should not be interruptible, whereas obsessive compulsive behaviours often are (see also Section 6.1 'Epileptic Seizures'). Furthermore, it is also common for primary behavioural issues to have a more distinct pattern in terms of when they occur, such as in response to certain stimuli or in the presence (or absence) of a specific person. In contrast, neurological behavioural disturbances are more commonly random and unpredictable.

A very specific form of behavioural disturbance is the so-called *rapid eye movement* (REM) *sleep disorder*, in which dogs can develop abnormal behaviour patterns during REM sleep (see Video 9). This may include violent movements, barking and growling, chewing, biting, or howling. These episodes can develop at any age and may occur during daytime naps as well as during night-time sleep. In one study, 78% of cases responded to oral potassium bromide administration, indicating the possibility that this may be a seizure disorder (Schubert et al. 2011). A recent paper found an association between REM sleep disorder and dogs recovering from tetanus (Shea et al. 2018).

6.3.2 Neuroanatomic Localisation

An animal's level of consciousness and behaviour are governed by both intrinsic and extrinsic factors to the CNS. For a normal level of consciousness, neurons in the ascending reticular activating system (ARAS) of the brainstem and the thalamus (processing centre) must all be functioning normally. The ARAS lies deep within the brainstem and receives all kinds of sensory information from the body, before projecting this information into the thalamus. The thalamus is then responsible for diffusely stimulating the entire cerebral cortex. Therefore, lesions affecting the deeper parts of the brainstem or the thalamus may cause a reduced level of consciousness.

An animal's behaviour is governed more by the cerebral cortex, with the sensory cortex being responsible for the animal's perception of its environment. This explains why animals with unilateral cerebral cortical lesions may circle or turn their heads towards the side of the lesion; the cerebral cortex receives information from the contralateral side of the body, therefore the animal will circle or turn towards the side of its environment which it is still able to perceive (see Chapter 4). The limbic system, consisting of regions within the thalamus, the deep cerebral cortex, and parts of the brainstem such as the amygdala, hippocampus, and hypothalamus, is responsible for emotional and visceral responses and behaviour, and perhaps the more 'hard-wired' behaviours such as copulation and sleep/wake cycles.

6.3.3 Diagnostic Approach to Altered Mentation

A reduced level of consciousness indicates a potential intracranial lesion, most often affecting the brainstem (ARAS) or thalamus. However, it is very important to remember that extracranial disease may also result in reduced consciousness. A recent, large retrospective study of dogs and cats that presented to an emergency clinic because of stupor or coma revealed that although the commonest cause was head trauma, a significant percentage of these animals were suffering from some kind of systemic disease, in particular hypoglycaemia (Parratt et al. 2018). For this reason, the initial approach to any animal presenting with altered mentation should consider both intracranial and extracranial possibilities.

1. Clinical history

As in most situations, the first step should be acquiring a relevant clinical history. Depending on the degree of concern, this may be more or less shortened according to time available. However, several key questions must be answered.

a. General history

Apart from the usual questions concerning appetite, drinking, vaccination, travel status, antiparasitic treatments, and so on, there are a number of key questions relating to the presentation of altered mentation.

1. *Is there any possibility of trauma?* If the patient involved is feline, the answer may be 'possibly' or 'not sure'. For most canines, the owner can be more certain that this is not the case. In either case, if the patient is obtunded rather than stuporous or comatose then it is reasonable to allow time for a complete history taking and examination. If the patient is presented with a more severely depressed mentation and a history of possible head trauma, action may need to be taken more rapidly to deal with the possibility of brain injury.
2. *Is there any possibility of intoxication?* In any case of altered mentation, consideration must be given to the possible ingestion of recreational drugs such as cannabis. Careful questioning around the owners' dog-walking habits may reveal the possibility that the dog has scavenged discarded cannabis-containing material. Owners may be reluctant to admit to the possession of illegal recreational drugs in the home, so this line of questioning must be carried out in a sensitive way in order to gain maximum information.

3. *Is the animal in otherwise good health, or is it currently receiving medications?* In particular, care should be taken with animals which are diabetic and receiving insulin, as an overdose leading to hypoglycaemia may lead to a presentation of altered mentation. Endocrine disorders, such as hypothyroidism and hypoadrenocorticism, may also lead to an obtunded level of mentation. An animal which is in significant pain may occasionally present in an apparent state of mild obtundation (e.g. orthopaedic pain from osteosarcoma or severe osteoarthritis, visceral pain secondary to pancreatitis, spinal pain from chronic intervertebral disc disease).

b. Specific neurological history

1. *Onset* – When did the problem start? Was it an acute onset of mentation change, or has it come on more gradually? Did anything specifically seem to precipitate the change (such as possible trauma or toxin ingestion)? Did the owner notice any other changes accompanying the change of mentation which may indicate systemic disease?

2. *Progression* – Since the owner first noticed their pet's reduced consciousness, has the problem remained static, got worse, improved, or does it wax and wane?

3. *Pain* – Does the owner perceive their animal to be in pain? Determining whether an animal has a headache, particularly from physical examination, can be very difficult. In many cases of intracranial disease, it is likely that a state of obtundation may be brought about by head pain rather than specific effects on the anatomical structures responsible for maintaining alertness. Therefore, gaining the owner's insight, questioning whether there has been any vocalisation for instance, or any anorexia or even nausea, may assist the veterinarian in understanding the presence or absence of pain in this situation.

4. *Response to medication* – If the animal has been seen before, did it receive any medications and, if so, did they lead to any improvement? Again, this question must be phrased correctly in order to gain the appropriate response, since owners will often reply that a medication was not beneficial because, even if there was an obvious initial improvement, the effect was not permanent. In particular, a response to corticosteroids may indicate the presence of brain oedema or inflammation, or even that the animal may be hypoglycaemic or suffering from hypoadrenocorticism. A response to analgesics may support a suspicion of headache or some other pain leading to the animal's mentation change.

2. Signalment

The age of the animal may give a clue that a certain disease category is more likely to explain the clinical presentation than another, for example increasing age leading to an increased suspicion of intracranial neoplasia. Animals which present with obtundation at a very young are more likely to be suffering from a metabolic disease or perhaps even a congenital problem.

An awareness of certain breed predilections is always helpful when trying to establish an appropriate list of differential diagnoses (see Chapter 2). In the case of obtundation, the Cavalier King Charles Spaniel and Greyhound have been shown to be over-represented in cases of stroke; smaller terrier breeds are more commonly affected by immune-mediated inflammatory disease of the brain (meningoencephalitis of unknown origin, MUO), with Chihuahuas, Yorkshire Terriers and Pugs suffering from specific forms such as necrotic meningoencephalitis (NME) in the case of Pugs and Chihuahuas, and necrotic leucoencephalitis (NLE) in the case of Yorkshire Terriers; Chihuahuas are predisposed to hydrocephalus; Yorkshire Terriers are prone to portosystemic shunting and hepatic encephalopathy; and Boxers are predisposed to intracranial neoplasia. There are also many other breed-specific degenerative conditions which may lead to an altered mentation, although rarely in the absence of other neurological signs.

3. Physical examination

A full general physical examination should be performed in all cases of altered mentation. Specific attention should be paid to the cardiorespiratory system, since raised ICP may lead to changes in breathing patterns and/or cardiovascular parameters. These changes are rare, however, and usually only occur in extreme states. More importantly, examining for evidence of systemic disease such as anaemia, pyrexia, and abdominal pain may give vital clues as to the cause of the patient's altered mental state. Checking for evidence of lymphadenopathy, for any signs of unknown trauma, and at the same time observing the animal's response to being examined can also be rewarding. Careful examination for evidence of petechiae or ecchymoses, or overt bruising, is also important, since coagulopathy or trauma may have led to intracranial haemorrhage. Where possible and when time allows, fundoscopic examination should be performed to look for signs of retinal haemorrhage, which could indicate hypertension or a coagulopathy, and optic disc swelling, which can occur with raised ICP.

4. Neurological examination

A complete neurological examination is ideal in all cases of suspected neurological disease, but the clinician will sometimes need to modify this approach because the animal is uncooperative, is unable to perform all aspects of the examination, or due to time constraints. This rarely limits the possibility of making at least some sort of neuroanatomical localisation, which is the purpose of the examination. As stated in Chapter 3, an understanding of the possible and/ or likely neuroanatomical localisations for any given presentation means that the examination can, if needed, be tailored towards identifying the presence or absence of key deficits.

In cases of altered mentation, as already stated, the potential neuroanatomical localisations for primary neurological disease are intracranial and may involve either the brainstem or forebrain. Therefore, the focus of the neurological examination should be on performing tests which may identify potential disease in these locations.

Mentation: This is the reason for the presentation. However, the clinician should continuously observe the patient throughout the consultation in order to form an opinion about the true state of the animal's mentation, allowing for the effects of stress and anxiety.

Gait and posture: The animal may have normal posture or may have low head carriage, or potentially head tilt or turn. An attempt should be made to observe the animal's gait. Most obtunded animals should be physically able to walk, although many will refuse to do so (especially cats). Owners often have video clips of their animal taken in the home environment, which may be helpful in these situations. Many cases of forebrain disease have a surprisingly normal gait, even in the presence of relatively large lesions, but there may be evidence of tetra- or hemiparesis, compulsive pacing, or circling. In brainstem disease, there is often moderate to severe ataxia, again with hemi- or tetraparesis. Circling may also be apparent, especially if there is any vestibular involvement. Generalised weakness may be present in cases of systemic disease, which may be difficult to distinguish from genuine tetraparesis.

Postural reactions: The author finds the paw replacement test to be the most consistent and reliable when looking for evidence of proprioceptive deficits. However, other tests, such as hopping, can also be very useful when looking for subtle deficits (see Chapter 3). Remember that proprioceptive responses require the entire nervous system to be functioning, and therefore they are a sensitive but non-specific part of the neurological examination. In general, with asymmetrical brain lesions, forebrain disease will lead to contralateral postural reaction deficits, whereas brainstem disease causes ipsilateral deficits. As with other parts of the examination, great care must be taken when interpreting postural reaction testing, since a severely obtunded or painful animal may show apparent deficits which are not caused by a proprioceptive failure, but by a reluctance to perform the test.

Cranial nerves: The reader should refer again to Chapter 3 for a full explanation of how to perform a cranial nerve examination with the minimum of stress and 'hands-on' testing. For obtunded animals in particular, maximum use of observational skills should be made to gain information regarding the cranial nerves. If forebrain disease is suspected, the menace response and nasal planum nociception tests should always be performed if possible, since these are both conscious responses that require forebrain involvement. All other cranial nerve tests involve brainstem reflexes, and abnormalities may therefore point to a structural brainstem lesion. In the case of structural disease, one may see deficits in consecutive cranial nerves on the same side of the brain; deficits which point to isolated cranial nerve problems, particularly if bilateral, are more likely to indicate peripheral nerve disease.

Spinal reflexes: In cases of altered mentation, this is potentially the least useful part of the neurological examination. One would not expect deficits of spinal reflexes in cases of intracranial disease, unless the disease is multifocal and also involves the spinal cord intumescences. However, if an animal appears genuinely weak then the pedal withdrawal reflexes should always be assessed, since occasionally a peripheral localisation (such as botulism or acute fulminating myasthenia gravis) may present with an apparently obtunded mentation.

Palpation: In the majority of cases, palpation for the presence of pain will be unrewarding, but it should always be carried out in order to exclude the possibility that the animal's altered mentation is actually caused by chronic or severe pain.

6.3.4 Obtundation
1. Neuroanatomical localisation
As already stated, the two possible neuroanatomic localisations for primary neurological causes of altered mentation are the forebrain and the brainstem. The results of the neurological examination may confirm the likelihood of one of these locations, but it is also possible, particularly in the case of forebrain disease, that the remainder of the neurological examination is normal. In this case, the clinician must remain open to the possibility of extracranial disease, whilst also being aware that intracranial disease is not ruled out by such a neurological examination.

2. Differential diagnoses
Broadly speaking, the possible causes of intracranial disease are similar for both forebrain and brainstem, and therefore the differential diagnoses will be similar in the case of either neuroanatomical localisation. Additional information from the clinical history and signalment should allow the clinician to formulate a list of likely and possible differential diagnoses for intracranial disease. These may include vascular disorders (e.g. stroke), inflammatory or infectious disease (e.g. meningoencephalitis of unknown origin), head trauma, anomalies (e.g. hydrocephalus), metabolic (e.g. hepatic encephalopathy, hypoglycaemia, shock), neoplastic disorders, and degenerative disorders (e.g. storage diseases).

3. Formulating a plan
The decision whether to start with in-house investigations or to immediately refer for further investigation by a specialist is one which requires discussion with the owner, and in many cases referral may not be an option for financial or logistical reasons. Immediate referral should be considered, if possible, in cases where the neurological examination reveals clear evidence for an intracranial structural lesion. The one exception to this may be in situations where a vascular

cause (e.g. stroke) is highly suspected from the clinical history and/or physical examination findings, in which case further in-house investigation of potential underlying cases may be justified.

If the remainder of the neurological examination is normal, it is certainly reasonable to consider further investigations in-house, which may be similar to those recommended in cases of seizures (see Section 6.1 'Epileptic Seizures'). Investigations that could be performed might include:

- *Haematology, serum biochemistry, and urinalysis.*
- *Blood pressure testing.* If this is persistently elevated, an ACTH stimulation test may be justified, especially with supporting clinical and biochemical features of hyperadrenocorticism.
- *Bile acid stimulation testing +/− serum ammonia*, particularly if hepatic encephalopathy and a portosystemic shunt is suspected.
- *Thyroid function testing* – total thyroid hormone (T4), free T4, TSH.
- *Fructosamine, glucose, and insulin levels* if an insulinoma is suspected.
- *A coagulation profile and testing for Angiostrongylus vasorum* if a disorder of blood clotting is suspected.
- *Infectious disease testing* dependent on the species and relative risk of exposure – *T. gondii* in cats and dogs, *N. caninum* or canine distemper virus in dogs, FeLV, FIV, and feline coronavirus in cats.
- *Urine metabolic screening* if an inborn error of metabolism is suspected (e.g. young animal with progressive neurological disease).
- *Toxicology* for known or suspected toxin exposure.
- *Thoracic radiography, abdominal ultrasonography,* or *thoracic and abdominal CT* – particularly if neoplasia is likely.

If a diagnosis of systemic disease is confirmed, then treatment should be directed at resolving the underlying disease and then assessing whether this leads to an improvement in the animal's mentation. Where in-house investigations do not reveal the diagnosis, referral for potential advanced imaging of the brain and CSF analysis should always be offered, since it is possible to have a large intracranial structural lesion in the forebrain with minimal effects on the neurological examination.

4. Raised intracranial pressure (ICP)

In any case with an obtunded level of mentation, consideration should be given to the possibility of raised ICP; signs may include a reduced level of consciousness, altered brainstem reflexes (especially pupillary light reflexes and vestibulo-ocular reflexes), and altered motor function. This topic will be covered more extensively in Chapter 7, but it is important to be aware that mild rises in ICP may only lead to obtundation with minimal other signs. Direct or indirect measurement of ICP is difficult and in a first-opinion practice without access to advanced imaging and specialist monitoring equipment, diagnosis may only ever be presumptive. If advanced imaging is not available, treatment should ideally be directed at correcting the underlying disease suspected to be responsible for the abnormal mentation. However, careful monitoring should be performed, particularly in cases of suspected stroke, head trauma, or inflammatory disease, and if the animal's neurological status appears to be deteriorating then specific treatment may normally be safely instigated with the purpose of reducing a suspected ICP elevation. In emergency or rapidly deteriorating situations, this entails administering a bolus of either hypertonic saline or mannitol. Dose rates may be found in the Chapter 7 section on head trauma; it is always important to follow administration with adequate crystalloid fluid therapy to avoid systemic dehydration.

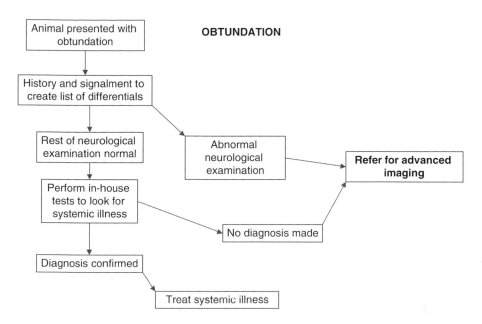

Approach to cases of obtundation in practice.

The following section is aimed at providing advice and guidance in situations where further referral is not an option and where the diagnosis is unclear or can only be suspected.

For treatment of specific medical conditions, the reader is directed to consult an appropriate textbook on internal medicine.

5. Treatment of specific suspected causes of obtundation
a. Stroke
Cerebrovascular disease (ischaemic stroke) most commonly presents as an acute onset of cerebellar/vestibular dysfunction resulting from involvement of the vas-

cular supply to the cerebellum. However, if a cerebral artery is occluded and the forebrain is affected, then stroke may result in a peracute onset of altered mentation and frequently asymmetrical neurological deficits. If referral for advanced imaging to confirm the diagnosis is not possible, then investigations and treatment should be directed at identifying and correcting any underlying predisposing factors. If the animal has presented with significant obtundation, the possibility of raised ICP should always be considered.

Correction of underlying factors:

1. *Coagulopathy*: If the animal has an unknown antiparasiticide status and/or tests positive for the presence of *A. vasorum,* an appropriate antiparasitic treatment should be administered. If rodenticide ingestion is suspected, this should be further investigated and treated with administration of vitamin K as appropriate. Other suspected coagulopathies, such as immune-mediated thrombocytopenia, will require further investigations for diagnosis and instigation of immunosuppressive therapy if confirmed.
2. *Hypertension*: In cases where significant systemic hypertension is identified (MAP persistently greater than 180 mmHg), use of an antihypertensive medication such as amlodipine should be considered. Factors predisposing to hypertension include chronic renal disease and hyperadrenocorticism, and these should be appropriately investigated and treated if identified.

It is important to bear in mind that hypertension can affect the brain in two ways; firstly, it may predispose to haemorrhagic stroke, but secondly it can also lead to a specific hypertensive encephalopathy which may present with obtundation as the main or only clinical sign. Diagnosis of hypertensive encephalopathy can be difficult, and in some cases the diagnosis is presumptive based on response to antihypertensive medication. Animals usually improve rapidly with resolution of the hypertension, and the prognosis is relatively favourable.

b. Hydrocephalus

If hydrocephalus is suspected to be the most likely cause of altered mentation based upon the physical appearance, age, and breed of the animal, and if systemic illness has been excluded and advanced imaging for confirmation is not possible, then starting medical treatment may be appropriate. The focus of such treatment is reduction in the production of CSF. The most effective medication at achieving this, and the only one with good evidence for efficacy, is corticosteroid. Therefore, initiating treatment with prednisolone at a starting dose of 0.5 mg/kg twice daily may be reasonable. In mild cases, the prognosis can be good, with significant improvement in the animal's demeanour following initiation of steroid therapy. A recent paper found little difference in outcome between dogs treated medically and surgically for congenital hydrocephalus, with roughly half of dogs having a positive outcome in both the medically and surgically treated groups (Gillespie et al. 2019).

It is important to remember that corticosteroids have multiple effects, and in cases where diagnosis is presumptive and not confirmed by advanced imaging +/− CSF analysis, there is always the possibility that one may be dealing with a different disease process (e.g. sterile inflammatory brain disease). Infectious disease of the CNS is rare and therefore, whilst still a risk, deterioration due to the potentially immunosuppressive effect of corticosteroid is unlikely. It should also be considered that the use of corticosteroid may complicate or even preclude the possibility of making a diagnosis if referral were subsequently pursued; the presence of inflammatory cells in the CSF may be reduced or altered, and previous corticosteroid administration may alter the changes observed on brain MRI.

c. Cannabis intoxication

If intoxication with cannabis, or a similar recreational drug, is suspected from the clinical history and presenting signs, treatment is largely supportive. A large recent study found that ataxia and obtundation were the most common presenting signs in dogs with a known history of marijuana intoxication, with almost half of cases also showing acute dribbling urinary incontinence (Meola et al. 2012).

As for most suspected intoxications, treatment involves reducing exposure by inducing emesis if it is considered safe and ingestion has occurred within 30–60 minutes. Administration of activated charcoal to reduce further absorption, and potentially administration of intravenous lipid emulsion can be performed as cannabinoids are extremely lipophilic. Supportive care involves the use of intravenous fluid therapy and general nursing to ensure animals are kept clean, dry, and warm. Specific medications which may be helpful can include anxiolytics, such as acepromazine or butorphanol, and antiepileptic medications if seizures occur, such as diazepam or phenobarbitone. The prognosis is generally good, with most affected animals recovering within 1–2 days.

d. Neoplasia

If intracranial neoplasia is suspected based upon the signalment, history, and neurological examination but cannot be confirmed with advanced imaging, owners must be aware of the potential for a guarded prognosis (for example, a 10-year-old Boxer Dog with seizures and slowly progressive intracranial signs, including obtundation). Extracranial disease (e.g. insulinoma) should always be excluded first, and thoracic radiographs +/− abdominal ultrasound can be performed to look for evidence of primary neoplastic or metastatic disease. If these investigations are normal and it is firmly established that referral is not possible, then palliative treatment with corticosteroids can be considered. Prednisolone at a dose of 0.5 mg/kg twice daily may be effective in the short to medium term by reducing any peritumoural oedema and may also provide some analgesic effect if a structural intracranial lesion is present. In addition, specific analgesics such as paracetamol, gabapentin, and tramadol may also be useful. Antiepileptic medications should be used if there is a history of epileptic seizures. Prognosis remains guarded, with the median survival time for dogs with intracranial neoplasia treated symptomatically being around 2 months (Hu et al. 2015).

6.3.5 Coma and Stupor

1. Differential diagnoses

Any animal that presents in a state of coma or stupor represents a clinical and neurological emergency. It is therefore important to have an understanding of the potential causes of coma and stupor. A relatively large study published in 2018 provided an overview of the causes that were identified in one emergency referral centre (Parratt et al. 2018); the most common identified cause was head trauma, with hypoglycaemia, shock, and systemic disease also being relatively common.

The general approach to achieving a list of differential diagnoses is the same as described above for obtundation. However, for animals presenting in a state of stupor or coma, the clinical history taking may need to be more rapid due to the potential emergency nature of the situation, and the performance of a complete neurological examination may be more difficult since assessment of gait and postural reactions is unlikely to be possible. A complete physical examination should always be performed to investigate the potential for systemic disease and since cardiorespiratory abnormalities are more likely in cases of significant head trauma.

2. Formulating a plan

Initial patient assessment using the modified Glasgow Coma Scale (MGCS), as described in (Box 6.3.1), has been proposed as a means to provide an initial objective assessment and to provide a baseline from which monitoring can be performed.

One study has correlated the MGCS on admission with survival in dogs suffering from head trauma, with a 50% survival to 48 hours in dogs with a score of 8 (Platt et al. 2001). However, there are some considerations with the use of this scale: there is clearly a degree of subjectivity regarding the brainstem reflexes, and even the motor activity may be difficult to consistently categorise since it may be variable, and true decerebrate rigidity (mentioned in level 5) could also be described well by the situation corresponding to level 2 of motor activity. Furthermore, the use of the terms 'depression', 'delirium', and 'semicomatose' does not fit well with the terminology and descriptions currently accepted within veterinary neurology and, again, an allowance for observer interpretation must be made. The scale does, however, provide some level of objectivity in the monitoring of animals presented with suspected head trauma and is a method of monitoring response to treatment interventions.

Box 6.3.1 Modified Glasgow Coma Scale.

	Score
Motor activity	
Normal gait and spinal reflexes	6
Hemiparesis, tetraparesis, or decerebrate activity	5
Recumbent, intermittent extensor rigidity	4
Recumbent, constant extensor rigidity	3
Recumbent, constant extensor rigidity with opisthotonus	2
Recumbent, hypotonia, depressed, or absent spinal reflexes	1
Brainstem reflexes	
Normal PLR and vestibulo-ocular reflexes	6
Slow PLR and normal to reduced vestibulo-ocular reflexes	5
Bilateral unresponsive miosis with normal to reduced vestibulo-ocular reflexes	4
Pinpoint pupils with reduced to absent vestibulo-ocular reflexes	3
Unilateral, unresponsive mydriasis with reduced/absent vestibulo-ocular reflexes	2
Bilateral unresponsive mydriasis with reduced/absent vestibulo-ocular reflexes	1
Level of consciousness	
Occasional periods of alertness and responsive to environment	6
Depression or delirium, capable of responding but response may be inappropriate	5
Semi-comatose, responsive to visual stimuli	4
Semi-comatose, responsive to auditory stimuli	3
Semi-comatose, responsive only to repeated noxious stimuli	2
Comatose, unresponsive to repeated noxious stimuli	1

In-house investigations that may be considered in cases with stupor or coma are very similar to those described for obtundation. It should be remembered that cases of coma and stupor caused by primary intracranial disease are more likely to be suffering from elevated ICP, and therefore controlling this in order to maintain cerebral blood flow may be vital to the prognosis. Management of head trauma in dogs and cats is described in Chapter 7 and the reader is referred to this chapter for a more detailed understanding of the approach to traumatic brain injury.

For other possible causes of coma and stupor, the major differential diagnoses are the same as for obtundation, with systemic illness being a major consideration. Therefore, routine blood tests, urinalysis, and blood pressure measurement should be performed in every case. Supportive care, restoration of circulating blood volume in cases of shock, maintaining systemic blood pressure, and occasionally the use of hyperosmolar solutions aimed at reducing ICP may all be important in such cases. Ultimately, the prognosis is dependent on the underlying aetiology, but successful management of cases presenting as stuporous or comatose requires both an understanding of possible aetiologies and a recognition of the physiological factors which can play a role in maintenance of adequate cerebral blood flow. Referral to an establishment where adequate critical care can be provided, alongside advanced imaging and monitoring, should always be considered when possible, as long as the animal is considered stable enough to travel.

6.3.6 Behavioural Abnormalities

If an animal presents with an abnormal quality of mentation or behaviour there are some key considerations, as previously discussed. There must be an attempt to evaluate whether the problem is primarily neurological or is actually behavioural (i.e. a psychological or obsessive compulsive disorder which may have causes and treatments lying outside of the scope of experience of the neurologist or general practitioner). If this is thought likely or possible, and the rest of the physical and neurological examination is normal, then referral to a suitably qualified veterinary behaviourist may be the best solution.

If the behavioural abnormality is episodic or paroxysmal in nature, then there may be the possibility that it is a manifestation of focal seizure activity. In this case, the same approach as for seizure investigation should be followed (see Section 6.1 'Epileptic Seizures'). Videos of the episodes may also be particularly useful in such cases.

However, if the behavioural abnormality is thought to represent a true neurological disorder then this may imply forebrain disease. In this situation, the diagnostic approach to obtundation is appropriate and should be pursued. If the neurological examination is consistent with a structural forebrain lesion, then an attempt should always be made to refer the animal for further investigations and advanced imaging.

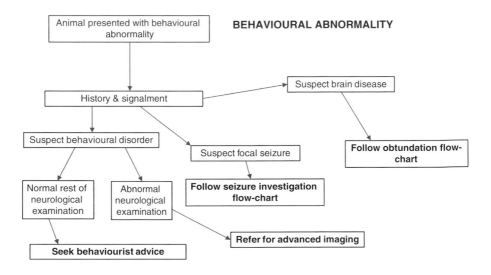

Approach to cases of behavioural abnormality in practice.

6.4   Blindness

Edward Ives

Blindness can be defined as complete, or near complete, vision loss that results in an inability to perceive objects within the field of view. It may affect one or both eyes and can be caused by a multitude of disorders affecting the eyeball itself, or the neuroanatomic structures that transmit visual information from the retina to the visual cortex in the occipital lobe of the brain. Animals often present with a history of sudden onset blindness. However, it may be difficult to judge from the clinical history whether the vision loss was genuinely acute, or whether it was a culmination of a chronic, progressive process that was only apparent to the owner once all vision was lost.

6.4.1   Is Vision Loss the Cause of the Presenting Complaint?

When an animal presents with a history of suspected vision loss, the first consideration should always be whether the animal is genuinely blind or whether the clinical signs represent a different cause. Dogs or cats may bump into objects or stumble when walking for reasons other than vision loss, and it is therefore essential that vision loss is confirmed before formulating a diagnostic plan.

Mimics of vision loss may include:

- *Ataxia of all limbs* resulting in falling, stumbling and bumping into objects. This may be observed secondary to vestibular disease, cerebellar disease, or spinal cord lesions.
- *A reduced level of mentation* secondary to a brainstem lesion, diffuse forebrain disease, or severe systemic disease.
- *Reduced or absent menace responses*, without vision loss, as a result of facial paralysis or cerebellar disease; menace responses may also appear reduced in animals that are stressed at the time of examination and can be particularly difficult to elicit in some normal cats (see Chapter 3) (Quitt et al. 2018).

6.4.2   How to Assess Vision

As summarised in Chapter 3, vision can be assessed in a number of ways.

- *Observation of the animal* navigating an unfamiliar environment.
- *Setting up an obstacle course* for a dog or cat to walk around.
- *Visual tracking* of an object that is dropped within the field of view, such as a small piece of cotton wool (see Video 38). This object should not have a strong smell or make a sound when it is dropped.
- *Menace response testing* (see Video 1a) – if the palpebral reflex is normal, confirming an ability to blink, then an absent menace response would be most

consistent with a complete, or near complete, vision loss in the eye being tested. This is particularly appreciable if the vision loss is unilateral, as the response in the blind eye can be compared to the normal response in the visual eye (see Video 28).

The pupillary light reflex (PLR) and dazzle reflex are subcortical reflexes that screen the function of the retina and optic nerves, but their integrity does not rely upon cerebrocortical perception of the visual image. These reflexes can, therefore, be normal in an animal that is clinically blind if the lesion responsible is restricted to the thalamus or visual cortex and spares the optic nerves. The reader is referred to Chapter 3 for further discussion of these reflex tests.

6.4.3   Lesion Localization

If blindness is confirmed or highly suspected, based upon the tests summarised above, then the site of the lesion responsible should be determined before a diagnostic plan is made. The first consideration should be whether there are any abnormalities on ophthalmic examination that could explain the vision loss.

1. Ophthalmic disease

Normal vision relies upon light reaching the surface of the eye, passing through the transparent structures of the eyeball, and stimulating the retinal photoreceptors. Passage to the visual cortex then occurs for processing and perception of this visual information. From a clinical perspective, the retina will be included in the ophthalmic category and post-retinal blindness will be considered separately.

Ophthalmic disease can result in vision loss as a consequence of the following.

- Light being unable to reach the retina (i.e. loss of transparency of the cornea, aqueous humour, lens, or vitreous humour):
    - corneal ulceration and oedema
    - cataract formation and lens opacification
- Retinal damage, detachment, or degeneration:
    - post-traumatic retinal detachment
    - hypertensive retinopathy
    - toxic retinopathy (e.g. fluoroquinolones, ivermectin in cats)
    - glaucoma-induced retinal damage
    - progressive retinal atrophy (PRA)
    - sudden acquired retinal degeneration syndrome (SARDS) (see Box 6.4.1).

Referral to a veterinary ophthalmologist should be considered in any animal with suspected vision loss, even if your ocular and retinal examinations appear generally unremarkable. This ensures that an ophthalmic condition is not missed before the possibility of neurologic disease is considered. Normal functioning of the retina can also be confirmed using electroretinography (ERG) if indicated.

Box 6.4.1 Sudden Acquired Retinal Degeneration Syndrome (SARDS)

SARDS is an acute retinal disorder that results in sudden vision loss, initially without abnormalities on fundoscopic examination (Komáromy et al. 2016). It can therefore mimic a central nervous system (CNS) lesion that is resulting in post-retinal blindness. An abnormal electroretinogram is required to differentiate SARDS from causes of post-retinal blindness (e.g. optic neuritis), reinforcing the importance of referral to an ophthalmologist with access to such equipment before assuming the presence of a CNS lesion. The pathogenesis of SARDS is poorly understood and up to 40% of dogs will show concurrent systemic signs of polyuria, polydipsia, polyphagia, and weight gain (Komáromy et al. 2016). Some dogs will also show abnormalities on haematology, serum biochemistry, and urinalysis, such as a stress leucogram, thrombocytosis, hypercholesterolaemia, elevated hepatic enzymes, isosthenuria, and proteinuria. The presence of these signs may increase the index of suspicion for SARDS; however, they are very similar to the changes observed in association with hyperadrenocorticism. Therefore, a hormonally active pituitary macroadenoma that is compressing the adjacent optic chiasm/tracts should also be considered. The median age of dogs with SARDS is reported to be 9 years old, with an over-representation of female dogs, smaller dog breeds (<10 kg), Dachshunds, and Miniature Schnauzers (Heller et al. 2017). The presence of conjunctival hyperaemia and retinal vascular attenuation on ophthalmic examination can also be suggestive of SARDS (Montgomery et al. 2008). A previous study did not find a statistical difference in the age or sex distribution between dogs with SARDS and those with neurologic disease as a cause for acute blindness (Montgomery et al. 2008). However, an acute onset of blindness in a young dog may reduce the index of suspicion for SARDS and increase suspicion for optic neuritis. Assessment of the pupillary light reflex using both red and blue light can also be helpful to distinguish SARDS from disorders involving the optic nerve and/or chiasm. This test is termed the chromatic pupillary light reflex (cPLR). The cPLR will be absent using both red and blue light in dogs with acute blindness secondary to an optic nerve lesion. This is in contrast to dogs with SARDS, in which the pupils will remain dilated in response to red light but will constrict when a blue light source is used (Grozdanic et al. 2007).

Retinal examination, or more specifically assessment of the optic nerve head, is unique in that it is the only non-invasive test that allows direct visualisation of the CNS. The index of suspicion for neurological disease can therefore be increased on the basis of a thorough retinal examination. However, retinal examination may be normal, even in the presence of significant optic nerve or CNS disease, if the affected region is post-retinal.

If the eyeball itself appears normal and retinal examination is unremarkable, then a lesion affecting the neuroanatomic structures between the back of the eyeball and the visual cortex is most likely. This is termed 'post-retinal blindness' or 'amaurosis'. The term 'central blindness' has been used to suggest a cortical lesion that results in vision loss, in which the PLR should be intact. However, this term can be misleading as the optic nerves also form part of the CNS. Therefore, a 'central blindness' could more accurately be thought of as anything post-retinal.

2. Post-retinal blindness

The visual pathway between the retina and visual cortex is summarised in Figure 6.4.1. A lesion affecting one or more of the following structures can therefore result in reduced or absent vision in one or both eyes:

- *Optic nerves.*
- *Optic chiasm* – the majority of optic nerve fibres cross at the optic chiasm (c.75% in dogs, c.65% in cats), with a smaller proportion continuing to the ipsilateral thalamic nuclei.
- *Optic tracts* between the optic chiasm and the lateral geniculate nuclei in the thalamus.
- *Lateral geniculate nuclei in the thalamus.*
- *Optic radiation* travelling in the white matter tracts of the cerebral hemispheres (corona radiata).
- *Visual cortices in the occipital lobes of the forebrain* – the occipital lobes form the caudodorsal part of the cerebral cortex, lying immediately rostral and dorsal to the cerebellum. The right visual field is predominately represented within the left visual cortex, and vice versa.

In order to localise a post-retinal lesion further, the following questions should be considered:

- Is the vision loss unilateral or bilateral?
- Is the PLR normal in the affected eye(s)?
- Are there any other neurological deficits consistent with a forebrain lesion?

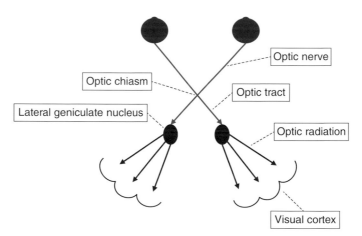

Figure 6.4.1 The visual pathway in dogs and cats. The right visual field is predominately represented within the left visual (occipital) cortex, and vice versa. The degree of decussation of the optic nerve fibres at the optic chiasm varies between species (dog c.75%, cat c.65%).

a. Is the vision loss unilateral or bilateral?

Unilateral vision loss would most commonly result from either:

- an optic nerve lesion on the same side as the blind eye (ipsilateral)
- a forebrain lesion (thalamus, optic radiation, and/or visual cortex) on the contralateral side to the blind eye (as the majority of optic nerve fibres decussate at the optic chiasm).

Bilateral vision loss could result from:

- a disease process affecting both optic nerves concurrently (e.g. optic neuritis, ischaemic optic neuropathy)
- a lesion or mass in the region of the optic chiasm where the visual pathways from both eyes are in close association (e.g. meningioma, pituitary macroadenoma)
- diffuse or bilateral forebrain disease (e.g. hepatic encephalopathy, hydrocephalus, inflammatory brain disease, cerebrocortical hypoxia).

b. Is the PLR normal in the affected eye(s)?

The neurologic pathway tested by the PLR is summarised in Figure 6.4.2. There is a common pathway for vision and the PLR up the level of the optic tracts. At this point, the pathway for vision continues to the lateral geniculate nuclei in the thalamus (see Figure 6.4.1) and the PLR pathway branches off to the pretectal nuclei in the midbrain. A lesion affecting the common pathway before this branching point will result in both blindness and an absent direct PLR in the blind eye. A lesion that affects the visual pathway *after* this point may result in blindness, but the PLR will remain normal in both eyes. This pathway is discussed further in Section 6.5 'Abnormalities of Pupil Size'.

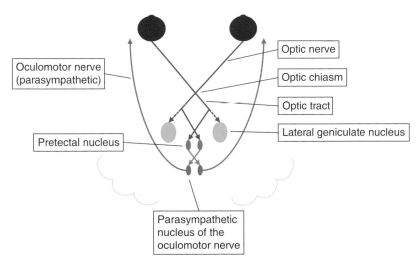

Figure 6.4.2 The pathway tested by the pupillary light reflex (PLR).

By using the PLR, post-retinal blindness can therefore be separated into lesions that affect the following.

- Optic nerve(s), optic chiasm and proximal optic tract(s):
    - *Menace response absent in the affected eye(s).*
    - *Direct PLR absent in the affected eye(s).*
    - *Dazzle reflex absent in the affected eye(s).*
    - *For bilateral blindness, both pupils will be fully dilated.*
    - *In the case of unilateral blindness, both pupils may appear similar in size as enough light will enter the visual eye to result in constriction of the contralateral pupil. If the visual eye is covered then the pupil of the blind eye will passively dilate to full mydriasis (see Section 6.5 'Abnormalities of Pupil Size' for further discussion).*
- Forebrain (thalamic or cortical):
    - *Menace response absent in the affected eye(s).*
    - *PLR and dazzle reflex normal in the affected eye(s) and both pupils will be an appropriate size for the external light level.*

Unfortunately, not all cases conform to our attempts to understand and over-simplify the neurological system; some animals will appear clinically blind and have an intact PLR on examination, but further investigations will reveal a lesion affecting the retina, optic nerves, or optic chiasm. This is most likely to be caused by an incomplete lesion that is damaging a sufficient number of optic nerve axons to result in near complete vision loss, but enough axons remain functional to elicit reflexive pupil constriction in response to bright light.

c. Are there any other neurological deficits consistent with a forebrain lesion?

Neurological deficits that would add support for a lesion at the level of the thalamus, subcortical white matter, or visual cortex include:

- *Compulsive circling*: most frequently towards to side of the lesion, and therefore away from the side of the blind eye (i.e. absent menace response in the right eye, circling to the left).
- *Proprioceptive deficits* in the thoracic and pelvic limbs ipsilateral to the side of the blind eye.
- *Reduced nasal nociception* in the nostril ipsilateral to the side of the blind eye.
- *An onset of seizures* coincident with the onset of blindness.
- *A reduced level of mentation*, particularly in cases of bilateral cortical blindness.

6.4.4 Clinical Approach

The clinical approach to an animal presenting with suspected vision loss is summarised below:

1. Confirm unilateral or bilateral vision loss as the cause for the presenting complaint

- Vision appears normal in the consultation – consider other causes for the presenting complaint (e.g. lethargy, ataxia), or a waxing/waning disease process (e.g. hepatic encephalopathy).
- Blindness confirmed on clinical assessment (obstacle course, visual tracking, menace response testing) – go to step 2.

2. Perform a full ophthalmic and retinal examination

- Ophthalmic examination reveals a possible cause for reduced vision (e.g. corneal ulceration/oedema, cataract formation, retinal lesions):
  - ○ investigate and manage in practice if appropriate
  - ○ consider referral to a veterinary ophthalmologist if possible.
- Ophthalmic examination appears normal – go to step 3.

3. Perform a full neurological examination

a. Neurological examination otherwise normal

Refer to a veterinary ophthalmologist to further exclude ophthalmic disease before considering referral to a veterinary neurologist for advanced imaging of the head.

If an animal presents with a clinical history of acute, bilateral vision loss and there are no abnormalities found on ophthalmic or neurological examinations, then two possibilities should be considered:

- This animal suffers from SARDS – see Box 6.4.1.
- There is a post-retinal lesion that is currently sparing other neurological functions. This is most commonly seen with disorders that affect the optic nerves/optic chiasm. In a case series of four dogs and three cats with acute blindness as the only neurological deficit at presentation, a lesion was observed on MRI in six out of seven cases (Seruca et al. 2010). All of these cases had a normal ophthalmic examination and electroretinogram prior to advanced imaging of the head. One case was diagnosed with bilateral optic neuritis and five cases with intracranial neoplasia (two meningiomas in the region of the optic chiasm, two nasal tumours with intracranial extension, and one pituitary tumour). CNS disease should therefore always be considered as a cause for blindness, even in the absence of other neurologic deficits, and this study emphasises the importance of advanced imaging to achieve a definitive diagnosis if referral is an option.

If referral is not an option, then a diagnostic approach to these cases in general practice could include:

- *Haematology, serum biochemistry and urinalysis* to further investigate possible inflammatory, metabolic, or systemic disease. As summarised in Box 6.4.1, certain biochemical changes may also be seen in dogs with SARDS.

- *Blood pressure testing.*
- *Thyroid hormone testing,* particularly in cats.
- *Infectious disease testing* (e.g. *T. gondii* serology in dogs and cats, FeLV and FIV testing in cats, and *N. caninum* serology and CDV testing in dogs).
- *Ultrasound of the retrobulbar space* through a closed eyelid.
- *Nasal radiography* to screen for a nasal tumour with possible intracranial extension, particularly if there is a history of epistaxis or reduced nasal airflow on examination.
- *Thoracic radiography and abdominal ultrasonography* to screen for neoplastic disease in other body cavities (e.g. lymphoma, metastatic disease). This can be particularly useful in cats, for which lymphoma is an important differential diagnosis.
- *Computed tomography (CT)* is increasingly available in general practice and can be used to image the head and other body cavities. However, magnetic resonance imaging (MRI) remains preferred over CT for imaging of the optic nerves and brain in light of its superior soft tissue resolution. Referral for assessment by a neurologist, and MRI +/− CSF analysis if indicated, should therefore always be offered to an owner prior to performing CT in practice. This ensures that funds are available to perform the test that is most likely to achieve a definitive diagnosis. The lower cost of CT means that it can be a useful test if the costs associated with referral and MRI are prohibitive.
- *Monitoring the clinical course of the disease without treatment.* The appearance of neurological deficits over time would support a progressive intracranial lesion as a cause for blindness. If the clinical signs remain static and the animal is suspected as having SARDS, then many dogs can still live a good quality of life in the long-term.

b. Additional neurological deficits are found on examination that support an intracranial lesion as a cause for blindness

Refer to a veterinary neurologist if possible.

The list of differential diagnoses in these cases will depend upon the species, the signalment, and whether the vision loss is unilateral or bilateral.

- Unilateral blindness in an older dog or cat that has a concurrent history of altered mentation, circling, or seizures: this would be most consistent with a focal asymmetric, intracranial lesion (e.g. neoplastic mass).
- Unilateral or bilateral blindness in a young or middle-aged, small breed dog with concurrent neurological deficits (e.g. Pug, Yorkshire Terrier, Chihuahua, Boston Terrier, French Bulldog): this could indicate an underlying inflammatory disorder, with meningoencephalitis of unknown origin (MUO) being most common if infectious disease testing is negative.
- Bilateral blindness in a young animal with a dull mentation, domed skull, and bilateral ventrolateral strabismus: this could indicate underlying hydrocephalus, but hepatic encephalopathy should also be considered in these cases.

- Post-anaesthetic cortical blindness may be observed in dogs or cats following anaesthetic complications that result in cerebral hypoxia (e.g. cardiorespiratory arrest). However, it has also been reported in cats following routine anaesthesia during which a spring-loaded mouth gag was used, such as dentistry or endoscopy. It has been hypothesised that use of a mouth gag results in compression of the maxillary arteries which, unlike in the dog, provide the majority of cerebral blood flow in cats (Martin-Flores et al. 2014). In a study of 20 cats with post-anaesthetic cortical blindness, a mouth gag had been used in 16 cases; 85% had other neurological deficits in addition to blindness, 70% of cats had a documented recovery of vision, and 59% of the cats that had additional neurological deficits showed a full recovery (Stiles et al. 2012).

If referral to a veterinary neurologist is not possible, then the same tests listed above for animals with a normal neurological examination should be considered. The choice of which tests to perform will depend upon the list of differential diagnoses. If the clinical signs are progressive, and further investigations have been unrewarding or cannot be performed for economic reasons, then the option of starting a prednisolone trial could be considered. The limitations of this approach should always be thoroughly discussed with the owner before starting treatment, particularly regarding the possibility of clinical deterioration if an undiagnosed infectious disease is present, or the likelihood of a poor response to treatment. An initial dose of 0.5–1 mg/kg prednisolone once or twice daily could be used, dependent on the ranked list of differential diagnoses (e.g. 0.5 mg/kg once or twice daily for neoplasia, 1 mg/kg twice daily for meningoencephalitis of unknown origin). Concurrent seizures, if present, should always be managed using antiepileptic medications, as discussed in Section 6.1 'Epileptic Seizures'.

6.5 Abnormalities of Pupil Size

Edward Ives

In the healthy dog or cat, pupil size is determined by the environmental light levels and emotional status of the individual. Both pupils should be equal in size and respond in the same manner to these stimuli.

- A bright environment will stimulate active pupil constriction to optimise vision and avoid being dazzled. This is mediated via the parasympathetic nervous system.
- The pupils will passively dilate in low environmental light levels to maximise the amount of light reaching the retina.
- Stimulation of the sympathetic nervous system in response to stress, pain, or exercise will result in active pupil dilation as part of the 'fight or flight response'.

Box 6.5.1 Terminology

- Pupil dilation is termed 'mydriasis' and pupil constriction is termed 'miosis'.
- A dilated pupil is therefore termed 'mydriatic' and a constricted pupil 'miotic'.
- The term 'anisocoria' is used to describe unequal pupil size, with one pupil being either inappropriately miotic or mydriatic.
- Internal ophthalmoparesis/ophthalmoplegia refers to weakness/paralysis of the iris sphincter and ciliary body muscle secondary to loss of parasympathetic innervation by the oculomotor nerve. This results in a mydriatic pupil.
- External ophthalmoparesis/ophthalmoplegia refers to weakness/paralysis of the extraocular muscles that are responsible for eyeball movement.

---

1. Active pupil constriction in response to light

   As discussed in Section 6.4 'Blindness', there is a common neurological pathway for both vision and pupil constriction up to the level of the optic tracts (Figure 6.5.1). The majority of optic tract fibres are destined for the visual area of the cerebral cortex, via the lateral geniculate nuclei of the thalamus. However, around 20% of the optic tract fibres branch away to the pretectal nuclei, which reside at the boundary of the thalamus and midbrain. Axons from the pretectal nuclei stimulate the parasympathetic nuclei of the oculomotor (III) nerves. These parasympathetic fibres leave the midbrain to join the motor fibres of the oculomotor nerve. The oculomotor nerves run along the floor of the skull through the middle cranial fossa, either side of the pituitary gland, and leave the skull via the orbital fissures. The pre-ganglionic parasympathetic fibres contained within the oculomotor nerve synapse with post-ganglionic ciliary nerve axons at the ciliary ganglion in the retrobulbar space. These post-ganglionic parasympathetic fibres innervate the constrictor muscles of the pupil.

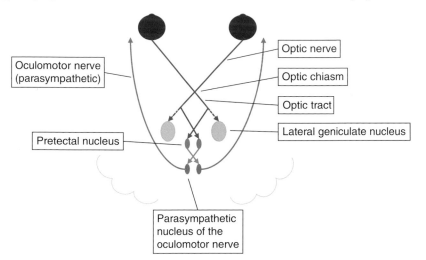

Figure 6.5.1 The pathway for active pupil constriction in response to light. This is the same pathway that is tested by the pupillary light reflex (see Section 6.4 'Blindness').

This is the entire pathway that is tested by the pupillary light reflex (PLR). Partial decussation at both the optic chiasm and pretectal nuclei means that there is bilateral representation of information at the level of the optic tracts, pretectal nuclei, and oculomotor nuclei. This results in constriction of both pupils, even if light only enters one eye. Constriction of the pupil of the stimulated eye is termed the 'direct PLR' and constriction of the contralateral pupil is termed the 'consensual PLR'. However, the use of the terms 'direct' and 'consensual' can sometimes be confusing when reading clinical records, as it can be unclear as to which eye is being stimulated and which pupil is being referred to. For this reason, the results of PLR testing should be described in terms of which eye is receiving light and which pupil constricts. For example, the left pupil constricts when light is shone into both the left and right eyes, but the right pupil does not constrict when light is shone into either eye – this situation would be most consistent with a lesion affecting the parasympathetic fibres in the right oculomotor nerve.

Lesions affecting a multitude of anatomical structures (transparent structures of the eyeball, retina, optic nerves, optic chiasm, optic tracts, midbrain, parasympathetic fibres of the oculomotor nerves, iris constrictor muscles) could all result in a failure of pupil constriction, a pathological mydriasis, and/or an abnormal PLR. However, by careful assessment of vision, menace responses, and PLR testing in both eyes, the most likely site of the lesion can be identified. A list of differential diagnoses can then be formulated, and the decision regarding whether to refer, who to refer to (e.g. ophthalmologist or neurologist), or what further investigations would be most useful in practice can be made.

2. Active pupil dilation in response to sympathetic stimulation

   The sympathetic innervation to each eye represents a long, ipsilateral pathway that can be divided into three main sections (Figure 6.5.2).

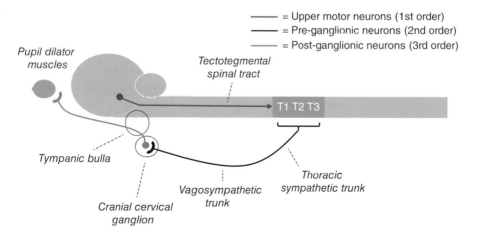

Figure 6.5.2 The neurologic pathway for active pupil dilation in response to sympathetic stimulation ('fight or flight response').

- *The upper motor neurons (also termed 'first-order' neurons)* originate in the hypo-thalamus and midbrain. They travel down the brainstem and cervical spinal cord in an ipsilateral bundle of nerve fibres called the 'tectotegmental spinal tract'. These axons synapse with the cell bodies of the pre-ganglionic sympathetic neurons in the grey matter of the T1–T3 spinal cord segments.
- *The pre-ganglionic ('second-order') neurons* originate in the intermediolateral grey matter of the T1–T3 spinal cord segments and leave the spinal cord in the T1–T3 ventral nerve roots. The sympathetic fibres separate from the ventral nerve roots before the level of the brachial plexus and ascend through the cranial thorax as the thoracic sympathetic trunk. They then join the vagus nerve to form the vagosympathetic trunk within the carotid sheath. Synapse with the post-ganglionic sympathetic neurons occurs in the cranial cervical ganglion, which lies adjacent to the tympanic bulla.
- *The post-ganglionic ('third-order') neurons* are the final neurons in the pathway. The precise route that these fibres take to the smooth muscles of the eyelids, iris, and periorbita has not been fully elucidated, and may involve multiple routes. However, it is thought that they travel in close association with the tympanic bulla, before running with the ophthalmic branch of the trigeminal nerve via the retrobulbar space.

This long sympathetic pathway to the eye means that lesions affecting the brain, cervical spinal cord, cranial thorax, neck, tympanic bulla, and/or retrobulbar space can all result in a failure of pupil dilation and unopposed pupil constriction (miosis).

6.5.1   Bilateral Mydriasis

Bilateral pupil dilation would be appropriate in a dark environment; however, if both pupils appear inappropriately dilated for the external light levels then it is important to consider both non-neurological and neurological causes for pathologic mydriasis. Increased sympathetic stimulation (e.g. excitement, stress, or fear) is a very common cause of bilateral, symmetric pupil dilation during clinical examination. The PLR may also appear bilaterally reduced unless a very bright light is used. Examination in bright sunlight can help to demonstrate appropriate pupil constriction in these cases, but care should always be taken when interpreting the clinical significance of bilateral, symmetric mydriasis in a stressed animal that otherwise appears normal.

1. Non-neurological causes

- *Bilateral glaucoma* – The index of suspicion should be increased by concurrent ophthalmic abnormalities such as scleral congestion or discomfort on gentle retropulsion of the eyeballs.
- *Previous application of a topical parasympathetic blocking agent into both eyes (e.g. atropine, tropicamide)* – This should be supported by a history of such application.

- *Bilateral iris atrophy* – The application of 0.1% pilocarpine eye drops can help to differentiate age-related atrophy of the iris constrictor muscles from denervation secondary to an oculomotor nerve lesion. This direct parasympathomimetic agent will stimulate pupil constriction if there is denervation hypersensitivity of the iris constrictor muscles. In the case of iris atrophy, these muscles will remain mechanically unable to contract even when stimulated pharmacologically, and the pupils will therefore remain dilated.
- *Bilateral blindness resulting from an ophthalmic lesion* (e.g. bilateral cataract formation, bilateral retinal lesion such as SARDS).

2. Neurological causes

- *Bilateral blindness involving the visual pathway between the retina and the branching of the optic tracts to the pretectal nuclei* – Affected animals will have difficulty navigating around obstacles, will not visually track objects dropped silently in front of them, and the PLR, dazzle reflex, and menace response will be absent in both eyes. Assuming that there are no concurrent trigeminal or facial nerve lesions, the palpebral reflexes should be normal and spontaneous blinking should be observed. Differential diagnoses could include a bilateral optic nerve lesion (e.g. optic neuritis) or a lesion affecting the optic chiasm (e.g. pituitary macroadenoma). A lesion that affects the visual pathway from the level of the lateral geniculate nuclei to the visual cortex, sparing the earlier components (e.g. retina, optic nerves, optic chiasm, optic tracts), can result in blindness but will not affect the pupil size or PLR.
- *A disorder that affects both parasympathetic oculomotor nuclei in the midbrain (e.g. thiamine deficiency, increased intracranial pressure [ICP]), or that affects the parasympathetic fibres in both oculomotor nerves (e.g. mass situated in the middle cranial fossa, dysautonomia, botulism)* – The PLR will be absent in both eyes, but the vision should be normal and the menace responses intact bilaterally unless there is concurrent involvement of the optic nerves. Affected animals may appear dazzled in a bright environment as a result of excessive light entering via the inappropriately dilated pupils.
- *Ingestion of belladonna plant species containing atropine* – This will block the effect of acetylcholine released from the parasympathetic oculomotor nerve fibres, resulting in bilateral mydriasis. The PLR will be absent in both eyes, but vision will be normal.

6.5.2 Bilateral Miosis

1. Non-neurological causes

- *Bilateral corneal lesions resulting in reflex pupil constriction (e.g. ulceration).*
- *Bilateral uveitis.*

- *Previous application of a topical parasympathomimetic agent into both eyes (e.g. pilocarpine)* – This should be supported by a history of such application.
- *Following opioid administration in dogs (e.g. buprenorphine, methadone, fentanyl)* – This is particularly apparent following high doses of opiates, or in animals that are individually sensitive to such agents (Stephan et al. 2003). Opiate administration can also result in sedation and cardiorespiratory depression which, in conjunction with bilateral miosis, could mimic primary intracranial disease and increased ICP.

2. Neurological causes

- *Appropriate response to a bright environment.*
- *Bilateral stimulation of the parasympathetic oculomotor nuclei (e.g. increased ICP or diffuse forebrain lesions that result in disinhibition of the oculomotor nerves)* – This will be accompanied by other neurological deficits reflecting significant intracranial pathology, such as an altered level of mentation, tetraparesis, a poor gag reflex, or a reduced vestibulo-ocular reflex.
- *Organophosphate or carbamate toxicity* – These agents inhibit the enzyme acetylcholinesterase, resulting in an increased level of acetylcholine at the neuromuscular junction (NMJ) and stimulation of the pupil constrictor muscles.
- *Bilateral loss of sympathetic innervation to the pupil dilator muscles (bilateral Horner syndrome)* – This is rarely observed but has been reported in association with extensive cervical spinal cord lesions, diabetes mellitus, bilateral trigeminal nerve disorders, and as an idiopathic condition (Carpenter et al. 1987; Holland 2007). Concurrent bilateral enophthalmos, third eyelid protrusion, and ptosis should allow bilateral Horner syndrome to be distinguished from other causes of bilateral miosis.

6.5.3 Anisocoria

Anisocoria is the term used to describe a difference in the size of the left and right pupils. The most common reason for this difference is that one pupil remains normal whilst the contralateral pupil is either inappropriately dilated (unilateral mydriasis) or inappropriately constricted (unilateral miosis). Therefore, the first step in the approach to anisocoria should be to identify which pupil is the abnormal one. This differentiation can be more difficult than it initially sounds, but a simple and effective way is to assess pupil size in both dark and bright environments:

- An inappropriately dilated pupil will be most obvious in a bright environment. This will accentuate the difference between the abnormal pupil, which fails to appropriately constrict, and the normal pupil, which will still constrict in response to light.

- An inappropriately constricted pupil will be more obvious in a dark environment, as it will fail to dilate when compared to the normal contralateral pupil.

Other important tests to perform include assessment of vision, menace responses, pupillary light reflexes, and observation for other neurological deficits that would indicate dysfunction of either the oculomotor nerve or sympathetic nerve supply to the eyes (e.g. abnormal strabismus, eyelid position).

In simple terms, an inappropriately dilated pupil (mydriasis) will result from either:

- a loss of the ability to constrict the pupil (i.e. a parasympathetic oculomotor nerve lesion)
- or, increased activity of the pupil dilator muscles (i.e. stimulation or disinhibition of the sympathetic innervation to the eye).

Likewise, an inappropriately constricted pupil (miosis) will result from either:

- an inability to dilate the pupil (i.e. loss of sympathetic innervation to the eye)
- or, increased activity of the pupil constrictor muscles (i.e. stimulation or disinhibition of the parasympathetic fibres of the oculomotor nerve).

Other than the notable exceptions of epileptic seizures and certain movement disorders (see Sections 6.1 'Epileptic Seizures' and 6.2 'Movement Disorders'), clinical neurology most commonly deals with *loss of function* in the form of neurological 'deficits'. This is also true for anisocoria, in which unilateral mydriasis most commonly results from loss of parasympathetic innervation to the pupil constrictor muscles, and unilateral miosis results from loss of sympathetic innervation to the pupil dilator muscles. A logical approach to these two scenarios is summarised below.

1. Unilateral mydriasis

As for bilateral mydriasis, it is essential to consider non-neurological causes for unilateral mydriasis as these may be commonly encountered in general practice. Such conditions include unilateral glaucoma, iris atrophy (Grahn and Cullen 2004), and previous application of a mydriatic agent into the affected eye (e.g. atropine or tropicamide).

Unilateral blindness results in only mild anisocoria as sufficient light will enter the visual eye to elicit a consensual PLR. This will maintain a near-normal pupil size in the blind eye. If the visual eye is covered, then the blind eye will passively dilate and become mydriatic. Light directed into the visual eye will result in constriction of both pupils, whereas neither pupil will change in size if light is directed into the blind eye.

In the absence of a non-neurological cause, unilateral mydriasis most commonly results from ipsilateral dysfunction of the oculomotor nerve (parasympathetic fibres). This is termed internal ophthalmoparesis/ophthalmo-plegia and presents as a visual eye with a dilated pupil that fails to constrict when light is shone into either eye. The contralateral pupil should, however, still constrict when light is shone into the affected eye.

In addition to parasympathetic fibres, the oculomotor nerve also has a motor component. These fibres innervate the levator palpebrae superioris muscle contributing to elevation of the upper eyelid and innervate the extraocular muscles responsible for eyeball movement. The motor fibres can be affected at the same time as the parasympathetic fibres, resulting in ptosis, a resting ventrolateral strabismus, and an inability to move the eyeball dorsally, ventrally, or medially (O'Neill et al. 2013). These signs of motor dysfunction are termed external ophthalmoparesis/ophthalmoplegia. The parasympathetic fibres lie superficial to the motor fibres in their course to the eye, meaning that they can be affected in isolation before motor involvement is observed. This may be seen in association with slowly expanding masses within the middle cranial fossa.

Differential diagnoses to consider for a suspected, unilateral parasympathetic oculomotor nerve lesion should include:

- A unilateral midbrain lesion that is affecting the ipsilateral parasympathetic nucleus of the oculomotor nerve (e.g. neoplasia, infarction, focal inflammatory lesion, head trauma) (Webb et al. 2005). In light of the small size of this nucleus, adjacent neuroanatomic structures are likely to also be affected, resulting in concurrent neurological deficits, such as ipsilateral hemiparesis, proprioceptive deficits, and a reduced level of mentation.
- A lesion in the middle cranial fossa that is compressing the oculomotor nerves as they run along the floor of the cranial vault towards the eye (e.g. pituitary macroadenoma, meningioma, germ cell neoplasia, lymphoma, abscess/granuloma) (Larocca 2000) (Figure 6.5.3). Lesions in this location may affect other cranial nerves that run in close association with the oculomotor nerves, including the trochlear nerve, abducens nerve, and all three branches of the trigeminal nerve. This will result in a combination of ipsilateral clinical signs termed 'cavernous sinus syndrome', such as loss of facial sensation, masticatory muscle atrophy, and complete paralysis of all extra-ocular muscles (Guevar et al. 2014; Jones et al. 2018).
- A primary oculomotor nerve lesion (e.g. lymphoma, malignant nerve sheath tumour).
- A retrobulbar lesion (e.g. neoplasia, abscess, trauma) – lesions in this location may also affect the optic nerve, resulting in blindness of the affected eye, an absent menace response, and absent constriction of the contralateral pupil when light is shone into the affected eye.
- Idiopathic oculomotor neuropathy – unilateral mydriasis, with or without external ophthalmoplegia, has been reported as an idiopathic condition in dogs (Tetas Pont et al. 2017). Flat-coated Retrievers appear over-represented. MRI can reveal enlargement and contrast enhancement of the affected oculo-

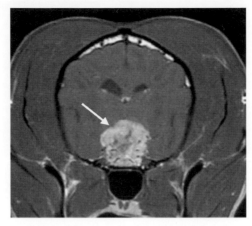

Figure 6.5.3 A transverse T1-weighted MRI at the level of the pituitary gland and inter-tha-lamic adhesion following the administration of intravenous contrast media in a 12-year-old, male neutered Border Terrier with a clinical history of lethargy and unilateral, right-sided mydriasis. The neurological examination was otherwise normal. The lesion localised to the parasympathetic component of the right oculomotor nerve. Magnetic resonance imaging of the brain demonstrated a large, strongly contrast-enhancing, extra-axial mass in the region of the pituitary fossa that was suspected to represent a pituitary macroadenoma. The mydriasis observed in this case was secondary to compression of the adjacent right oculomotor nerve as it ran rostrally through the middle cranial fossa on its way to the eye.

motor nerve, prompting suggestion that this may represent an idiopathic oculomotor neuritis. This condition is non-progressive and is associated with a good prognosis. A retrospective study of 14 dogs with suspected idiopathic oculomotor neuropathy reported an improvement in 50% of dogs over a median follow-up time of 25 months (five dogs without treatment and two dogs with systemic corticosteroid treatment) (Tetas Pont et al. 2017).

Rare neurological causes for unilateral mydriasis:

- Cerebellar lesions can result in ipsilateral or contralateral mydriasis dependent on the cerebellar nucleus affected (Figure 6.5.4). The vision and palpebral reflexes will be normal in these cases, but the menace response may be absent. Additional signs to indicate cerebellar dysfunction will usually be present, such as hypermetria, ataxia, an intention tremor, or central vestibular syndrome.
- Overstimulation/irritation of the sympathetic nerve supply to the eye. This is termed 'Pourfour du Petit syndrome' and has been reported in cats with otitis media and in cats following mild, iatrogenic trauma to the middle ear cavity (Boydell 2000). In these cases, the pupil should still be able to constrict to some degree in response to a bright light source as the optic and oculomotor (parasympathetic) pathways remain intact. This condition may precede a loss of sympathetic function that will result in Horner syndrome in the affected eye.

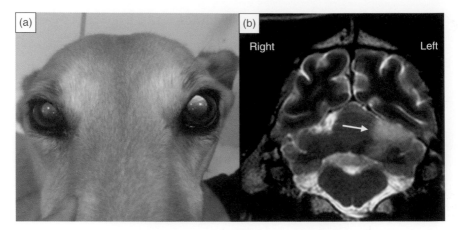

Figure 6.5.4 (a) Anisocoria with left mydriasis in an 8-year-old, female neutered Greyhound with a clinical history of acute onset, non-progressive ataxia of all limbs and a left head tilt. (b) A transverse T2-weighted MRI at the level of the cerebellum and medulla oblongata in the affected dog demonstrating a well-defined, 'wedge-shaped' hyperintensity affecting the cerebellar cortex and fastigial nucleus on the left side (white arrow). The clinical history and imaging findings in this case were consistent with a cerebrovascular accident (ischaemic stroke). With thanks to Joe Fenn DipECVN, Royal Veterinary College, UK, for the photo and MRI.

Box 6.5.2 Oculomotor Nerve Dysfunction in Cats

Isolated oculomotor nerve dysfunction is a rare clinical sign in cats, with neoplastic disease being the most common cause. A recent retrospective study from a referral institution reported 12 cats with internal ophthalmoparesis/ophthalmoplegia (unilateral in 9 cats and bilateral in 3 cats) (Hamzianpour et al. 2018). An abnormal mentation was recorded in 9 cats and additional neurologic deficits were present in 10 of the 12 cats. A mass lesion was observed on advanced imaging of the head in all 10 cases in which it was performed, and the remaining 2 cats were diagnosed with multicentric lymphoma following abdominal ultrasound and biopsy. The prognosis was poor in all cases, with a median time from diagnosis to euthanasia of 3.5 days (range 0–80 days).

Clinical approach to unilateral mydriasis

1. Confirm that the mydriatic pupil is the abnormal pupil by examination in a bright environment and PLR testing.
2. Have any topical medications been recently applied that could cause mydriasis (e.g. atropine, tropicamide)?
3. Perform an ophthalmic examination to assess for primary ocular disorders that could result in mydriasis (e.g. glaucoma, iris atrophy), or evidence of retrobulbar disease that could be affecting the oculomotor nerve.
   - Refer to an ophthalmologist or further work-up in practice as appropriate.
4. If the eye otherwise appears normal, then a neurological cause for unilateral mydriasis is most likely:

- Perform a menace response to assess vision in the affected eye.
- If vision is normal, then an ipsilateral parasympathetic oculomotor nerve lesion is most likely. The affected pupil will not constrict when light is shone into either eye, but the normal pupil will still constrict when light is shone into the affected eye. Clinical signs consistent with external ophthalmoplegia may also be present (e.g. ptosis, resting ventrolateral strabismus).
- A pilocarpine response test (0.1% pilocarpine eye drops) can be performed to further exclude iris atrophy. Constriction of the pupil following pilocarpine application would be consistent with oculomotor nerve dysfunction and denervation of the pupil constrictor muscles.

5. Perform a full neurological examination:
    - Assess for other neurological deficits that would be consistent with a lesion affecting the parasympathetic nucleus of the oculomotor nerve in the midbrain (e.g. tetraparesis or hemiparesis, proprioceptive deficits, reduced level of mentation, other cranial nerve deficits).
    - Concurrent involvement of cranial nerves IV, V, and VI, with or without other neurologic deficits, could indicate a lesion in the region of the middle cranial fossa.
    - Idiopathic oculomotor neuropathy should be considered in dogs with unilateral mydriasis and no other neurologic deficits on examination. However, internal ophthalmoplegia may be the sole clinical sign in the early stages of progressive disease (e.g. neoplasia) and, if funds allow, idiopathic oculomotor neuropathy should never be assumed without exclusion of other causes.

6. Refer for advanced imaging of the head – MRI is the gold standard due to its superior soft tissue resolution when compared to CT. However, CT may reveal the underlying cause if an extra-axial middle cranial fossa mass is highly suspected (e.g. meningioma, pituitary macroadenoma, nasal adenocarcinoma with intracranial extension).

7. If referral is not an option, then further investigations can be performed in practice:
    - Screening for involvement of other body systems or body cavities: haematology, serum biochemistry, urinalysis, thoracic radiography, abdominal ultrasonography. This is recommended in cats due to the relatively high incidence of lymphoma in this species compared to dogs; this is frequently a systemic disease process that may be diagnosed by sampling other, more accessible, regions of the body (e.g. lymph nodes, liver, spleen).
    - Infectious disease testing: *T. gondii* serology in dogs and cats, *N. caninum* serology in dogs, FeLV, FIV and feline coronavirus testing in cats.
    - Monitoring of the clinical course without treatment, particularly if there is a high clinical suspicion of idiopathic oculomotor neuropathy in a dog.

Owners should always be warned of the possibility of an underlying progressive disease process and that the prognosis may be poor if additional neurological deficits are subsequently observed.

2. Unilateral miosis

If non-neurological causes are excluded (e.g. uveitis, painful ocular conditions), then the most common cause for unilateral miosis is loss of sympathetic innervation to the smooth dilator muscles of the pupil. This results in unopposed pupil constriction and a miotic pupil that fails to dilate fully in a dark environment. The affected pupil may constrict further in response to bright light as the parasympathetic fibres in the oculomotor nerve are unaffected.

In addition to the dilator muscles of the pupil, the sympathetic nervous system also provides innervation to the smooth muscles of the eyelids, periorbita, and blood vessels of the head. Therefore, a combination of clinical signs termed 'Horner syndrome' is commonly observed following loss of sympathetic innervation to the eye (Kern et al. 1989; Morgan and Zanotti 1989) (Figure 6.5.5):

- *ipsilateral miosis*
- *a narrow palpebral fissure* – drooping of the upper eyelid (ptosis) and decreased smooth muscle tone in the lower eyelid

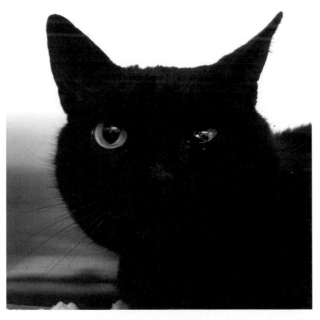

Figure 6.5.5 Horner syndrome in a 5-year-old cat with left-sided otitis media. Note the narrow palpebral fissure in the left eye, protrusion of the left third eyelid, and left-sided miosis relative to the normal right eye.

- *third eyelid protrusion* – observed secondary to loss of tone in the periorbital smooth muscle and subsequent passive retraction of the eyeball
- *enophthalmos* – often mild or clinically inapparent
- *loss of sympathetic vascular smooth muscle tone on the affected side of the head,* resulting in peripheral vasodilation, hyperaemia, warmth of the ipsilateral pinna, and mild scleral congestion.

Partial Horner syndrome, associated with miosis alone, is uncommon but can occur following partial avulsion of the roots of the brachial plexus (e.g. avulsion of the T1 nerve root sparing the T2 and T3 nerve roots).

Unilateral Horner syndrome is rarely a problem for the affected animal, but it should alert the clinician to the presence of a sympathetic lesion somewhere in the long and convoluted pathway from the brain to the eye. This syndrome represents a prime example of why a thorough clinical history, general clinical examination, and neurological examination are essential to correctly localise the site of the lesion. The presence of concurrent clinical signs or neurological deficits can greatly assist in achieving an accurate neuroanatomic localisation, which can then be used to guide further investigations. The neuroanatomic localisation can be divided into the three parts of the sympathetic pathway described above.

a. Upper motor neuron (first-order) lesion: brain and C1–C8 spinal cord segments (Figure 6.5.6)

Concurrent neurological deficits will be present in cases with a first-order lesion as adjacent neuroanatomical structures are invariably affected. These deficits will depend upon the lesion location but could include a change in the level of mentation, seizures, other cranial nerve deficits, a change in drinking (e.g. hypothalamic lesions), tetraparesis, ipsilateral hemiparesis/hemiplegia, and ipsilateral proprioceptive deficits.

Differential diagnoses to consider in these cases should include head trauma, neoplasia, meningoencephalomyelitis (infectious or sterile), fibrocartilaginous embolic myelopathy, cervical intervertebral disc extrusion, and spinal fracture/luxation.

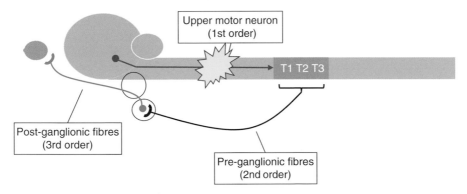

Figure 6.5.6 Lesion localisation for an upper motor neuron (first-order) Horner syndrome.

b. Pre-ganglionic (second-order) lesion: T1–T3 spinal cord segments, T1–T3 nerve roots, cranial thorax, and neck (Figure 6.5.7)

A lesion that affects the cell bodies of the second-order neurons residing within the grey matter of the T1–T3 spinal cord segments will result in Horner syndrome, together with lower motor neuron paresis of the ipsilateral thoracic limb (reduced limb muscle tone, weak withdrawal reflex), and upper motor neuron paresis of the ipsilateral pelvic limb (delayed/absent proprioception, normal muscle tone, intact patellar and withdrawal reflexes). Horner syndrome and concurrent lower motor neuron paresis of the ipsilateral thoracic limb, without involvement of the pelvic limbs, can be seen secondary to disorders affecting the T1–T3 ventral nerve roots (e.g. avulsion of the roots of the brachial plexus, peripheral nerve sheath tumour [PNST]).

Horner syndrome is frequently the only neurological deficit observed in cases with lesions affecting the thoracic sympathetic trunk or vagosympathetic trunk in the neck. Thorough cervical palpation should always be performed in these cases, assessing for bite wounds, evidence of previous venepuncture, or masses (e.g. thyroid adenocarcinoma, lymphoma) (Melián et al. 1996). Thoracic radiography may also be useful to assess for cranial mediastinal masses. Iatrogenic trauma to the pre-ganglionic sympathetic fibres can be seen as a post-surgical complication following thyroid surgery, ventral slot surgery, thoracotomy, or chest drain placement (Boydell et al. 1997).

c. Post-ganglionic (third-order) lesion: from the level of the tympanic bulla to the eye, via the trigeminal nerve (Figure 6.5.8)

Recognition of concurrent vestibular syndrome and/or facial paralysis, without other neurological deficits, would be highly suggestive of a lesion in the region of the tympanic bulla (e.g. otitis media, neoplasia). Horner syndrome may also be observed as a post-surgical complication following total ear canal ablation or ventral bulla osteotomy (Spivack et al. 2013).

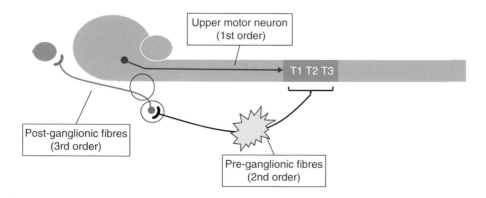

Figure 6.5.7 Lesion localisation for a pre-ganglionic (second-order) Horner syndrome.

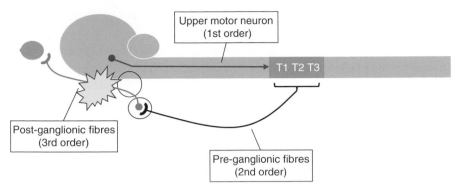

Upper motor neuron
(1st order)

T1 T2 T3

Post-ganglionic fibres
(3rd order)

Pre-ganglionic fibres
(2nd order)

Figure 6.5.8 Lesion localisation for a post-ganglionic (third-order) Horner syndrome.

Retrobulbar disease that damages the sympathetic nerve fibres behind the eye is often accompanied by exophthalmos or mechanical strabismus (e.g. abscess, neoplasia). The optic and oculomotor nerves can also be affected in these cases, resulting in blindness and/or a mid-range pupil that can neither dilate nor constrict.

Disorders affecting the trigeminal nerve may result in concurrent damage to the sympathetic fibres that run in close association with this nerve to the eye (Carpenter et al. 1987). Clinical signs of trigeminal nerve dysfunction include ipsilateral masticatory muscle atrophy, weak/absent palpebral reflex in the ipsilateral eye as a result of loss of facial sensation, and a dropped jaw in the case of bilateral lesions.

Box 6.5.3 Idiopathic Horner Syndrome

This is a relatively common condition that has been estimated to affect up to 55% of dogs and 40% of cats presenting with Horner syndrome (Kern et al. 1989, Morgan and Zanotti 1989). Male Golden Retrievers appear to be over-represented (Boydell 2000). It is a diagnosis of exclusion with no identifiable cause being found on diagnostic investigations. This syndrome was previously reported as an idiopathic pre-ganglionic (second-order) lesion; however, a recent publication reported a post-ganglionic (third-order) lesion in 8 of 10 Golden Retrievers assessed (Simpson et al. 2015). This conclusion was made on the basis of pharmacologic testing using topical phenylephrine. All of these cases were unilateral and showed complete resolution over 11–20 weeks. The aetiopathogenesis of idiopathic Horner syndrome remains unknown but suggestions include autoimmune demyelination, direct trauma to the pre-ganglionic axons as they ascend the neck, or a vascular aetiology related to the close proximity of the internal carotid artery and sympathetic axons.

Clinical approach to unilateral miosis

1. Confirm that the miotic pupil is the abnormal pupil by examination in light and dark environments.

2. Have any topical medications be recently applied that could cause miosis (e.g. pilocarpine)?

3. Perform an ophthalmic examination to assess for retrobulbar disease or primary ocular disorders that could result in miosis (e.g. uveitis, ocular discomfort).
   - Refer to an ophthalmologist or further work-up in practice as appropriate.

4. If the eye otherwise appears healthy, then a neurological cause for miosis is most likely. Horner syndrome is the most common neurological cause for unilateral miosis and would be supported by concurrent ptosis, third eyelid protrusion, and enophthalmos.

5. Perform a full clinical and neurological examination
   - Assess for other neurological deficits that would be consistent with either an upper motor neuron (first-order) Horner syndrome, or damage to the T1–T3 spinal cord segments/nerve roots (e.g. reduced level of mentation for brainstem lesions, tetraparesis, hemiparesis, proprioceptive deficits, ipsilateral thoracic limb monoparesis).
   - In the absence of other neurological deficits to indicate a brainstem localisation, a lesion in the region of the tympanic bulla would be most likely if there is a Horner syndrome with concurrent vestibular syndrome and/or facial paralysis. Otitis media is a common cause of Horner syndrome with concurrent vestibular syndrome and/or facial paralysis in cats.

6. If other neurological deficits are present, then referral for further neurological assessment and advanced imaging is advised. If referral is not possible, then the options for further diagnostic investigations and management in general practice will depend upon the neuroanatomic localisation and your differential diagnoses. The reader is referred to Sections 6.10 'Paresis, Paralysis, and Proprioceptive Ataxia' and 6.11 'Monoparesis and Lameness' for further discussion on the approach to spinal cord lesions and monoparesis. Tympanic bulla radiography and/or myringotomy could be performed if there is a high clinical suspicion of a tympanic bulla lesion (e.g. otitis media).

7. If the neurological examination is otherwise normal, then a pre-ganglionic lesion in the cranial thorax / neck or a post-ganglionic lesion are most likely.
   - Perform thorough palpation of the cervical region for any lesions that could affect the sympathetic nerve fibres as they ascend the neck.
   - A phenylephrine response test could be used to guide whether a pre- or post-ganglionic lesion is most likely (Box 6.5.4).

8. If a pre-ganglionic lesion is suspected, then appropriate further investigations could include thoracic radiography, ultrasound examination of the neck, or advanced imaging (e.g. CT) of the thorax and neck. Referral for further neurological examination, with a view to advanced imaging if indicated, should always be discussed with an owner at this time.

9. Monitoring the clinical course without treatment is not an unreasonable option if funds are not available for further investigations and the animal is otherwise well. This is particularly the case if there is a high clinical suspicion

Box 6.5.4 The Phenylephrine Response Test

Phenylephrine is a direct sympathomimetic agent that can be used to confirm sympathetic denervation of the pupil dilator muscles by stimulating dilation of the affected pupil. The time to pupil dilation following topical application of 1% phenylephrine eye drops into the affected eye has been suggested to guide the distinction between a pre-ganglionic and post-ganglionic lesion:

- pupil dilation in <20 minutes most consistent with a post-ganglionic lesion (<5–8 minutes if 10% drops are used)
- pupil dilation in 20–45 minutes more consistent with a pre-ganglionic lesion.

This test is not required if there are concurrent neurological deficits that would confirm either an upper motor neuron (first-order) lesion or damage to the T1–T3 spinal cord segments/nerve roots (e.g. hemiparesis, ipsilateral thoracic limb monoparesis).

The phenylephrine response test should only be used as a guide to the neuroanatomic localisation and the results should always be combined with other clinical findings and the results of further investigations. The test requires denervation hypersensitivity of the pupil dilator muscles to have occurred, which may take 7–14 days, therefore the results may not be reliable before this time.

of idiopathic Horner syndrome (e.g. in a male Golden Retriever) (see Box 6.5.3). In this instance, owners should always be warned of the possibility of an underlying disease process that may have a poor prognosis if clinical progression is subsequently observed.

6.6 Cranial Nerve Dysfunction

Edward Ives

Cranial nerve deficits are frequently encountered in general practice and can have a multitude of clinical presentations from unilateral dysfunction of a single cranial nerve, to involvement of multiple cranial nerves +/– the lower motor neurons to the limbs and trunk. A logical approach is therefore essential in order to accurately localise the lesion and plan further investigations.

There are 12 pairs of cranial nerves that, with the exception of the olfactory (I) and optic (II) nerves, have cell bodies that lie within corresponding brainstem nuclei. A peripheral, axonal component connects each nucleus to either the receptor organ for sensory functions, or to the effector muscle or gland for motor functions. Cranial nerve dysfunction can therefore be termed 'central' if a lesion affects the neuronal cell bodies in a brainstem nucleus, or 'peripheral' if it affects the receptor organ, effector muscle, NMJ, or the cranial nerve axons after they have left the brainstem. As will be discussed for vestibular dysfunction in Section 6.7 'Vestibular Syndrome', this distinction is important as different disease processes, with potentially different treatments and prognoses, will be more likely to affect the central component compared to peripheral component.

The initial considerations in the approach to any case with cranial nerve dysfunction should be:

1. Is only one cranial nerve affected, or are multiple nerves affected?
   - The involvement of multiple cranial nerves on the same side, particularly if their nuclei reside close to each other in the brainstem, should increase the index of suspicion for a central lesion (e.g. trigeminal (V), facial (VII), and vestibulocochlear (VIII) nerves).
   - However, there are also regions outside the brain where specific cranial nerves lie in close anatomical association. A certain combination of cranial nerve deficits may therefore be highly suggestive a particular peripheral localisation, such as in the region of the tympanic bulla if the facial nerve, vestibulocochlear nerve, and sympathetic fibres to the head are affected, or the middle cranial fossa if there is concurrent involvement of the oculomotor (III), trochlear (IV), trigeminal (V), and abducens (VI) nerves.
2. Are the clinical signs unilateral or bilateral?
   - Unilateral paresis or paralysis of a single muscle is most likely to reflect a lesion affecting the cranial nerve (nucleus or axons), rather than the NMJ or muscle itself. Whilst individual cranial muscles can be affected by myopathies or junctionopathies, this involvement is usually bilateral and symmetric.
   - Bilateral dysfunction of one or more cranial nerves should increase the index of suspicion for a peripheral lesion, particularly if the level of mentation remains bright and there are no proprioceptive deficits. A central lesion that is large enough to damage the brainstem nuclei on both sides would be expected to affect adjacent neuronal pathways, resulting in concurrent neurological deficits (e.g. stupor/coma, tetraparesis, proprioceptive deficits in all limbs).
3. Are there any other neurological deficits that would be consistent with a brainstem neuroanatomic localisation (e.g. tetraparesis, hemiparesis, proprioceptive deficits, an abnormal level of mentation)?
4. Are there any other clinical signs to suggest a generalised neuromuscular disorder?
   - Dependent on whether this represents a peripheral neuropathy, myopathy, or junctionopathy, other clinical signs could include exercise intolerance, a stiff gait in all limbs, generalised muscle atrophy, reduced limb muscle tone, and reduced/absent spinal reflexes. The approach to neuromuscular disease is further discussed in Section 6.12 'Neuromuscular Weakness'.

This section will focus on an approach to disorders affecting the two most commonly affected cranial nerves in general practice: the trigeminal (V) and facial (VII) nerves. Dysfunction of the olfactory (I) nerve results in an inability to smell, termed anosmia. However, this is difficult to appreciate clinically, particularly if partial or unilateral, and would rarely occur or be recognised in isolation. Dysfunction of the optic (II) and oculomotor (III) nerves is discussed further in Sections 6.4 'Blindness' and 6.5 'Abnormalities of Pupil Size', respectively. Deficits relating to trochlear (IV) or abducens (VI) nerve dysfunction are rarely observed in isolation, resulting in different forms of resting strabismus as discussed in Chapter 3. The reader is referred to Section 6.7 'Vestibular Syndrome' for a summary of the approach to vestibulocochlear (VIII) nerve dysfunction. Dysfunction of the vagus (X) nerve, resulting in megaoesophagus or laryngeal paralysis, and the hypoglossal (XII) nerve, resulting in paresis of the tongue, are also discussed at the end of this section.

6.6.1 Trigeminal Nerve

The trigeminal nerve is the fifth cranial nerve and contains both motor and sensory fibres. It is comprised of three main branches.

- The ophthalmic branch, providing sensory information from the skin overlying the medial canthus of the eye, cornea, nasal septum, and frontal region.
- The maxillary branch, providing sensory information from the skin overlying the muzzle, upper lips, lateral canthus of the eye, and top of the head.
- The mandibular branch, providing sensory information from the skin overlying the mandible, and motor innervation to the muscles of mastication (temporalis, masseter, pterygoids, and rostral digastricus).

From a clinical perspective, dysfunction of the trigeminal nerve may result in two primary abnormalities on the neurological examination.

- Loss of facial sensation, with the region affected dependent on the branches involved (e.g. medial canthus of the eye if the ophthalmic branch is affected). This is most frequently recognised as a reduced/absent palpebral reflex in an animal that can still voluntarily blink, assuming that there is normal facial nerve function. Marked neurogenic keratitis may occur following loss of sensory innervation to the cornea, and this can be the primary reason for presentation in some cases.
- Denervation of the masticatory muscles if either the trigeminal motor nucleus in the pons or the motor axons in the mandibular branch are affected. If the lesion is unilateral, this will be clinically apparent as rapid denervation atrophy of the masticatory muscles on the affected side (Figure 6.6.1). These animals will still be able to close their mouth and eat normally, as sufficient strength will remain in the masticatory muscles on the unaffected side. An inability to

keep the mouth closed against the force of gravity ('dropped jaw') will only be seen if the motor components in both trigeminal nerves are affected (i.e. bilateral denervation).

1. Unilateral trigeminal nerve dysfunction

The most common cause of unilateral trigeminal nerve dysfunction in dogs is a trigeminal peripheral nerve sheath tumour (PNST). A presumptive trigeminal PNST was diagnosed in 48% of dogs presenting with unilateral masticatory muscle atrophy in one study (Milodowski et al. 2018). The degree of unilateral masticatory muscle atrophy observed in these cases is often marked (Figure 6.6.1). This asymmetric involvement of the masticatory muscles would not be expected for a primary myopathy, which usually result in bilateral and symmetric muscle loss. Ipsilateral loss of facial sensation may also be observed if the trigeminal sensory fibres are affected. Trigeminal PNSTs can be relatively slow-growing neoplasms, but they will frequently progress along the nerve to invade the brainstem at the level of the pons. Additional neurological deficits can be observed at this stage, including involvement of other cranial nerve nuclei in the near vicinity (e.g. facial, vestibulocochlear, glossopharyngeal, vagus), a reduced level of mentation, ipsilateral hemiparesis, and ipsilateral proprioceptive deficits.

Differential diagnoses for a unilateral trigeminal PNST are listed below.

- A brainstem lesion involving the motor nucleus of the trigeminal nerve (e.g. inflammatory/infectious, another form of extra-axial mass lesion, intra-axial

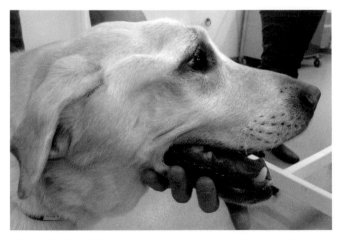

Figure 6.6.1 Marked, right-sided atrophy of the masseter and temporalis muscles in a 10-year-old Labrador Retriever with a peripheral nerve sheath tumour affecting the motor fibres of the right trigeminal nerve. Note the prominent zygomatic arch secondary to loss of the surrounding musculature.

neoplasia). The presence of additional neurological deficits that are consistent with a brainstem lesion should alert the clinician to the possibility of a central rather than peripheral lesion.

- Trauma to one or more branches of the trigeminal nerve (external or iatrogenic).
- A different form of neoplasia that is involving the peripheral component of the trigeminal nerve (e.g. lymphosarcoma, particularly in cats).
- Unilateral inflammation of the trigeminal nerve (trigeminal neuritis). This diagnosis would require biopsy confirmation as it may be difficult to distinguish inflammation from neoplastic infiltration as the cause for nerve enlargement on advanced imaging. A study has reported that dogs with trigeminal neuritis are more likely to show diffuse nerve enlargement without a mass effect, compared to the solitary or lobulated masses with displacement of the adjacent neuropil observed in cases with PNST (Schultz et al. 2007).

Diagnosis of a trigeminal PNST, and the other less common causes of unilateral masticatory muscle atrophy, requires advanced imaging of the head (Figure 6.6.2). This can also be used to evaluate the proximity of a suspected PNST to the brainstem, which may guide the likely rate of clinical progression. A recent association between trigeminal nerve lesions on MRI and the presence of asymptomatic, ipsilateral middle ear effusion has also been reported

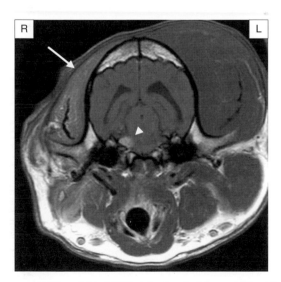

Figure 6.6.2 A transverse T1-weighted MRI at the level of the caudal midbrain/pons following the administration of intravenous contrast media in a 7-year-2-month-old, female neutered Staffordshire Bull Terrier with a 4-week history of progressive, right-sided masticatory muscle atrophy. The neurological examination was otherwise normal. Note the marked, right-sided masticatory muscle atrophy with fibrous and fat replacement (white arrow). The right trigeminal nerve is strongly contrast-enhancing, enlarged (4 mm compared to 1.5 mm on the contralateral side) and is exerting a mild mass effect on the pons (arrow head).

(Kent et al. 2013; Wessmann et al. 2013). This is suggested to result from denervation of the tensor veli palatini muscle, failure of dilation of the Eustachian tube, and reduced drainage of the middle ear (Kent et al. 2015). Thoracic and abdominal imaging can be performed in general practice to screen for neoplasia elsewhere in the body, particularly if there is a high clinical suspicion of lymphoma. However, this may be unrewarding as metastasis is uncommon for primary tumours of the trigeminal nerve.

Surgical resection of trigeminal PNST is performed in humans and has been reported in dogs (Bagley et al. 1998; Schmidt et al. 2013). However, the location of these neoplasms deep within the head means that primary surgical management is rarely performed in veterinary medicine at the current time. Trigeminal PNSTs also appear to be poorly responsive to chemotherapy. Palliative medical management may therefore be chosen until an animal's quality of life becomes adversely affected. This is usually observed when the brainstem becomes compressed by the expanding mass, or if there are complications associated with loss of facial sensation (e.g. keratitis, self-trauma). A survival time ranging from 5 to 21 months was reported for untreated dogs with a presumptive diagnosis of trigeminal PNST in one study (Bagley et al. 1998).

Two recent studies have reported the use of focused stereotactic radiation therapy for trigeminal nerve sheath tumours in dogs. The median disease-specific survival was 745 days in one study (range 99–1375 days, $n = 6$), with no acute adverse effects reported (Hansen et al. 2016). The second study compared 15 dogs treated with stereotactic radiation therapy to 10 dogs not receiving treatment (Swift et al. 2017). All dogs in this study had neoplastic extension into the brainstem at the time of diagnosis. Of the 15 dogs treated with stereotactic radiation therapy, one had improved masticatory muscle atrophy, and six had poor ocular health after treatment. Neurologic signs improved in 4/5 dogs with intracranial signs. The difference in mean survival time between the two groups was not statistically significant but the study was limited by both sample size and selection bias (mean 95% CI for unirradiated dogs was 44–424 days and mean 95% CI for dogs receiving stereotactic radiation therapy was 260–518 days).

2. Bilateral trigeminal nerve dysfunction

Bilateral dysfunction of the trigeminal motor fibres presents as a loss of masticatory muscle tone and an inability to close the mouth, colloquially known as a 'dropped jaw'. Animals will often have a history of drooling and abnormal prehension of food, but they remain able to move their tongue and swallow if food can get to the pharyngeal region. An important differential diagnosis for a dropped jaw is an *unwillingness* to close the mouth rather than an *inability* to close to the mouth. This may be observed secondary to painful conditions such as masticatory myositis, temporomandibular joint disease, craniomandibular osteopathy, retrobulbar lesions, dental disease, oropharyngeal foreign bodies, or tongue lesions.

If an unwillingness to close the mouth is excluded, then a full neurological examination should be performed to localise the lesion to either the peripheral, axonal component of both trigeminal nerves, or to the trigeminal motor nuclei in the brainstem (pons). As discussed previously, a central lesion that is large enough to affect both trigeminal motor nuclei should be accompanied by other neurological deficits, such as tetraparesis, ataxia of all limbs, proprioceptive deficits, a reduced level of mentation, or other cranial nerve deficits.

In the absence of other neurological deficits, bilateral trigeminal dysfunction most commonly represents a peripheral lesion. Horner syndrome may be observed in some cases if the sympathetic fibres that run in close association with the trigeminal nerves are also affected. In a retrospective study of 29 dogs that were unable to close their mouths due to flaccid paresis/paralysis of the masticatory muscles, an idiopathic trigeminal neuropathy was diagnosed in 26 dogs based on complete resolution of the clinical signs and a lack of any long-term neurological disease (Mayhew et al. 2002) (see Box 6.6.1). The remaining three dogs were diagnosed with lymphosarcoma, *N. caninum* infection, and polyneuritis of unknown origin following post-mortem examination. Lymphosarcoma should always be considered in cats as idiopathic disease appears to be less common in this species. Bilateral trigeminal neuropathy has also been reported secondary to immune-mediated inflammation of the dura mater (pachymeningitis) (Roynard et al. 2012). This likely represents involvement of the trigeminal nerves as they exit the brainstem via its surrounding meninges. Dogs with this condition usually present with additional neurological deficits, such as blindness and mentation change. Obtaining a full travel history is also important in all cases, as the early stages of rabies may rarely present as a dropped jaw if there has been a bite to the face.

Box 6.6.1 Idiopathic Trigeminal Neuropathy

This condition is suspected to represent an autoimmune demyelinating neuritis. The extent of bilateral masticatory muscle atrophy observed in these cases depends on the degree of axonal loss but is usually mild. Idiopathic trigeminal neuropathy is the most common cause of flaccid paresis/paralysis of the masticatory muscles in dogs, and Golden Retrievers appear to be over-represented (Mayhew et al. 2002). Loss of facial sensation has been reported in around a third of cases, concurrent Horner syndrome in 10% of cases, and facial nerve deficits in 10% of cases as part of a suspected inflammatory cranial polyneuropathy. Idiopathic trigeminal neuropathy should self-resolve without treatment over 3–4 weeks, with a mean time to recovery of 22 days reported by one study (Mayhew et al. 2002). Assisted feeding with balls of wet food is often required over this time, or an oesophagostomy tube can be placed in more severely affected cases. Ocular lubrication should be used in cases with sensory dysfunction. Corticosteroid therapy has not been reported to influence the clinical course of this condition.

a. Clinical approach to bilateral trigeminal neuropathy

1. Exclude an unwillingness to close the mouth and confirm an inability to close the mouth as a result of loss of jaw tone.
2. Perform a full neurological examination. Referral for advanced imaging would be advised if there are concurrent neurological deficits consistent with a central lesion.
3. If there are no additional neurological deficits, then the option of referral should still be discussed. If referral is not an option, then further investigations that could be performed in general practice would include serological testing for *N. caninum* in dogs, and screening for lymphoma affecting other body systems (especially in cats). It is not unreasonable to make a presumptive clinical diagnosis of idiopathic trigeminal neuropathy in a dog that is otherwise well. However, further investigations should always be advised if there is no clinical improvement over 2–4 weeks, or if other neurological deficits are observed at any time.

b. Bilateral masticatory muscle atrophy

A disorder that affects the motor fibres in both trigeminal nerves may result in bilateral masticatory muscle atrophy, but this is invariably accompanied by loss of jaw tone and an inability to close the mouth (see above). Bilateral masticatory muscle atrophy *without* a loss of jaw function most frequently occurs secondary to disorders affecting the masticatory muscles themselves. This can present as an isolated masticatory myopathy, or as part of a more generalised polymyopathy (Evans et al. 2004).

The masticatory muscles appear particularly susceptible to atrophy resulting from systemic disease processes or secondary to corticosteroid excess. This is often more noticeable than the accompanying atrophy of the appendicular muscles. Therefore, hyperadrenocorticism, exogenous steroid therapy, and systemic conditions that result in cachexia (e.g. neoplasia, cardiac failure, systemic inflammatory disease, malnutrition, maldigestion, malabsorption) should always be considered in cases with bilateral masticatory muscle atrophy. Age-related atrophy of the masticatory muscles, termed sarcopenia, can also be observed and may be related to enhanced autophagocytosis with ageing (Pagano et al. 2015).

In the absence of systemic disease or corticosteroid excess, the most common cause of bilateral masticatory muscle atrophy (without loss of jaw tone) is inflammation and destruction of the masticatory muscles. This may form part of a generalised myopathy affecting skeletal muscles throughout the body (e.g. idiopathic polymyositis, *N. caninum* myositis (Figure 6.6.3)). However, it is more commonly observed as an isolated, sterile inflammatory condition called masticatory myositis (Evans et al. 2004; Paciello et al. 2007; Shelton et al. 1987) (see Box 6.6.2).

Box 6.6.2 Masticatory Myositis

This is a suspected autoimmune condition that results in damage to the Type II-M myofibres that are unique to the masticatory muscles (Paciello et al. 2007, Shelton et al. 1987). This results in two phases.

- *An acute phase* – swollen painful masticatory muscles, raised submandibular lymph nodes, reluctance to eat/open mouth +/– exophthalmos secondary to swelling of the masticatory muscles behind the eyes.
- *A chronic phase* – bilateral masticatory muscle atrophy with fibrous replacement, often in conjunction with enophthalmos and third eyelid protrusion secondary to loss of muscle mass behind the eyes.

Masticatory myositis is most frequently observed in young adult, large breed dogs, with the German Shepherd Dog and Hungarian Vizsla appearing over-represented (Tauro et al. 2015). An atypical form has been reported in three 12-week-old Cavalier King Charles Spaniel littermates (Pitcher and Hahn 2007). Masticatory myositis has also been reported in a mixed breed cat presenting with trismus (Blazejewski and Shelton 2018).

Diagnosis:

- Clinical signs – bilateral masticatory muscle swelling or atrophy dependent on whether the animal presents in the acute or chronic phase. The acute phase may be mild and short and can be missed by some owners. Therefore, masticatory myositis should not be excluded if there is no prior history of muscle swelling or discomfort.
- Exclusion of other causes for bilateral masticatory muscle atrophy (cachexia, mal-nutrition, hyperadrenocorticism, exogenous corticosteroid therapy).
- Serum biochemistry – elevated serum muscle enzymes may be observed (creatine kinase [CK], AST, ALT).
- Serum Type II-M antibody titre – this test will result in a definitive diagnosis if ele-vated; however, the serum titre may be normal during the chronic phase or after steroid therapy. One study reported a positive result in 65% of affected cases (Evans et al. 2004).
- Muscle biopsy – this can confirm the diagnosis by demonstrating inflammatory infil-trates (primarily lymphocytes), muscle necrosis, and by excluding the presence of infectious agents.
- Infectious disease testing – *N. caninum* (Figure 6.6.3), *T. gondii, Leishmania infantum* (Vamvakidis et al. 2000).
- Magnetic resonance imaging – symmetric, heterogeneous hyperintensity within the masticatory muscles is observed in the acute phase, followed by atrophy and T1W muscle hyperintensity in the chronic phase (Cauduro et al. 2013). The computed

Box 6.6.2 (Continued)

> tomographic appearance of masticatory myositis has also been reported in dogs (Reiter and Schwarz 2007).
>
> - Electromyography – abnormal spontaneous myofibre activity in the affected muscles under general anaesthesia. This test is most useful to assess for involvement of other skeletal muscle groups in the case of a generalised polymyopathy.
>
> **Treatment:**
>
> - Immunosuppressive doses of prednisolone are the most common treatment for masticatory myositis, starting at 1 mg/kg per os twice daily for 2–4 weeks, followed by a steady tapering to 0.5 mg/kg per os every other day. Relapsing clinical signs may be observed as the dose is reduced.
> - The use of adjunctive immunosuppressive agents, such as cyclosporine or azathioprine, can be used in dogs that do not adequately respond to prednisolone alone. These can also be useful as steroid-sparing agents, particularly in large dogs that may not tolerate high oral doses of prednisolone.
> - Chronic muscle loss may result in permanent muscle atrophy and dysphagia. It is therefore advised to encourage jaw movements to minimise the risk of fibrosis and restricted jaw movements in the long term (e.g. chew toys).

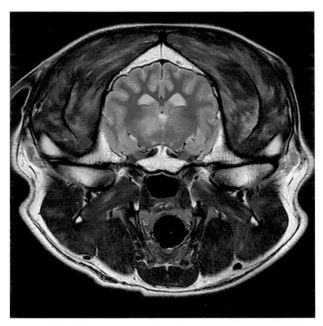

Figure 6.6.3 A transverse T2-weighted MRI at the level of the thalamus in a dog with myositis of the masticatory muscles resulting from *Neospora caninum* infection. Note the multifocal hyperintense lesions throughout the masticatory muscles, particularly affecting the temporalis muscles bilaterally. This dog also presented with hypermetria and ataxia of all limbs secondary to protozoal meningoencephalitis affecting the cerebellum (see Section 6.8 'Cerebellar Dysfunction').

6.6.2 Facial Nerve

The facial nerve is the seventh cranial nerve and it has three primary functions:

1. motor innervation to the muscles of facial expression
2. parasympathetic innervation to the mandibular and sublingual salivary glands, lacrimal glands, and lateral nasal glands
3. special sensation of taste from the rostral two thirds of the tongue – loss of this function is difficult to appreciate clinically.

Clinical signs of facial nerve dysfunction can therefore include:

- Ipsilateral drooping of the upper and lower lips. The lip commissure on the affected side will be lower than the normal side when a dog is panting.
- Drooping of the ear on the affected side in dogs without a rigid auricular cartilage. Animals with a rigid auricular cartilage will be unable to move the affected ear back against the head when excited or nervous (Figure 6.6.4).
- Drooling from the affected side of the mouth, food and salivation accumulation, and secondary halitosis.
- Absent spontaneous blinking, an absent palpebral reflex, and absent menace response on the affected side. Retraction of the eyeball and subtle third eyelid protrusion may still be observed at the time of palpebral reflex and menace response testing. This confirms intact facial sensation and vision, respectively.
- Exposure keratitis secondary to loss of spontaneous blinking, especially in brachycephalic breeds.

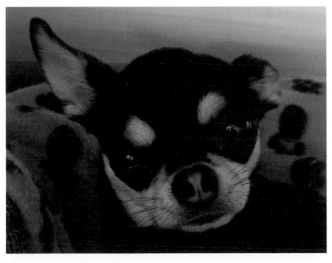

Figure 6.6.4 Right-sided facial paralysis in a Chihuahua with inflammatory brain disease. Note the narrow palpebral fissure on the right side and the inability to voluntarily retract the right ear against the head compared to the normal left side.

- Ipsilateral neurogenic keratoconjunctivitis sicca (KCS) secondary to loss of tear production if the parasympathetic fibres to the lacrimal glands are affected (Box 6.6.3).
- Hyperkeratosis of the ipsilateral nasal planum (xeromycteria) if the parasympathetic fibres to the lateral nasal glands are affected (Figure 6.6.5).

These clinical signs can be unilateral or bilateral and result from a lesion at any point along the course of the facial nerve(s), from the motor and parasympathetic nuclei in the brainstem to the target muscles/glands. Junctionopathies and myopathies may also result in facial paresis, which will usually be bilateral and associated with other clinical signs of generalised neuromuscular weakness. As for trigeminal nerve dysfunction, a full neurological examination is important to distinguish between a central and peripheral lesion localisation.

1. Central lesions

Central (brainstem) lesions resulting in facial paralysis are less frequently observed in practice compared to peripheral lesions. Differential diagnoses include vascular events (e.g. ischaemic stroke), neoplasia, and inflammatory or infectious disorders. These lesions will usually be accompanied by other neurological deficits, such as an altered level of mentation, other cranial nerve deficits, tetra-/hemiparesis, or ataxia of all limbs. However, it is important to remember that whilst the presence of these signs confirms a central lesion, their absence does not exclude one. Extra-axial,

---

Box 6.6.3 Neurogenic Keratoconjunctivitis Sicca (Neurogenic 'Dry Eye')

This condition may be observed in combination with facial nerve paralysis or it can occur in isolation as an idiopathic disorder (Matheis et al. 2012). Tear production is often markedly reduced, with Schirmer tear test values in the range of 1–5 mm/min in the affected eye(s) (normal >15 mm/min). Ipsilateral hyperkeratosis of the nasal planum (xeromycteria) may also be seen secondary to denervation of the lateral nasal glands in cases with concurrent facial paralysis (Figure 6.6.5). An important differential diagnosis for neurogenic keratoconjunctivitis sicca (KCS) should always be immune-mediated KCS, as the pathogenesis and treatment of these conditions differ. Firstly, immune-mediated KCS should not be associated with a concurrent facial nerve paralysis. Secondly, treatment of immune-mediated KCS involves the application of topical cyclosporine to restore tear production by regulating immune-mediated destruction of the lacrimal glands. This treatment will not be effective for neurogenic KCS other than by providing a very expensive lubricant. Treatment of neurogenic KCS involves the regular application of ocular lubrication to avoid keratitis and corneal ulceration. Administration of 1% pilocarpine eye drops *by mouth* has also been reported to treat neurogenic KCS, starting with one drop per 10 kg body weight twice daily until either restoration of tear production is observed or there are adverse effects of treatment (vomiting, diarrhoea, salivation). The idiopathic form of neurogenic KCS may self-resolve over a period of 3–4 months (Matheis et al. 2012).

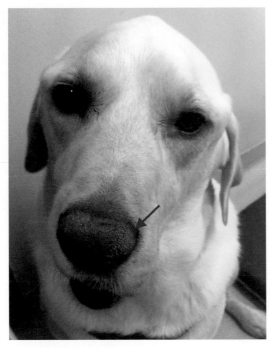

Figure 6.6.5 Left-sided xeromycteria in a dog with left-sided facial paralysis and peripheral vestibular syndrome. Note the hyperkeratosis of the left side of the nasal planum (arrow) compared to the normal right side, and also the mild left head tilt and drooping of the left upper lip.

intracranial masses in the region of the internal acoustic meatus can sometimes result in facial paralysis and/or vestibular dysfunction without other signs of brainstem involvement. A definitive diagnosis of central disease requires referral for advanced imaging of the head +/− CSF analysis. Screening of the thorax and abdomen for distant neoplasia can also be performed, particularly if there are progressive clinical signs and/or referral is not an option. Blood pressure testing, haematology, serum biochemistry, and urinalysis should be performed to investigate possible predisposing factors for cerebrovascular disease if there is consistent clinical history (e.g. an acute, non-progressive, non-painful, lateralised central lesion).

2. Peripheral lesions

Disorders that affect the peripheral component of the facial nerve(s) are more commonly observed in general practice compared to central lesions. These conditions may result in unilateral or bilateral clinical signs, with possible differential diagnoses including:

- *Infectious*: Otitis media/interna is a common cause of facial paresis/paralysis, particularly in cats. Concurrent vestibular syndrome and/or Horner syndrome may be observed (Figure 6.6.6).

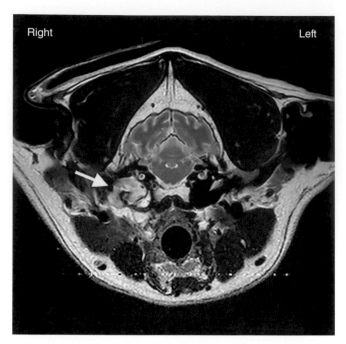

Figure 6.6.6 A transverse T2-weighted MRI at the level of the tympanic bullae in an 8-year-5-month old, male neutered Pyrenean Mountain Dog with a 1-week history of right facial paralysis, a right head tilt, and pain on opening the mouth. The MRI demonstrates heterogeneous, hyperintense material filling the right tympanic bulla (arrow), focal osteolysis of the bulla wall, and extension into the para-aural soft tissues. Note the difference when compared to the normal, gas-filled, hypointense tympanic bulla on the left side. A final diagnosis of bacterial otitis media and para-aural abscessation was made following myringotomy and the dog was treated surgically by total ear canal ablation (TECA) and lateral bulla osteotomy.

- *Traumatic*: External trauma (e.g. petrous temporal bone fracture) or iatrogenic trauma (e.g. following bulla osteotomy surgery).
- *Metabolic*: Hypothyroidism has been associated with facial paralysis in dogs but the evidence to support this association remains inconclusive (Jaggy and Oliver 1994).
- *Neoplasia*: PNST, lymphosarcoma, local invasion by adjacent neoplasia (e.g. affecting the tympanic bulla).
- *Idiopathic facial neuropathy*: This is a diagnosis of exclusion that is further described in Box 6.6.4.
- As part of a *generalised neuromuscular disorder*, such as polyneuropathy (e.g. polyradiculoneuritis) or junctionopathy (e.g. botulism, myasthenia gravis). Bilateral facial paresis/paralysis will be apparent in these cases.

The option of referral for further assessment should always offered to the owner of an animal with facial paralysis. MRI is the imaging modality of choice

---

Box 6.6.4 Idiopathic Facial Neuropathy

Idiopathic facial neuropathy is the most common cause of facial paralysis in dogs, reported in up to 75% of cases (Kern and Erb 1987). Cocker Spaniels and Cavalier King Charles Spaniels appear over-represented. There is usually an acute onset of unilateral or bilateral clinical signs, and the neurological examination is consistent with a peripheral lesion localisation. In unilateral cases, the contralateral side may subsequently become affected. Studies have reported that 40–70% of dogs may show concurrent vestibular signs (head tilt, ataxia, nystagmus), which is suggested to reflect the close proximity of the facial and vestibulocochlear nerves where they enter and exit the skull via the internal acoustic meatus (Smith et al. 2012). This condition has been termed 'facial and vestibular neuropathy of unknown origin' (FVNUO). A recent study of dogs with FVNUO reported that only 31% of dogs showed complete resolution of clinical signs: 38% showed long-term vestibular signs, 15% had permanent facial paralysis, 46% developed hemifacial contracture, and 15% showed relapse (Jeandel et al. 2016).

Idiopathic facial neuropathy may be analogous to a condition called Bell's Palsy in humans, in which a link has been found to human herpes simplex virus infection. There has been no definitive association found between idiopathic facial neuropathy and viral infection in dogs to date. However, it has been suggested that canine herpes virus-1 infection may be associated with idiopathic vestibular disease and other 'idiopathic' cranial neuropathies (Parzefall et al. 2011). The clinical signs of idiopathic facial neuropathy may self-resolve over 1–3 months, but this may simply reflect fibrosis and restoration of a more normal facial symmetry (hemifacial contracture), rather than a true return of voluntary motor function. Frequent ocular lubrication may be required to reduce the risk of exposure keratitis in an animal that cannot blink. There is currently no evidence to support the use of corticosteroids to accelerate the rate of recovery or to improve the chance of a functional recovery in affected dogs. Further work is required to assess whether a sub-set of dogs may benefit from this treatment and how these cases can be distinguished at the time of diagnosis from those that are unlikely to benefit.

---

as it can be used to exclude a central lesion and can also be used to support a diagnosis of idiopathic facial neuropathy. Enlargement and/or contrast enhancement of the affected facial nerve may be observed in idiopathic cases, with the presence of contrast enhancement potentially associated with a reduced chance of self-resolution (Varejão et al. 2006). Volumetric interpolated breath-hold examination magnetic resonance imaging (VIBE-MRI) has been shown to offer better visualisation of the facial nerve when compared to routine MRI sequences for the investigation of idiopathic facial neuropathy (Smith et al. 2012). A CT scan of the head could be performed if there is a high clinical suspicion of middle ear pathology. Electromyography and nerve conduction studies can be performed if there are other neurological deficits that are consistent with a generalised neuromuscular disorder.

In cases with a suspected peripheral cause for facial nerve paralysis, diagnostic investigations that could be performed in general practice include:

- otoscopic examination +/− myringotomy for cytology, culture, and sensitivity
- tympanic bulla radiography
- serum biochemistry, including total thyroid hormone (T4) and TSH concentrations in dogs
- if referral is not possible and further investigations are unrewarding, then a presumptive diagnosis of idiopathic facial neuropathy could made in a dog with consistent clinical signs, non-progressive disease, and that is otherwise well (Box 6.6.4).

6.6.3 Vagus Nerve
The vagus nerve is the tenth cranial nerve and has sensory, motor, and autonomic functions:

- sensory innervation from the larynx, pharynx, and thoracic and abdominal viscera
- motor innervation to the oesophagus, larynx (recurrent laryngeal branch), and pharynx (together with motor fibres of the glossopharyngeal [IX] nerve)
- parasympathetic innervation to all of the thoracic and abdominal viscera, other than those of the pelvic region.

The most common clinical signs associated with vagus nerve dysfunction are laryngeal paralysis, dysphagia, and regurgitation associated with oesophageal dysmotility (megaoesophagus).

1. Laryngeal paralysis
Laryngeal paresis/paralysis can be a congenital or an acquired condition (Box 6.6.5). It may be the sole clinical sign in some cases but often reflects a more generalised disease process. Typical clinical signs of laryngeal dysfunction include:

- *dysphonia* – most commonly reported by the owner as a change in the tone or strength of the bark
- *inspiratory stridor* – secondary to a failure to abduct the laryngeal cartilages during inspiration
- *exercise intolerance*, particularly during periods of hot weather – this may be severe enough to result in collapse
- *coughing*, particularly when drinking, secondary to an inability to adduct the laryngeal cartilages to protect the upper airway; these animals are at risk of aspiration pneumonia, particularly if there is concurrent pharyngeal weakness.

Box 6.6.5 Congenital Laryngeal Paralysis

Congenital laryngeal paralysis has been reported in a number of dog breeds and should be suspected in animals presenting at <1 year of age. Commonly affected breeds include Bouvier des Flandres, Siberian Huskies, Rottweilers, Pyrenean Mountain Dogs, Dalmatians, Russian Black Terriers, Bull Terriers, and Miniature Schnauzers (Braund et al. 1994; Gabriel et al. 2006; Mahony et al. 1998; von Pfeil et al. 2018). Laryngeal paralysis may also present in young animals as part of a more widespread degenerative disease process (e.g. inherited encephalomyelopathy-polyneuropathy in Rottweiler puppies) (Granger 2011). The clinical signs of laryngeal dysfunction in these cases may precede those of progressive tetraparesis and ataxia. Therefore, the possibility of a progressive, degenerative disease process should always be considered in puppies with laryngeal paralysis, and owners should be counselled accordingly before arytenoid lateralisation is performed (de Lahunta et al. 2015). A late-onset form of hereditary laryngeal paralysis, which is also associated with generalised neuropathic signs, has been reported in the Leonberger (Granger 2011; Shelton et al. 2003).

An important differential diagnosis for laryngeal paresis/paralysis is local structural disease affecting the larynx and/or pharynx, such as trauma, neoplasia, inflammation, infection, or obstruction by a foreign body. This possibility should always be excluded by thorough cervical palpation and laryngoscopic examination prior to performing further investigations. Confirmation of laryngeal paresis/paralysis can be made by direct observation of laryngeal function under a light plane of sedation or anaesthesia. Abnormal movement of the laryngeal cartilages can also be observed using ultrasound.

Laryngeal paralysis may result from:

- *A central lesion that is affecting the motor nucleus of the vagus nerve (nucleus ambiguus) in the caudal brainstem* – neoplastic and inflammatory lesions are most commonly responsible, with advanced imaging of the brain +/– CSF analysis usually required for a diagnosis.
- *A disorder that is affecting the vagus nerve and/or its recurrent laryngeal branch* – the vagus nerve is a long nerve that exits the back of the skull through the tympano-occipital fissure and runs to the larynx via the neck and cranial mediastinum. Potential causes of vagal nerve dysfunction include trauma (e.g. bite wound), iatrogenic damage during cervical surgery, retropharyngeal infections, thyroid neoplasia, and neuronal degeneration. A detailed clinical history and examination of the cervical region can assist in the exclusion of these possible causes.
- *A primary myopathy or junctionopathy that is affecting the skeletal muscles of the larynx* – this may be observed as focal laryngeal involvement, but more commonly forms part of a generalised neuromuscular disease. Differential diagnoses include idiopathic polymyositis, myasthenia gravis, and botulism. The clinical suspicion for each condition will depend upon the concurrent clinical signs and biochemical changes (e.g. elevated muscle enzymes for

polymyositis). Electrodiagnostic testing may be useful to confirm involvement of other muscle groups in these cases.

Laryngeal paralysis is most commonly encountered in middle-aged or older, large breed dogs. It can present in isolation but is more frequently associated with additional neurological deficits that reflect a diffuse polyneuropathy, termed 'laryngeal paralysis-polyneuropathy syndrome' (LPP) (Bookbinder et al. 2016; Braund et al. 1989; Jeffery et al. 2006; Thieman et al. 2010). Labrador Retrievers appear to be over-represented with this condition. Laryngeal paralysis-polyneuropathy (LPP) results in clinical signs of laryngeal paralysis and sciatic nerve dysfunction, including a plantigrade posture, poor hock flexion when walking, reduced pelvic limb withdrawal reflexes, and pelvic limb proprioceptive deficits. The oesophagus may also be affected, resulting in megaoesophagus (see below). It is postulated that the long length of the recurrent laryngeal and sciatic nerves predisposes them to this condition, as the neuronal cell bodies become unable to maintain such a long axon in later life.

Idiopathic laryngeal paralysis is a diagnosis of exclusion in adult dogs that present without other neurological deficits. The early stages of LPP, before the onset of sciatic nerve dysfunction, should always be considered in these cases. Hypothyroidism has been anecdotally associated with laryngeal paralysis in dogs, and thyroid function testing (total T4 and TSH levels) can be performed to exclude this potentially treatable condition (Jaggy and Oliver 1994).

Laryngeal paralysis appears to be rare in cats but has been reported as a unilateral or bilateral condition (Macphail 2014). Unilateral laryngeal paralysis may remain subclinical, and therefore undiagnosed, in cats given their relatively inactive nature compared to dogs. Idiopathic laryngeal paralysis has been reported in cats but neoplastic infiltration, particularly by lymphoma, should always be considered in this species.

Treatment of laryngeal paralysis is required if the clinical signs of stridor, coughing, and exercise intolerance are impacting significantly on an animal's quality of life. This involves surgical lateralisation of the arytenoid cartilage to improve air flow through the larynx (Monnet 2016). Owners should always be warned of the increased risk of aspiration following surgery, particularly in cases with concurrent pharyngeal dysphagia or megaoesophagus (Wilson and Monnet 2016). They should also be made aware that pre-operative exercise intolerance may persist following surgery, particularly in those with a progressive polyneuropathy; dogs with LPP will show an inevitable decline in their pelvic limb gait secondary to sciatic nerve dysfunction over a period of months to years.

A logical approach to a case with suspected laryngeal paralysis should include the following considerations. A short list of differential diagnoses can usually be formulated by combining the clinical history and signalment of the animal together with the results of a thorough general physical examination and neurological examination.

1. Exclude a local structural cause for the clinical signs and confirm laryngeal paralysis.
2. What was the age of the animal at the onset of clinical signs (see Box 6.6.5)?
3. Is there a history of toxin exposure? Laryngeal paralysis has been reported following lead or organophosphate intoxication. Additional clinical signs, specific to the particular toxin, would be expected in these cases, such as weight loss, gastrointestinal signs, seizures, ataxia, and blindness for lead toxicity, and miosis, salivation, gastrointestinal signs, muscle fasciculations, restlessness, or weakness for organophosphate exposure.
4. Is there a history of recent cervical surgery (e.g. thyroid surgery, ventral slot decompression)?
5. Are there any other neurological deficits that would be consistent with a brainstem neuroanatomic localisation? These would include a depressed level of mentation, hemiparesis/tetraparesis, proprioceptive deficits, and other cranial nerve deficits such as facial paralysis, vestibular syndrome, or pharyngeal dysphagia.
6. Are there any other neurological deficits that would be consistent with a generalised neuromuscular disorder? These could include generalised muscle atrophy, exercise intolerance, megaoesophagus, lower motor neuron tetraparesis, and reduced/absent spinal reflexes.

2. Megaoesophagus

Megaoesophagus is the term used to describe oesophageal dilatation, which is frequently accompanied by reduced oesophageal motility and regurgitation of undigested food. As for laryngeal paralysis, megaoesophagus may be secondary to local structural disease, or it may be non-structural resulting from abnormal innervation of the oesophageal musculature. The canine oesophagus is predominately comprised of striated skeletal muscle, meaning that it may be affected by generalised neuromuscular disorders such as polymyopathies and myasthenia gravis.

a. Classification

Local structural disorders resulting in megaoesophagus include intra- and extraluminal masses, obstruction by foreign bodies, oesophageal strictures, hiatal hernia, vascular ring anomalies, and oesophagitis. These disorders frequently result in focal dilation of the oesophagus cranial to the level of obstruction. This is in contrast to non-structural causes, which more frequently result in generalised dilation and dysmotility.

Non-structural megaoesophagus can be classified as:

- Congenital, idiopathic megaoesophagus in animals presenting within 6 months of weaning (at less than around 8 months of age) and for which an underlying cause cannot be found (Boudrieau and Rogers 1985).
- Acquired megaoesophagus – this category can be further subdivided into:
    - Idiopathic acquired megaoesophagus in animals first displaying clinical signs at >8 months of age for which an underlying cause cannot be

found. An idiopathic disorder affecting the sensory innervation of the oesophagus is suspected in these cases. This condition may account for up to 75% of all canine cases with acquired, non-structural megaoesophagus (Boudrieau and Rogers 1985; Nakagawa et al. 2019). However, the incidence of idiopathic disease may be overestimated in older studies as recent advances in both knowledge and the diagnostic tools available mean that an underlying disease process may now be identified in many of these cases.

– Secondary acquired megaoesophagus in animals presenting at any age for which an underlying cause is identified on diagnostic investigations. These animals frequently present with other neurological deficits and/or clinical signs consistent with the presence of an underlying disease process.

b. Clinical signs

The classical clinical sign associated with megaoesophagus is regurgitation of undigested food. This process involves minimal abdominal effort and is usually observed shortly after eating. However, it may be delayed by minutes to several hours in some cases. In order to distinguish regurgitation from gagging or vomiting, it is vital to obtain a thorough clinical history from the owner or observe an episode first-hand. Gagging is typically associated with pharyngeal abnormalities and is observed at the time of swallowing. Vomiting most commonly occurs in association with gastrointestinal disease and is an active process involving abdominal effort. It is also frequently associated with nausea, the vomitus may be partially or completely digested, and often contains bile. However, it can be difficult to distinguish vomiting from regurgitation in many cases, as some animals with oesophageal disorders may appear nauseous and salivate profusely at the time of regurgitation. Weight loss is commonly observed in dogs with megaoesophagus, secondary to frequent regurgitation and reduced calorie intake.

c. Diagnosis and neuroanatomic localisation

The presence of megaoesophagus can be confirmed on conscious, plain thoracic radiography, with a left lateral view being preferred (Figure 6.6.7). Oesophageal dilation may be observed as an incidental finding in animals that have received sedation or a general anaesthetic for imaging. Therefore, care should always be taken in the interpretation of thoracic radiographs in these cases. The use of a barium swallow to highlight oesophageal dilation is not recommended, as animals with megaoesophagus are prone to aspiration, potentially resulting in a chemical pneumonitis.

The neuroanatomic localisation for secondary acquired megaoesophagus can be divided as follows:

• A central lesion that is affecting the motor nucleus of the vagus nerve (nucleus ambiguus) in the caudal brainstem – this is an uncommon cause of acquired

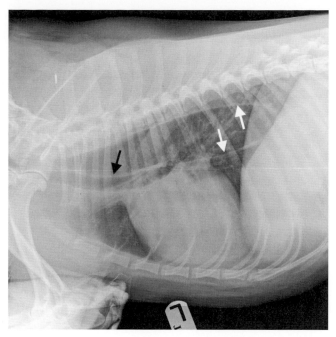

Figure 6.6.7 Left lateral thoracic radiograph in a dog with generalised acquired megaoesophagus secondary to myasthenia gravis. Note the well-defined, linear, soft tissue opacity created by summation of the ventral oesophageal wall and dorsal tracheal wall, termed a 'tracheal stripe sign' (black arrow). Note also the sharp, soft tissue interface from the thoracic inlet to the ventral aspect of the T6 vertebra created by the dorsal wall of the dilated oesophagus contacting the paired longus colli muscles under the vertebral column, and the pair of thin, parallel, soft tissue opacity stripes that converge at the diaphragm representing the dorsal and ventral walls of the dilated oesophagus (white arrows).

megaoesophagus as bilateral vagal dysfunction is typically required to result in clinically significant oesophageal dilation. This would require a large lesion that involves the motor nuclei on both sides of the brainstem, with potentially fatal involvement of other neuroanatomical structures.

- Bilateral dysfunction of the peripheral component of the vagus nerves – megaoesophagus rarely occurs in isolation in these cases and is more commonly seen together with dysfunction of the pharynx, larynx, and/or appendicular muscles (e.g. paraneoplastic polyneuropathy, LPP syndrome).
- A primary myopathy or junctionopathy that is affecting the striated muscles of the oesophagus – this is the most common neuroanatomic localisation for secondary acquired megaoesophagus in dogs and cats. Myasthenia gravis is the most common diagnosis in dogs, which may be focal to the oesophagus or present as a generalised form (Haines 2019; Nakagawa et al. 2019; Yam et al. 1996). Other differential diagnoses include idiopathic polymyositis, infectious myopathies, hypoadrenocorticism, hypothyroidism, and botulism (Bartges and Nielson 1992; Fracassi and Tamborini 2011; Gaynor et al. 1997; Haines 2019;

Whitley 1995). The clinical suspicion for each condition will depend upon the concurrent clinical signs and biochemical changes (e.g. elevated muscle enzymes for myopathies). Electrodiagnostic testing may be useful for the diagnosis of generalised myopathies.

d. Diagnostic approach

The diagnostic approach to megaoesophagus is very similar to that for laryngeal paralysis:

1. Confirm the presence of megaoesophagus and exclude a local structural cause.
2. What was the age of the animal at the onset of clinical signs? Congenital idiopathic megaoesophagus is the most common cause of non-structural megaoesophagus in young animals, but a structural cause should always be considered first (e.g. vascular ring anomaly). Congenital myasthenia gravis should also be considered as a cause for secondary acquired megaoesophagus in a young animal.
3. Is there a history of toxin exposure? Megaoesophagus has been reported as a rare clinical sign associated with lead or organophosphate intoxication.
4. Are there any other neurological deficits that would be consistent with a brainstem neuroanatomic localisation?
5. Are there any other neurological deficits that would be consistent with a generalised neuromuscular disorder?
6. Are there any other clinical signs that could be consistent with an underlying endocrine disorder? These could include gastrointestinal signs and intermittent weakness/collapse for hypoadrenocorticism, or non-pruritic hair loss, weight gain, lethargy, and bradycardia for hypothyroidism.

If megaoesophagus is confirmed on conscious thoracic radiography, local structural disease has been excluded, and there are no additional neurological deficits to suggest a central lesion, then further investigations should include a complete blood cell count, serum biochemistry, and endocrine testing (total T4, TSH, basal cortisol). An ACTH stimulation test should be performed in animals for which hypoadrenocorticism cannot be excluded using a basal cortisol level alone (i.e. those with a basal cortisol <55 nmol/l) (Bovens et al. 2014). Serum muscle enzymes (CK, AST, ALT) can be used to investigate the possibility of a polymyopathy. This can be further excluded using electrodiagnostic testing +/− muscle biopsy. Myasthenia gravis is the most common cause of secondary acquired megaoesophagus in dogs, therefore nicotinic acetylcholine receptor (nAchR) antibody testing is a useful test in general practice. However, false negative results are possible in cases with focal or generalised disease and this should always be considered if there is otherwise a high clinical suspicion for this condition. Repeat testing can be performed after 2–4 weeks in these cases. Radiographic measurements do not appear useful in distinguishing dogs with megaoesophagus secondary to myasthenia gravis from those with megaoesophagus due to other causes (Wray and Sparkes 2006).

e. Management

The management of megaoesophagus should focus on correction of the underlying cause if possible. Megaoesophagus may be reversible in certain cases, such as those with hypothyroidism, hypoadrenocorticism, and in some cases of myasthenia gravis. However, megaoesophagus is frequently permanent, particularly in idiopathic cases.

Management of these cases involves careful feeding and provision of water to reduce the risk of aspiration and secondary pneumonia (Mace et al. 2012):

- Feed a high-quality, calorific food in small portions, multiple times a day. This reduces the volume of food eaten at any one time. Access to other sources of food and water away from meal times should ideally be prevented. The ideal consistency of food to reduce the risk of aspiration varies with the individual; some dogs tolerate balls of wet food best, whereas others cope better with soaked kibble or a slurry of food.
- Mild cases may be fed from a height using elevated food and water bowls. The animal can also be taught to stand with their front paws on a block to increase the height of the mouth relative to the stomach.
- More severe cases benefit from being held vertically for 20–30 minutes after eating, either in an owner's arms or by using a specially designed 'Bailey chair' for bigger dogs.
- A permanent gastrostomy tube can be placed for longer-term feeding in severely affected cases.
- Intermittent, at-home suctioning of oesophageal content has been reported to reduce the incidence of regurgitation and recurrent aspiration pneumonia in dogs with megaoesophagus (Manning et al. 2016).

A recent study has suggested that sildenafil citrate could represent a novel treatment option for dogs with congenital idiopathic megaoesophagus (Quintavalla et al. 2017).

6.6.4 Hypoglossal Nerve

The hypoglossal nerve is the twelfth cranial nerve. It provides motor innervation to geniohyoideus and to the intrinsic and extrinsic muscles of the tongue (styloglossus, hyoglossus, genioglossus). The neuronal cell bodies reside within a motor nucleus in the medulla oblongata of the caudal brainstem, and the axons exit the caudal aspect of the skull via the hypoglossal canal.

Hypoglossal nerve dysfunction presents as ipsilateral atrophy of the tongue. In chronic cases, the tongue may deviate towards to the affected side following denervation and contracture of the intrinsic tongue muscles. Bilateral lesions result in an inability to withdraw the tongue into the mouth and associated difficulty in the prehension of food and water. An important differential diagnosis for bilateral hypoglossal nerve dysfunction is tongue paresis/atrophy secondary to a primary myopathy affecting the tongue. This condition has been reported sporadically in Pembroke Welsh Corgis (Ito et al. 2009; Toyoda et al. 2010). The intrinsic tongue muscles may also be affected in dogs with generalised polymyositis; however, these dogs will typically show other clinical signs consistent with a generalised disease process (e.g. weight loss, generalised muscle atrophy, stiff gait, exercise intolerance, elevated muscle enzymes). Dysphagia secondary to a focal inflammatory myopathy and consequent dorsiflexion of the rostral part of the tongue has been recently reported as an isolated case in a young, female Pitbull Terrier cross-breed dog (Strøm et al. 2018). The tongue may also be affected as a component of the generalised neuromuscular weakness observed in cases with botulism.

The hypoglossal nerve is rarely affected in isolation and is more frequently affected by lesions that also involve adjacent cranial nerves. This may occur at the level of the brainstem nuclei, or where the individual nerves are closely associated as they exit the skull. These cranial nerves include the vestibulocochlear nerve (VIII), glossopharyngeal nerve (IX), and vagus nerve (X). Tongue atrophy and paresis may therefore be observed in combination with other neurological deficits, such as vestibular syndrome, pharyngeal dysphagia, laryngeal paralysis, or megaoesophagus. A depressed level of mentation, ipsilateral hemiparesis, tetraparesis, and/or ataxia of all limbs may be observed if the lesion involves the brainstem nuclei (Figure 6.6.8). These additional deficits would be absent if the lesion is situated outside the skull and is affecting the cranial nerve axons as they exit from their respective foramina. Radiography and/or ultrasonography of the caudal aspect of the skull can be performed in general practice

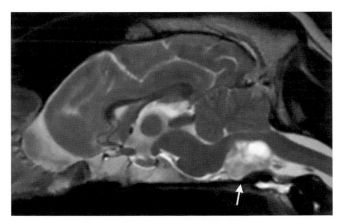

Figure 6.6.8 A mid-sagittal T2-weighted MRI in an 8-year-1-month old, female neutered Labrador Retriever with a 2-week history of lethargy, pacing, a low head carriage, dysphagia, and drooling from the left side of the mouth. Neurological examination revealed a depressed level of mentation, compulsive pacing, mild tetraparesis and ataxia of all limbs, delayed proprioception in all limbs, intact withdrawal reflexes in all limbs, a positional vertical nystagmus on head elevation, a poor gag reflex, and reduced tongue tone. The neuroanatomic localisation was to the brainstem. The MRI demonstrates an ovoid, broad-based, extra-axial mass lesion with a cystic component that is lying ventral to the medulla oblongata and is resulting in marked, dorsal deviation of the brainstem. This mass was suspected to represent a meningioma, but histopathology was not performed in this case to confirm the diagnosis.

if unilateral tongue paresis/atrophy is noted, with or without concurrent involvement of other cranial nerves. Referral for advanced imaging of the head and CSF analysis is recommended in animals with a suspected brainstem lesion. In contrast to the trigeminal and facial nerves, an idiopathic cause of hypoglossal nerve dysfunction has not been reported in dogs or cats, therefore a structural cause should always be investigated in these cases if possible.

6.7 Vestibular Syndrome

Paul M. Freeman

The vestibular system broadly consists of the sensory organs located in the inner ear (semi-circular canals, utricle, and saccule), the vestibulocochlear nerve, and the vestibular nuclei of the brainstem. A detailed description of the anatomical structures of the vestibular system is beyond the scope of this book but is available in many other texts for the interested reader. What is required for the general practitioner is an understanding of the functional anatomy and how this affects the clinical approach to vestibular disease (see Figure 6.7.1). For the purposes of formulating a sensible approach to differential diagnoses and prognosis, the vestibular system may be divided into peripheral and central components; the sensory organs of the inner ear and the vestibulocochlear nerve comprise the peripheral vestibular system, and the brainstem vestibular nuclei and associated cerebellar projections form the central vestibular system.

The vestibular nuclei in the brainstem project axons rostrally via the medial longitudinal fasciculus (MLF) to the nuclei of cranial nerves III, IV, and VI in order to control eyeball position and movement. Axonal projections also pass via the thalamus to the cerebral cortex to enable conscious perception of head and body position. Deeper fibres project to the vomiting centre of the medulla oblongata. Caudally, fibres from the vestibular nuclei form the medial and lateral vestibulospinal tracts, which are motor tracts that predominantly facilitate the ipsilateral extensor muscles. Through these fibres, they are responsible for maintaining weight-bearing and posture of the limbs, neck, and trunk.

In addition, the vestibulocochlear nerve projects directly to the cerebellum, and there are further connections between the cerebellum and the brainstem vestibular nuclei. The cerebellum is largely responsible for coordinating movement, and it also has a mainly *inhibitory* effect on the vestibular nuclei via ipsilateral projections. Finally, there are afferent fibres which travel from the dorsal nerve roots of the first three cervical spinal cord segments (C1–C3) to the vestibular nuclei that are thought to play a role in maintaining head and neck position. The basic anatomy and important connections to be aware of in order to understand the common reasons behind vestibular dysfunction are illustrated in Figure 6.7.1.

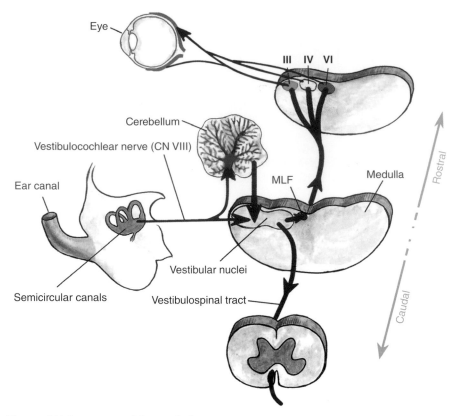

Figure 6.7.1 Anatomy of the vestibular system.

6.7.1 Clinical Signs of Vestibular Disease

In order to adequately assess and approach vestibular cases, it is important to understand the potential presenting signs of vestibular disease. An understanding of the functional anatomy of the vestibular system allows for a better appreciation of the various signs of vestibular dysfunction, and the possible neuroanatomical localisations when faced with such a case. The major signs of vestibular disease, some or all of which may be present in any case, are summarised below.

Head tilt (Figure 6.7.2) – This is when the horizontal axis of the head (through the eyes) is rotated relative to the sagittal plane of the animal. It must be differentiated from head turn, which is when the head is turned towards the body, but the horizontal axis remains perpendicular to the sagittal plane, as may be seen in forebrain disease. A head tilt almost always implies vestibular disease, although in some instances of painful otitis externa an animal may hold the head tilted to one side because of pain.

Vestibular ataxia – Vestibular ataxia involves the tendency to drift or fall towards the affected side, due to loss of normal extensor muscle tone. There may also be tight circling to that side (see Video 17). In cases of bilateral vestibular

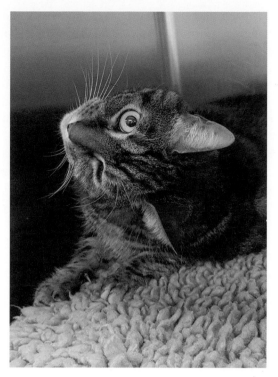

Figure 6.7.2 Head tilt. This cat is suffering from a left central vestibular syndrome and is displaying a particularly severe left head tilt. The gait was also severely affected, although the severity of the signs does not always correlate with the prognosis in vestibular syndrome.

disease, animals tend to crouch low and often show wide excursions of the head from side to side. The tail is often carried high in cats as a means of improving balance (see Video 27 and Figure 3.6).

Nystagmus – Nystagmus is involuntary or uncontrolled eye movement and is seen frequently as part of vestibular syndrome. Nystagmus can be induced in a *normal* animal by moving the head from side to side (the vestibulo-ocular reflex, or physiologic nystagmus). This ensures that the eyes are kept centrally positioned to maximise visual acuity. In cases with vestibular dysfunction, reduced vestibular output on the affected side when the head is not moving is 'interpreted' as movement of the head, causing the eyes to drift slowly towards the affected side, and then 'run away' rapidly from the side of the lesion. This is termed a 'jerk nystagmus' as it consists of these fast and slow phases (see Video 20). In bilateral disease, both the vestibulo-ocular reflex and any pathological nystagmus are absent, since there is symmetric loss of vestibular information bilaterally.

Nystagmus may be horizontal, rotatory, or vertical. When horizontal or rotatory, the slow phase is typically directed towards the affected side. The loss of unilateral vestibular signal that causes nystagmus is often rapidly superseded by visual compensation, and this can lead to resolution of the spontaneous nystagmus.

When vestibular disease is suspected but signs are subtle, an abnormal 'positional' nystagmus can sometimes be induced by placing the animal in an abnormal position (e.g. lying on its back looking up [see Figure 6.7.3], or by elevating the head) (see Video 25). Similarly, blindfolding an animal with vestibular disease will remove the ability to visually compensate and will often cause a marked deterioration in signs. See Chapter 3 for further discussion of how different characteristics of a nystagmus (e.g. direction or rate) can be used to guide the distinction between a suspected peripheral or central vestibular syndrome.

Strabismus – Strabismus is defined as an abnormal position of an eye. It may be either 'fixed', where the eye is permanently displaced, or 'positional', where the strabismus is elicited by changing the position of the head. In vestibular disease, animals will not have a fixed strabismus but may show a ventrolateral positional strabismus when the head is elevated (see Figure 6.7.4).

6.7.2   Diagnostic Approach to Vestibular Disease

In terms of producing the differential diagnosis list for cases with vestibular syndrome, an important distinction must first be made between a central and a peripheral neuroanatomic localisation. To this end, the neurological examination is of critical importance, and should be considered ahead of the signalment and clinical history in cases of vestibular syndrome.

1. Neurological examination

Mentation: In cases of peripheral vestibular disease, the level of mentation should be normal. The exception is in situations where the animal feels so disorientated and/or nauseous that they may become apparently depressed. In cases of central

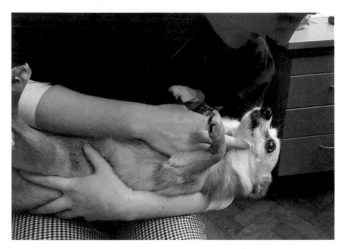

Figure 6.7.3 Attempting to induce nystagmus in an animal with subtle vestibular signs. Visual compensation means that many animals with a vestibular syndrome may lose the spontaneous nystagmus within a day or two; however, it is often possible to induce nystagmus in such cases by elevating the head or placing the affected animal on their back, as in this case.

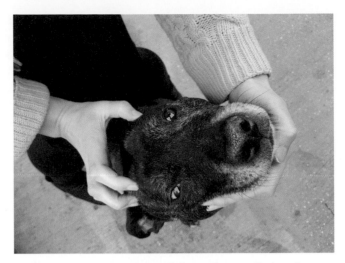

Figure 6.7.4 Strabismus. Animals with vestibular syndrome will often demonstrate a ventral or ventrolateral strabismus when the head is elevated, as in this case where the right eye is in an abnormal position associated with a right-sided vestibular syndrome.

disease, it is possible that any lesion which affects the vestibular nuclei of the brainstem may also affect the ascending reticular activating system (ARAS), leading to a reduced level of consciousness and genuine obtundation.

Gait and posture: A head tilt towards the affected side and vestibular ataxia (see Video 17) may be features of *both* peripheral and central vestibular disease. In some cerebellar lesions, the head tilt (and nystagmus) may point towards a lesion on the *opposite* side to that of the actual cerebellar lesion. This is termed a 'paradoxical vestibular syndrome' (see Section 6.8 'Cerebellar Dysfunction'). This is due to a loss of inhibition to the vestibular nuclei on the side of the cerebellar lesion, leading to a *relatively* reduced vestibular output on the opposite (contralateral) side to the lesion. It is usually obvious that there is a cerebellar lesion on the truly affected side due to the presence of asymmetrical hypermetria and/or other signs of cerebellar disease or postural reaction deficits (see Video 19). The veterinarian only needs to be aware of the possibility of a paradoxical vestibular syndrome to avoid a mistaken assumption that there may be multifocal lesions, which can lead to problems regarding formulating the list of differential diagnoses.

Postural reactions: These should be normal in cases with peripheral vestibular disease but can be abnormal in cases of central disease due to concurrent disruption of the ascending proprioceptive pathways within the brainstem. Deficits are usually ipsilateral to the side of the central lesion.

Cranial nerves: Nystagmus and/or positional strabismus may be expected in the early stages of most cases of peripheral or central vestibular syndrome (see above). Associated ipsilateral cranial nerve deficits, especially of those nerves that are anatomically close to cranial nerve VIII, may indicate a central (brainstem) localisation. However, it should be remembered that cranial nerve VII (the facial nerve) and the sympathetic nerves to the eye pass immediately adjacent to the tympanic bulla unseparated by bone from the cavity of the middle ear. Therefore, it is common for facial nerve paralysis and/or Horner syndrome to accompany peripheral vestibular syndrome in cases of otitis media/interna (see Sections 6.5 & 6.6 'Abnormalities of Pupil Size' and 'Cranial Nerve Dysfunction'). The clinician should take care not to misinterpret these signs as evidence of brainstem involvement in the absence of other key indicators, such as postural reaction deficits or changes in the level of mentation.

Spinal reflexes: Unless there is multi-focal disease, the spinal reflexes should be normal in cases with both peripheral and central vestibular syndrome as the C6–T2 and L4–S3 spinal cord segments will not be affected.

Palpation for pain: This is frequently normal except in the case of otitis media/interna, which may be a very painful condition, or in animals with inflammatory brain disease and referred neck pain.

In summary, the neuroanatomic localisation may be considered central if there is an abnormal level of mentation, multiple cranial nerve deficits, or postural reaction deficits. In the absence of these signs, or if there is concurrent vestibular syndrome, facial paralysis +/− Horner syndrome without postural reaction deficits, the localisation may be considered peripheral. This differentiation is crucial, but not always easy! It is also vital to consider that a central lesion is highly likely if there are concurrent postural reaction deficits or a convincingly altered level of mentation, but a central lesion can never be excluded in the absence of these signs (i.e. central disease can mimic peripheral disease but rarely vice versa) (Box 6.7.1).

Box 6.7.1

Top tip: Neither the severity of signs nor the acuteness of onset have any correlation with prognosis in vestibular disease. Some of the most acute and severe cases are idiopathic!

---

2. Differential diagnoses for peripheral vestibular disease (see also Section 6.6.2 'Facial Nerve')

- *Vascular*: unlikely.
- *Inflammatory/infectious*: otitis media/interna, inflammatory nasopharyngeal polyp, inflammatory neuritis.
- *Traumatic*: injury to tympanic bulla.
- *Toxic*: topical otitis treatments, aminoglycosides (topical or systemic).
- *Anomalous*: congenital vestibular syndrome; this has been described in a number of breeds including German Shepherd Dogs and Doberman Pinschers.
- *Metabolic*: hypothyroidism; as with facial neuropathy, the evidence that hypothyroidism can cause vestibular nerve dysfunction is weak, but there are

reports of vestibular signs responding to thyroid supplementation in dogs with a diagnosis of hypothyroidism.
- *Idiopathic vestibular syndrome* (see below).
- *Idiopathic cranial polyneuropathy*: occasionally a syndrome of apparently idiopathic polyneuropathy of cranial nerves is seen, where multiple cranial nerve deficits are found either unilaterally or bilaterally and all investigations are unrewarding. Prognosis appears good although occasionally some symptoms such as facial paralysis and head tilt may be permanent.
- *Neoplastic*: lymphoma, ceruminous gland adenocarcinoma, squamous cell carcinoma.
- *Degenerative*: no specific syndromes.

Hence it can be seen that if the neuroanatomic localisation is peripheral, by far the most likely causes are idiopathic or otitis media/interna. It should often be possible to eliminate 'anomalous'/'congenital' from signalment and 'toxic' from history taking. Hypothyroidism is a suggested cause of peripheral vestibular syndrome but is extremely rare without other significant signs of hypothyroidism in the author's experience. Neoplastic causes of peripheral vestibular syndrome are also rare in the absence of other signs.

3. Idiopathic (geriatric) vestibular syndrome
Idiopathic vestibular syndrome is the most common cause of vestibular disease in dogs. It may be seen in any age or breed of dog, as well as in cats, but is most commonly seen in older dogs. Clinical signs are acute or peracute, moderate to severe, and are consistent with a peripheral vestibular syndrome, including head tilt, nystagmus, and vestibular ataxia. The signs may be severe enough to render an affected animal unable to walk, and occasionally may cause nausea, vomiting, and associated anorexia. The diagnosis is achieved by excluding other possible causes of vestibular disease. However, as long as the clinician is reasonably certain from the general physical and neurological examinations that he or she is dealing with a peripheral vestibular syndrome rather than a central lesion, making a presumptive diagnosis of idiopathic vestibular syndrome without advanced imaging may be reasonable.

There is no specific treatment for idiopathic vestibular syndrome. Most dogs and cats improve within a few days, and many make a full recovery within 1–2 weeks. Occasionally, a suspected idiopathic vestibular syndrome may have a much longer and more chronic recovery, with the acute and severe signs improving but milder signs persisting or sometimes even waxing and waning. In this situation, referral for further investigation is advised in order to rule out a potential central vestibular disease, or a less common cause of peripheral disease such as neoplasia. Symptomatic treatment with antiemetics, such as maropitant, and occasionally even mild sedation with diazepam or acepromazine may prove useful in the most acute, severe phase.

4. Differential diagnoses for central vestibular disease

- *Vascular*: ischaemic or haemorrhagic stroke affecting the brainstem or thalamus.
- *Inflammatory/infectious*: meningoencephalitis of unknown origin, protozoal meningoencephalitis (Toxoplasma, Neospora), bacterial meningitis or empyema (potentially secondary to chronic otitis media/interna), viral meningoencephalitis (such as feline infectious peritonitis [FIP] and canine distemper virus [CDV]).
- *Traumatic*: traumatic brain injury (unlikely to present with central vestibular signs alone).
- *Toxic*: metronidazole toxicity (see Section 6.8 'Cerebellar Dysfunction').
- *Anomalous*: hydrocephalus, supracollicular fluid accumulation.
- *Metabolic*: hypothyroidism; again, central vestibular disease has been reported in dogs with hypothyroidism, but the mechanism for this is not understood and the evidence remains weak.
- *Neoplastic*: intracranial (e.g. glioma, meningioma), extracranial (e.g. lymphoma).
- *Nutritional*: thiamine deficiency; cats and dogs may occasionally be affected with thiamine deficiency, most commonly cats fed a diet containing raw fish which may contain thiaminase. Clinical signs include anorexia and lethargy, as well as neurological signs such as a central vestibular syndrome (often bilateral) and occasionally seizures. The onset may be acute or subacute, and diagnosis may be presumptive based on history and clinical signs. Blood thiamine levels may be measured although results are difficult to interpret. Many affected animals will show characteristic changes on brain MRI. Treatment involves correction of the diet and thiamine supplementation, with prognosis being good as long as treatment is initiated early enough.
- *Degenerative*: vestibular signs may be seen in neurodegenerative disorders, such as the lysosomal storage diseases. The signs are typically progressive and often multifocal, with involvement of other areas of the brain as well as in some cases other organs. These diseases are rare in general practice, but it is important to be aware of their existence and poor prognosis.

The most common causes of central vestibular disease are stroke, meningoencephalitis of unknown origin (MUO), and neoplasia, and therefore a suspicion of central disease should lead to a more guarded prognosis than for peripheral disease. In arriving at the most likely differential diagnoses, the signalment should increase the index of suspicion for the anomalous causes, and the history may help to eliminate metronidazole toxicity. Degenerative diseases should present as chronic progressive signs, usually in younger animals, unlike the three more common differential diagnoses. Stroke may be expected to have acute or peracute onset and then remain static or improve. MUO is likely to have an acute or subacute onset followed by often rapidly progressive signs, which may be multifocal. Neoplasia is usually chronic and progressive and is most commonly seen in older animals.

For a more detailed description of the potential conditions which may underlie a central vestibular syndrome please see also Section 6.8 'Cerebellar Dysfunction', since there is significant overlap between lesions that may lead to central vestibular syndrome and lesions that may cause a cerebellar syndrome.

6.7.3 Investigation of Vestibular Syndrome

Once the differential diagnoses are established, then a decision must be made whether to investigate further in-house, treat empirically based on most likely differentials, or refer for specialist examination +/− advanced imaging.

In a case of peripheral vestibular disease, this may be a relatively easy decision because the two most likely differential diagnoses are idiopathic vestibular syndrome and otitis media/interna. The main decision is therefore whether to investigate and/or treat for suspected otitis media/interna; this can often be based on the clinical history and physical examination, as well as radiography or CT of the tympanic bullae if available. If there is significant doubt regarding the possibility of otitis media/interna, or if there is uncertainty whether this is a peripheral or central lesion, then referral for specialist evaluation should be considered.

When central vestibular disease is suspected on the basis of the neurological examination, referral should always be offered to further investigate the most common causes. These conditions are likely to require advanced imaging and perhaps cerebrospinal fluid (CSF) analysis in order to obtain a diagnosis, and carry a guarded prognosis. The one exception to this may be in situations where a vascular cause (stroke) is strongly suspected from the history and/or physical examination findings; in these cases, further in-house investigation of potential underlying cases may be justified.

If referral is not an option, then a basic diagnostic work-up as for other potential intracranial disorders should be considered. The decision whether to initiate in-house investigations or immediately refer for further investigation by a specialist is, as already stated above, one which requires careful discussion with the owner, and in many cases referral may not be an option for financial or logistical reasons.

Investigations which may be performed include:

- *Haematology, serum biochemistry, and urinalysis.*
- *Blood pressure testing* – if this is persistently elevated an ACTH stimulation test may be justified, especially with supporting clinical and biochemical features of hyperadrenocorticism.
- *Thyroid function testing* – total thyroid hormone (T4), free T4, TSH.

- *A coagulation profile and testing for A. vasorum* if a disorder of blood clotting is suspected.
- *Infectious disease testing* dependent on the species and relative risk of exposure – *T. gondii* in cats and dogs, *N. caninum* or CDV in dogs, FeLV, FIV, and feline coronavirus in cats.
- *Urine metabolic screening* if an inborn error of metabolism is suspected (e.g. young animal with progressive neurological disease).
- *Radiography or CT of the tympanic bullae.*
- *Thoracic radiography, abdominal ultrasonography, or head, thoracic, and abdominal CT* – particularly if neoplasia is likely.

If a diagnosis of systemic disease is confirmed, then treatment should be directed at resolving the underlying disease and monitoring the progression of the vestibular signs. Where in-house investigations do not reveal the diagnosis, either continued monitoring or empirical treatment based on the most likely differential diagnoses may be considered.

6.7.4 Management of Vestibular Disease
1. Symptomatic treatment
Treatment is aimed at reducing any nausea with the use of antiemetics such as maropitant, and occasionally providing some anxiolytic therapy such as acepromazine or butorphanol if clinical signs are severe. It may be necessary to hospitalise a severely affected dog or cat with suspected idiopathic vestibular syndrome until the most severe signs have resolved and the animal is able to ambulate and is eating. Owners are often very distressed to see their pet in an acute severe vestibular state, and because most idiopathic cases occur in older animals they are sometimes inclined to assume that the prognosis is poor and request euthanasia. This should be resisted if the clinician is satisfied that the problem is most likely to be peripheral and represent an idiopathic vestibular syndrome.

2. Management of suspected stroke (see Section 6.3.4 'Obtundation')

3. Treatment of suspected intracranial neoplasia (see also Section 6.3.4 'Obtundation')
The prognosis and likelihood of achieving even short-term improvement with neoplasia in the brainstem is less than when palliatively treating tumours in the forebrain. If symptomatic treatment with corticosteroids is initiated in a case of suspected brainstem neoplasia that is causing central vestibular signs, improvement should be expected within a few days if it is going to occur at all; if this is not seen, and referral is not an option, then euthanasia should be considered.

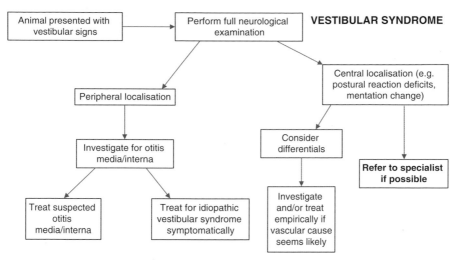

Approach to cases of vestibular syndrome in practice.

6.8   Cerebellar Dysfunction

Edward Ives

The cerebellum resides within the caudal fossa of the skull and lies dorsal to the pons and medulla oblongata of the brainstem. The primary functions of the cerebellum are:

- coordination and refinement of movements that are initiated by the motor centres of the cerebrum and brainstem
- regulation of posture and inhibition of extensor muscle tone
- coordination of postural reactions, such as hopping
- coordination of appropriate motor responses to visual and auditory stimuli (e.g. blinking of the eye in response to a menacing gesture).

The cerebellum also forms part of the central vestibular system and has a predominately inhibitory influence on the vestibular nuclei of the brainstem.

Disorders that affect the cerebellum do not influence whether a particular movement is initiated in the first place, but result in an inappropriate *rate, range,* and *force* of movement. This presents as unpredictable limb placement (ataxia), truncal swaying, and exaggerated, hypermetric limb movements, particularly if an animal is encouraged to walk up a kerb or climb steps (see Video 18). These hypermetric movements are characterised by excessive flexion of the limb during protraction, followed by forceful, erratic replacement of the paw back to the ground. This loss of coordination is termed 'dysmetria' and will also be appreciated when performing hopping tests, which will be delayed and exaggerated in the affected limbs. These clinical signs will involve all limbs for diffuse cerebellar lesions, or the ipsilateral thoracic and pelvic limbs for unilateral lesions. A loss of postural regulation may also result in a wide-based stance. In severe cases, the degree of ataxia may mean that an animal is unable to walk. However, as the cerebellum does not play a role in the initiation of movement, animals with cerebellar disease do not show paresis and will have preserved strength. The spinal reflexes will also be strong as the spinal cord segments involved in these reflexes remain unaffected.

Diffuse lesions affecting both cerebellar hemispheres may result in the oscillation of goal-orientated movements, termed an 'intention tremor' (Lowrie and Garosi 2016). This is most appreciable as a tremor of the head and neck during actions such as lowering the head towards a food bowl or reaching for a toy. Cerebellar dysfunction may also result in reduced/absent menace responses, but the vision, pupillary light reflexes, and palpebral reflexes will remain normal.

Severe, usually acute, lesions affecting the rostral cerebellum can result in a complete loss of inhibition of extensor muscle tone, termed 'decerebellate rigidity' (see Chapter 3). Affected animals will usually present in lateral recumbency with extended thoracic limbs, an extended neck posture (opisthotonus), and extended pelvic limbs that may be held flexed at the hips (Figure 6.8.1). This posture appears similar to the posture adopted by animals with diffuse cerebrocortical or midbrain lesions (decerebrate rigidity). However, as cerebellum does not play a role in the maintenance of wakefulness, the level of mentation will be unaffected by lesions that are isolated to the cerebellum. Therefore, animals in decerebellate rigidity will remain alert and responsive, whilst animals with decerebrate rigidity will have a severely altered level of mentation (stupor or coma). The close proximity of the cerebellum to the brainstem means that lesions affecting one of these structures may also influence the function of the other. This can result in combinations of neurological deficits that reflect both cerebellar and brainstem dysfunction, such as hypermetria, ataxia, and vestibular dysfunction together with hemi-/tetraparesis, paw replacement deficits, and/or cranial nerve deficits.

Cerebellar dysfunction, particularly if asymmetric, may be associated with clinical signs of vestibular syndrome (e.g. head tilt, nystagmus, drifting, and falling to one side). The underlying basis of any vestibular syndrome is an imbalance in the output from the vestibular nuclei in the brainstem; reduced output from the vestibular nuclei on one side relative to the other results in a head tilt and slow phase of a jerk nystagmus that are *towards* the side with reduced output. Unilateral disorders of the peripheral vestibular system, or those that affect the vestibular nuclei themselves, will result in reduced output from the ipsilateral vestibular nuclei. The direction of the resultant head tilt and slow phase of nystagmus will therefore be *towards* the side of the lesion. Certain regions of the cerebellum, such as the flocculonodular lobe, exert an inhibitory influence on the brainstem vestibular nuclei. A lesion that affects these regions, or the

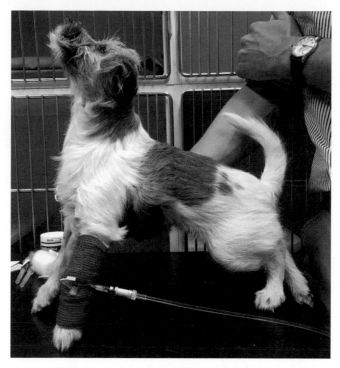

Figure 6.8.1 Decerebellate posture in a 2-year-old Jack Russell Terrier with meningoen-cephalitis of unknown origin, demonstrating increased extensor muscle tone in the thoracic limbs and an extended neck posture (opisthotonus). The pelvic limbs have more normal tone and are held partially flexed at the hip joints. This dog remained responsive to visual and auditory stimuli.

connections between the cerebellum and vestibular nuclei via the caudal cerebellar peduncle, will result in a loss of inhibition and an *increased* output from the ipsilateral vestibular nuclei. The subsequent imbalance between the output from the vestibular nuclei on each side of the brainstem will result in a head tilt and slow phase of a jerk nystagmus that are *away* from the side of the lesion (Figure 6.8.2). This is termed a 'paradoxical vestibular syndrome'. All the other neurological deficits that reflect cerebellar dysfunction will be ipsilateral to the side of the lesion (e.g. hypermetria, abnormal postural reactions, menace response deficit) (Figure 6.8.3). Dysfunction of the cerebellum does not always result in a paradoxical vestibular syndrome as this will depend on the region affected. Cerebellar lesions may therefore also result in a vestibular syndrome in which the direction of the head tilt or slow phase of the nystagmus are towards the side of the lesion.

As discussed in Chapter 3, cerebellar lesions can also disrupt the control of saccadic eye movements. This will present as abnormal spontaneous eye movements that lack the initial drift phase that is so distinctive for a nystagmus. These pathologic eye movements are termed saccadic oscillations. Opsoclonus is a form

(a)

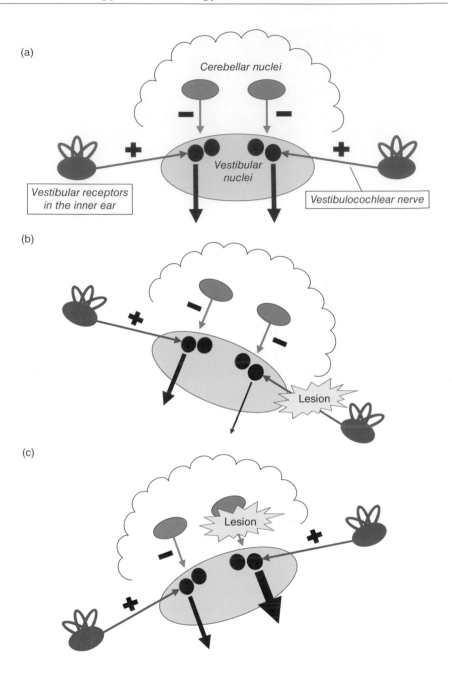

of saccadic oscillation that is characterised by rapid, multidirectional eye movements, and has been reported in animals with both cerebellar cortical degeneration and inflammatory disorders affecting the cerebellum (e.g. idiopathic generalised tremor syndrome) (Ives et al. 2018) (see Video 26).

Figure 6.8.2 Paradoxical vestibular syndrome. (a) In the normal animal with a static and horizontal head position, there is an equal and balanced input from the vestibular receptors in the inner ears to the brainstem vestibular nuclei. The output from the vestibular nuclei on both sides is therefore also equal (red arrows). The cerebellar nuclei exert a constant, inhibitory influence on the vestibular nuclei in the brainstem. (b) In the case of a peripheral vestibular lesion, there is loss of input from the vestibular receptors on the affected side compared to the contralateral side. This results in an imbalance in the output from the vestibular nuclei on each side of the brainstem; the reduced output on the affected side (smaller red arrow) results in a head tilt *towards* the side of the lesion as the extensor muscle tone in the ipsilateral neck muscles is reduced. (c) A cerebellar lesion may disrupt the normal inhibitory influence on the ipsilateral vestibular nuclei. This loss of inhibition results in an *increased* output from the brainstem vestibular nuclei on the affected side (large red arrow) compared to the unaffected side. This results in a head tilt that is *away* from the side of the lesion as there is a relative reduction in the extensor muscle tone in the contralateral neck muscles compared to the affected side.

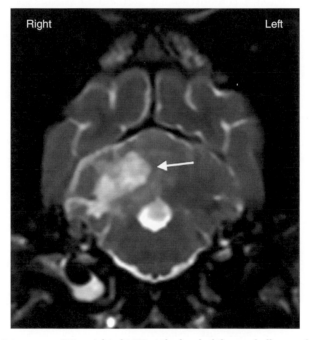

Figure 6.8.3 A transverse T2-weighted MRI at the level of the cerebellum and medulla oblongata in a 2-year-old, male neutered Pug with a 1-month history of a left head tilt and progressive balance loss. Neurological examination revealed a left head tilt, vestibular ataxia of all limbs, delayed proprioception and increased extensor muscle tone in the right thoracic and right pelvic limbs, and a reduced menace response in right eye. The neuroanatomic localisation was the right cerebellum, with a paradoxical vestibular syndrome explaining the left head tilt. The MRI demonstrated an ill-defined, intra-axial lesion affecting the right side of the cerebellum (arrow). Cerebrospinal fluid analysis revealed a mononuclear pleocytosis and infectious disease testing was negative. The dog showed a clinical improvement following the introduction of immunosuppressive medications, supporting a diagnosis of meningoencephalitis of unknown origin (MUO).

6.8.1 Differential Diagnoses

The presence of hypermetria, intention tremors, dysmetric hopping, and/or central vestibular dysfunction should alert the clinician to the possibility of a cerebellar lesion. The ranked list of differential diagnoses and subsequent clinical approach will then depend upon the signalment of the affected animal and the onset and progression of the disease. Disorders that may cause cerebellar dysfunction are discussed below and have been divided according to the VITAMIND mnemonic described in Chapter 5. This list is far from exhaustive, but it represents some of the more common disorders that may be observed in general practice.

1. Vascular

Cerebrovascular disease results from pathology affecting the blood supply to the brain (Boudreau 2018). It manifests clinically as an acute onset of non-progressive clinical signs, termed a cerebrovascular accident or 'stroke'. Cerebrovascular accidents affecting the blood supply to the cerebellum are not uncommon in dogs but have only been reported rarely in cats (Altay et al. 2011; Cherubini et al. 2007; Garosi et al. 2006; McConnell et al. 2005; Negrin et al. 2009; Negrin et al. 2018; Thomsen et al. 2016; Whittaker et al. 2018).

Cerebrovascular disease can be subdivided into the following categories:

- Ischaemia or infarction resulting from occlusion of the arterial supply to the region of the brain affected. This may be in the form of local thrombus formation or represent blood vessel occlusion by an embolus from a distant site (blood clot, neoplastic embolus, septic embolus, parasitic embolus).
- Haemorrhage secondary to disorders of coagulation or local disruption to the integrity of a vessel wall (artery or vein).
- Systemic hypertension resulting in hyperperfusion and cerebral oedema.

Ischaemic stroke is the most common form of cerebrovascular disease that affects the cerebellum, with Cavalier King Charles Spaniels and Greyhounds being over-represented in many case series (Kent et al. 2014; Thomsen et al. 2016). It typically presents as an acute onset of non-progressive, lateralised central vestibular syndrome, but ipsilateral hypermetria, loss of the menace response, and intention tremors can also be observed (Garosi et al. 2006; Thomsen et al. 2016). A concurrent medical condition may be identified in 50–60% of dogs with ischaemic stroke in general; the most frequently diagnosed conditions being chronic renal disease (protein-losing nephropathy) and hyperadrenocorticism (Garosi et al. 2005). Other reported conditions include diabetes mellitus, neoplasia, and hypothyroidism in dogs, and pulmonary disease, cardiomyopathy, and hyperthyroidism in cats (Whittaker et al. 2018). If ischaemic stroke is confirmed or suspected, then screening for an underlying predisposing factor is always important. This is because affected animals are significantly more likely to suffer recurrent events and have a poorer prognosis compared to animals for which an underlying medical condition cannot be identified (Garosi et al. 2005).

The diagnosis of ischaemic stroke requires advanced imaging of the brain (Figure 6.8.4). However, a high clinical suspicion can often be formed on the basis of the typical presentation of acute onset, lateralised, non-progressive clinical signs. Euthanasia of these animals at initial presentation may be requested by the owner, but if referral is not an option then monitoring without treatment is encouraged. A significant proportion of animals will show a gradual improvement over days or weeks and go on to make a functional recovery, even if they appear severely affected at initial presentation. The use of corticosteroids is not recommended and has the potential to worsen certain underlying medical

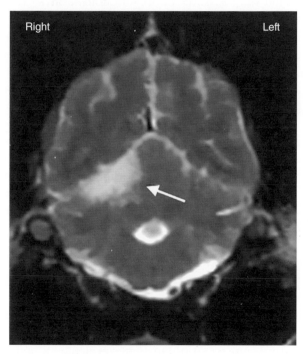

Figure 6.8.4 A transverse T2-weighted MRI at the level of the cerebellum and medulla oblongata in a 10-year-3-month old, male neutered Greyhound with a clinical history of acute onset, non-progressive balance loss. Neurological examination revealed falling to right side, ataxia of all limbs, and delayed and dysmetria hopping in the right thoracic and right pelvic limbs. The neuroanatomic localisation was the right central vestibular system (brainstem or cerebellum). Note the well-defined, hyperintense lesion affecting the cerebellar cortex on the right side. The clinical history and imaging findings in this case were most consistent with a territorial infarct involving the right rostral cerebellar artery. Urinalysis revealed a markedly elevated urine protein : creatinine ratio, with protein losing nephropathy and loss of antithrombin III being a likely predisposing factor for this ischaemic stroke. The dog's clinical signs showed a gradual improvement over a 6-week period.

conditions if present. Euthanasia should be considered if further investigations or referral are not possible, and there is a subsequent clinical deterioration that would suggest a progressive disease process (e.g. neoplasia).

Non-traumatic haemorrhagic lesions may also affect the cerebellum and can be primary or secondary in origin. Concurrent medical conditions that have reported in these cases include *A. vasorum*, intracranial neoplasia, metastatic neoplasia (e.g. hemangiosarcoma), hypertension, hypothyroidism, hyperadrenocorticism, and chronic kidney disease (Lowrie et al. 2012). The prognosis will depend upon the underlying cause but can be favourable in some dogs, particularly in those with *A. vasorum* infection or if no identifiable underlying cause is found. Hepatic disease and nephritis have been reported as concurrent medical conditions in cats with haemorrhagic infarcts (Altay et al. 2011).

Systemic hypertension may result in damage to susceptible organs, including the brain, eyes, and kidneys. This is most commonly associated with sustained elevations in systolic arterial blood pressure (>180 mmHg) or following acute elevations from the resting level. The clinical signs associated with hypertensive encephalopathy in animals more commonly reflect forebrain dysfunction, such as seizures, blindness, and an altered level of mentation (Brown et al. 2005, O'Neill et al. 2013). However, structures within the caudal fossa can also be affected, resulting in vestibular and cerebellar dysfunction. It may be difficult to determine whether hypertension represents the primary cause of the clinical signs observed, or whether it is secondary to another condition or clinical sign (e.g. stroke, neoplasia, stress, or seizures). Demonstration of persistent hypertension on repeat readings is therefore recommended in these cases. If a persistent hypertension is confirmed, then screening for underlying medical conditions is recommended, such as protein-losing nephropathy, hyperadrenocorticism, and phaeochromocytoma in dogs, or hyperaldosteronism in cats. Cases of essential or primary hypertension, in which a concurrent medical condition cannot be identified, are increasingly recognised in dogs and cats.

2. Inflammatory (sterile)

Inflammation of the CNS, in the absence of detectable infectious agents, is suspected to be autoimmune in origin and may involve the cerebellum and its overlying meninges (see Figure 6.8.3) (Hoon-Hanks et al. 2018). Definitive diagnosis of a specific, named condition requires histopathologic assessment of brain tissue. These conditions are therefore grouped under the broad term of 'meningoencephalitis of unknown origin' (MUO) pending biopsy or postmortem confirmation of a specific disorder (Cornelis et al. 2019). The most common form of MUO to affect the cerebellum in dogs is called granulomatous meningoencephalitis (GME). These conditions frequently result in multi-focal brain disease, with or without spinal cord involvement, and isolated cerebellar dysfunction is uncommon. Ante-mortem diagnosis of MUO requires consistent findings on MRI and CSF analysis, together with exclusion of infectious diseases.

Numerous treatment protocols for MUO in dogs have been reported. These most commonly involve the use of oral prednisolone together with an adjunctive immunosuppressive agent (e.g. cytosine arabinoside, cyclosporine, azathioprine). The prognosis appears highly variable, dependent on the individual case and short-term response to treatment.

Idiopathic generalised tremor syndrome is also suspected to represent an autoimmune condition. It is most commonly observed in young, small breed dogs and was previously termed 'little white shaker syndrome' due to the apparent over-representation of breeds such as West Highland White Terriers and Maltese Terriers. However, this condition may be observed in dogs of any breed or coat colour (Wagner et al. 1997). It has also been rarely reported in cats (Mauler et al. 2014). Affected animals present with low-amplitude, whole body tremors that are exacerbated by excitement or handling. The term 'idiopathic cerebellitis' has been used for this condition, as affected animals may also present with clinical signs referable to cerebellar dysfunction, such as hypermetria, vestibular dysfunction, and abnormal saccadic eye movements (opsoclonus). Diagnosis is made on the basis of clinical presentation and exclusion of other possible causes. Brain MRI is usually normal and CSF analysis may reveal evidence of mild inflammation. Treatment involves a tapering course of prednisolone starting at 1 mg/kg twice daily. Some dogs may relapse as the dose is reduced or stopped and require long-term therapy to maintain remission. Adjunctive immunosuppressive medications (e.g. cytosine arabinoside, azathioprine) may be useful in these cases to allow a reduction in the dose of steroid required to control the disease.

3. Infectious

Infectious meningoencephalitis may affect the cerebellum in both dogs and cats. It should therefore be considered as a differential diagnosis in any animal presenting with progressive signs of cerebellar dysfunction.

Feline coronavirus infection that results in feline infectious peritonitis (FIP) commonly affects the brainstem and cerebellum in cats. Affected cats may therefore present with clinical signs of ataxia, intention tremors, an altered level of mentation or vestibular dysfunction. *T. gondii* infection is an important differential diagnosis in any cat with CNS disease and can be screened for by serological testing. However, false positive results that reflect previous exposure to *T. gondii* rather than active infection are common, and a negative result may be more useful to lower the index of suspicion for this parasite. Bacterial meningitis resulting from cat bites over the caudal cranial fossa or extension of otitis media into the cranial vault can also affect the cerebellum in cats (Martin-Vaquero et al. 2011; Sturges et al. 2006). The clinical history and general clinical examination will often be supportive in these cases, with advanced imaging (CT or MRI) required for a definitive diagnosis. Otoscopy and myringotomy to collect samples for cytology and bacterial culture can be useful to diagnose otitis media. However, otoscopic examination may be normal in many cats with otitis media as infection frequently ascends from the pharynx via the Eustachian tube. This is in contrast to dogs, in which otitis media is most commonly secondary to otitis externa. Surgical management of both bacterial otitis media and intracranial abscessation has been advocated to improve the long-term outcome (Sturges et al. 2006). However, successful medical management of intracranial bacterial infection has been reported in cats and should be considered in animals for which surgery or referral are not an option (Cardy et al. 2017). See Figure 6.8.5 for a case example of a cat with an intracranial abscess involving the cerebellum after it was bitten on the head by another cat. Surgical

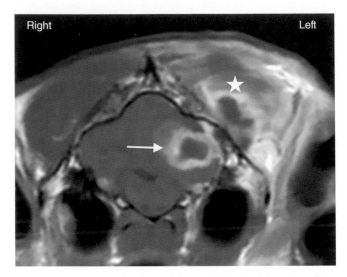

Figure 6.8.5 A transverse T1-weighted MRI following the administration of intravenous contrast media in a 6-year-old, male neutered, Maine Coon cat with a 4-day history of lethargy and progressive ataxia after returning home with wounds consistent with a cat fight. Physical examination revealed two puncture wounds on head, with the deepest being over the left occipital region. Neurological examination revealed a depressed level of mentation, marked ataxia of all limbs, falling to both sides, a poor menace response in the left eye, and a positional, vertical jerk nystagmus. The neuroanatomic localisation was brainstem and left cerebellum. The brain MRI revealed a left-sided, intra-axial, ring-enhancing, cavitated cerebellar lesion (arrow) that was exerting a mass effect on the adjacent brainstem. This lesion was communicating through a 4 mm left occipital bone defect with another cavitated lesion involving the soft tissues of the left temporal region (star). Other changes on the MRI scan included two small (1–2 mm) bone fragments depressed to lie within the caudal fossa, perilesional brain oedema, cerebellar herniation into the foramen magnum, focal meningitis, medial retropharyngeal lymphadenitis, and left temporal and right cervical myositis secondary to penetrating wounds. Surgical management was recommended in this case but was not possible due to economic limitations. The cat was initially treated with mannitol, a single injection of dexamethasone, and intravenous marbofloxacin and potentiated amoxicillin. The antibiotics were continued for 6 weeks and the cat made a complete recovery without relapse of clinical signs at 6-month follow-up.

management was recommended in this case but was not possible due to economic constraints. A complete clinical recovery was subsequently seen with medical management alone. Clinical deterioration in spite of treatment or relapsing clinical signs after cessation of antibiotic therapy are the primary concerns in these cases.

In utero infection by feline panleukopaenia virus can affect cerebellar cortical development in cats (Poncelet et al. 2013; Stuetzer and Hartmann 2014). This results in congenital cerebellar hypoplasia and affected kittens will display non-progressive clinical signs from the time they first attempt to walk. These clinical signs include coarse, low frequency (2–6 Hz) tremors, ataxia, hypermetria, and vestibular signs. Cats may compensate for this incoordination as they develop and can have a good quality of life if they are independently mobile. Ante-mortem diagnostic testing is usually normal and is primarily aimed at excluding other possible causes. There is no treatment for this congenital condition. Vaccination of pregnant queens with modified-live panleukopaenia virus vaccines should be avoided to reduce the incidence of this disorder.

Any infectious meningoencephalitis can theoretically affect the cerebellum in dogs, including bacterial, fungal, parasitic, and viral diseases (e.g. canine distemper virus, CDV). However, *Neospora caninum* appears to have a predilection for the cerebellum of adult dogs, resulting in progressive signs of cerebellar dysfunction (Garosi et al. 2010). This may occur in isolation or can be accompanied by additional deficits that reflect involvement of the spinal cord, peripheral nervous system, or other regions of the brain (Parzefall et al. 2014). The life cycle of *N. caninum* is incompletely understood but involves a canine definitive host and cattle as intermediate hosts. A history of exposure to farms or cattle may therefore raise the index of suspicion for this parasite. However, this is not always reported in the clinical history and dogs can harbour the parasite following transplacental transmission from mother to puppy. Immunosuppression related to systemic disease, or secondary to the use of immunosuppressive medications, may predispose to recrudescence of dormant parasitic stages in some dogs. Serological testing for *N. caninum* is recommended in all adult dogs that present with a history of progressive cerebellar dysfunction. Low positive serum antibody titres may indicate previous exposure but high serum titres (>1:800) are highly suggestive of active infection. Demonstration of parasite antigen by polymerase chain reaction (PCR) testing on CSF can confirm the diagnosis. The MRI appearance in adult dogs with neosporosis and cerebellar involvement is distinctive and is also highly suggestive for this condition (Figure 6.8.6). Clindamycin (10–15 mg/kg per os twice daily for a minimum of 2–3 months) and/or trimethoprim/sulphonamide can be used for treatment, but relapses are possible when treatment is stopped. Serum antibody titres can may remain high during and following treatment, which complicates their use for deciding when to stop therapy.

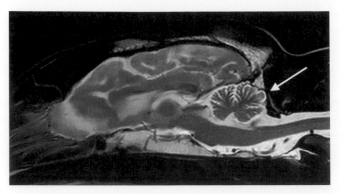

Figure 6.8.6 A mid-sagittal T2-weighted MRI in a 4-year-old, male neutered Greyhound with a 4-week history of progressive balance loss and a subsequent diagnosis of protozoal meningoencephalitis secondary to *Neospora caninum*. Neurological examination revealed a normal level of mentation, absent menace responses bilaterally, delayed and dysmetria hopping in all limbs, a wide-based stance, and hypermetria and ataxia affecting all limbs. Withdrawal reflexes were strong in all limbs and spinal palpation did not reveal any discomfort. The neuroanatomic localisation was diffuse cerebellar disease. Magnetic resonance imaging of the brain revealed marked cerebral and cerebellar atrophy, with thinning of the cortices and enlargement of the lateral ventricles. Note the markedly reduced size of the cerebellum, with an apparent increased volume of cerebrospinal fluid (CSF) surrounding the cerebellar folia (arrow). CSF analysis revealed a moderate, mixed (predominantly neutrophilic) pleocytosis. Serological testing for *Neospora caninum* was positive at >1:800 and PCR testing for *N. caninum* antigen in the CSF was positive.

4. Traumatic

Trauma to the cerebellum is uncommon but may result from blunt force trauma to the back of skull or bite wounds that puncture the occipital bones overlying the caudal cranial fossa. A clinical history and thorough general clinical examination will usually support a diagnosis of head trauma. The approach to head trauma as a potential neurological emergency is discussed in Chapter 7.

5. Toxic

Diffuse or multi-focal CNS disease may be observed following exposure to numerous toxins and cerebellar dysfunction is not uncommon in these cases. A thorough clinical history is therefore always important and should include questions regarding medications that the animal is currently receiving or other substances in the household that the dog or cat may have had access to. The most common neurotoxicity that presents with predominately cerebellar signs in dogs is metronidazole intoxication.

a. Metronidazole toxicity

Metronidazole is an antibacterial, anthelmintic, and antiprotozoal medication that is widely used in veterinary medicine, particularly in dogs with gastrointestinal disease. It is highly lipid soluble, which means that it can readily gain access to the CNS across the blood–CSF and blood–brain barriers. Serum concentrations peak within 1–2 hours of oral administration, with an elimination half-life of 4–6 hours in dogs. Previously recommended oral doses of metronidazole ranged from 10 to 25 mg/kg every 12 hours. A recently licensed veterinary formulation for the treatment of gastrointestinal infections caused by *Giardia* and *Clostridia* spp. in dogs and cats recommends a daily oral dose of 25 mg/kg every 12 hours. Clinical signs associated with metronidazole neurotoxicity include ataxia, hypermetria, increased extensor muscle tone, tremors, convulsions, and central vestibular syndrome (head tilt, vertical nystagmus). The pathophysiological mechanism of neurotoxicity is unknown but may be related to modulation of the receptor for the inhibitory neurotransmitter GABA within the cerebellum. A recent retrospective study of 26 dogs with metronidazole-induced neurotoxicity reported a median oral dose of 21 mg/kg twice daily (range 13–56 mg/kg twice daily) (Tauro et al. 2018). The median duration of treatment was 35 days (range 5–180 days). The authors of this study therefore recommended caution in administering metronidazole at oral doses >20 mg/kg twice daily. Diagnostic testing is generally unremarkable in affected animals, but MRI may rarely reveal symmetrical changes within the cerebellar medullary nuclei. Clinical signs should resolve when metronidazole administration is stopped. The median time to resolution of clinical signs was 3 days (range 1–26 days) in the study described above. The administration of diazepam to affected dogs (0.5 mg/kg per os every 8 hours for 3 days) has been recommended to shorten the recovery time in affected dogs; the recovery time for diazepam-treated dogs (1.6 days) was significantly shorter than that for untreated dogs (11 days) in a retrospective study of 21 cases (Evans et al. 2003). The mechanism of action for diazepam in these cases is potentially related to competitive reversal of metronidazole binding at the GABA receptor.

6. Anomalous

Anomalous disorders are most commonly observed in younger animals and include complete or near-complete absence of the cerebellum (aplasia), or a congenital reduction in cerebellar volume (hypoplasia). Congenital cerebellar hypoplasia has been reported in several breeds of dog, including Chow Chows, Irish Setters, and Wire-haired Fox Terriers. Clinical signs of cerebellar dysfunction are non-progressive in these animals and will be present from the time an animal first tries to walk. As discussed previously, in utero infection with certain viruses may be responsible for cerebellar hypoplasia in some puppies and kittens (e.g. feline panleukopaenia virus).

Other developmental abnormalities that may result in cerebellar dysfunction include epidermoid and dermoid cysts (Platt et al. 2016; Steinberg et al. 2007). These mass lesions represent entrapment of ectodermal tissue within the developing neural tube and are most commonly found in the region of the fourth ventricle, immediately ventral to the cerebellum. Enlargement of these cystic structures as the animal grows, together with the inflammatory response to their presence, results in progressive cerebellar disease in young to middle-aged animals. These cystic lesions mimic neoplasia and advanced imaging +/− biopsy is required for diagnosis.

7. Neoplastic

Primary tumours of the cerebellar parenchyma are rare in small animals but include medulloblastoma and gliomas. Extra-axial tumours arising from anatomical structures that are closely associated with the cerebellum are more common, such as meningiomas at the level of the cerebellomedullarypontine angle or choroid plexus tumours of the fourth ventricle. These tumours typically result in ipsilateral, asymmetric clinical signs of brainstem and cerebellar dysfunction. Advanced imaging is required for diagnosis, but the clinical suspicion of a neoplastic lesion should be increased in an older dog or cat with progressive clinical signs. Inflammatory or infectious diseases (e.g. neosporosis) are important differential diagnoses in these cases. A late onset form of cerebellar cortical degeneration should also be considered but, in contrast to neoplasia, degenerative disorders usually result in diffuse and symmetric cerebellar involvement (see below).

8. Degenerative

Clinical signs of cerebellar dysfunction may occur secondary to numerous degenerative disorders that affect the CNS. Evidence of more widespread neurological dysfunction is frequently observed in these cases (e.g. visual deficits, behaviour change, seizures, tetra/paraparesis). These disorders include inborn errors of metabolism that result in accumulation of cellular products within affected neurons and abnormal neuronal function. These conditions have been termed 'storage diseases' and primarily affect young pure-breed animals of specific breeds. However, the age at onset can be highly variable dependent on the breed and condition. Therefore, a degenerative disorder should always be considered in animals of any age that present with a chronic, progressive history of non-painful clinical signs, particularly if a known disorder has been reported in the same breed. Diagnosis may be achieved by a combination of urine metabolic screening, blood enzymatic testing, tissue biopsy, advanced imaging findings, and genetic testing (if available for a particular breed) (Sewell et al. 2012; Skelly and Franklin 2002). A list of degenerative conditions that may present with signs of cerebellar dysfunction is given below. Corneal clouding is a distinctive finding on the general physical examination for several of these conditions and would help to increase the index of suspicion if observed (e.g. mucopolysaccharidosis [MPS] II, MPS III, and GM1 gangliosidosis).

- *Mucopolysaccharidosis (MPS) II* – Labrador Retriever
- *MPS III* – Dachshund (adult onset), New Zealand Huntaway, Schipperke

- *Ceroid lipofuscinosis* (adult and juvenile forms dependent on the breed) – American Staffordshire Terrier, American Bulldog, Border Collie, Chihuahua, Cocker Spaniel, Dachshund, Dalmatian, English Setter
- *Glucocerebrosidosis* – Silky Terrier
- *Globoid cell leukodystrophy* – Beagle, Cairn Terrier, Irish Setter, Poodle, West Highland White Terrier, domestic shorthair cat
- *GM1 gangliosidosis* – Beagle, English Springer Spaniel, Portuguese Water Dog, Siberian Husky, domestic shorthair cat, Siamese cat
- *GM2 gangliosidosis* – German Shorthaired Pointer, Japanese Chin, Burmese cat, domestic shorthair cat, Korat cat
- *Niemann–Pick* – Balinese and Siamese cats (type A), domestic shorthair cat (type C).

a. Neuroaxonal dystrophy

Neuroaxonal dystrophy is a degenerative disease that is most widely recognised in the Rottweiler (Chrisman et al. 1984; Sisó et al. 2001; Lucot et al. 2018). However, it has also been reported in the Papillon, Spanish Water Dog, Chihuahua, Jack Russell Terrier, Collie, and domestic shorthair cats (Hahn et al. 2015; Nibe et al. 2007). Affected Rottweilers present with a history of chronic, progressive ataxia, hypermetria, and a wide-based stance at 1–2 years of age. Clinical progression is observed over months/years to include intention tremors, menace response deficits, and nystagmus. There is a gene test available in the Rottweiler, Papillon, and Spanish Water Dog but a definitive diagnosis can only be achieved post-mortem in other breeds (Hahn et al. 2015; Lucot et al. 2018). Diagnostic investigations are therefore primarily targeted at excluding other differential diagnoses such as *N. caninum* infection, meningoencephalitis of unknown origin, neoplasia (e.g. medulloblastoma), and anomalous conditions (e.g. epidermoid cyst). There is no effective treatment for this condition and the prognosis is poor.

b. Primary cerebellar cortical degeneration

Primary cerebellar cortical degeneration refers to degeneration of cerebellar neurons that have initially developed normally. An intrinsic cellular defect results in a reduced life span of the affected neurons, with the age at the onset of clinical signs dependent upon the onset of neuronal loss. This typically occurs between 3 and 12 months of age in affected dogs, but the onset of clinical signs may not be observed until 5–8 years old in certain breeds (e.g. Old English Sheepdog, Brittany Spaniel, Gordon Setter, Scottish Terrier, Labrador Retriever). Important differential diagnoses in these dogs include inflammatory, infectious, and neoplastic disorders. Primary cerebellar cortical degeneration has been reported in numerous breeds of dog, including the Kerry Blue Terrier, American Staffordshire Terrier, Scottish Terrier, Rough-coated Collie, Border Collie,

Labrador Retriever, Rhodesian Ridgeback, Golden Retriever, Beagle, and Cocker Spaniel, and has also been reported in cats (Bertalan et al. 2014, de Lahunta and Averill 1976, Urkasemsin et al. 2010, Inada et al. 1996, Olby et al. 2004). Clinical signs of cerebellar dysfunction are progressive and there are no effective treatments. Ante-mortem diagnostic testing is usually unremarkable and primarily aimed at excluding other differential diagnoses for which there may be a treatment. MRI may reveal reduced cerebellar volume in some cases, and a gene test is available for certain breeds (Henke et al. 2008; Inada et al. 1996; Kwiatkowska et al. 2013).

6.8.2 Clinical Approach to Cerebellar Disease

The clinical approach to any animal that presents with a neurological examination consistent with cerebellar dysfunction will depend upon many factors. These include the clinical history, the list of differential diagnoses, and the funds available for referral or further investigations. As for all neurological syndromes, there is no ideal 'recipe' for approaching these cases and some may fall between the broad categories summarised below. However, the clinical approach can be initially divided by onset, progression of clinical signs, and age of the affected animal.

1. Acute, non-progressive or improving clinical signs
- Rule out trauma using the clinical history and general clinical examination.
- Consider cerebrovascular disease, particularly if the neurological deficits are asymmetrical: Refer for advanced imaging to confirm the diagnosis if possible.
- Screen for underlying medical conditions: blood pressure testing, urinalysis (including urine protein : creatinine ratio), haematology, serum biochemistry, coagulation testing, *A. vasorum* testing, ACTH stimulation testing, total thyroid hormone and TSH levels, body cavity screening for neoplasia.

2. Chronic, non-progressive clinical signs in a puppy or kitten
- Congenital cerebellar aplasia or hypoplasia is most likely. The prognosis may be good if the animal is ambulatory and has a reasonable quality of life.

3. Acute, progressive clinical signs in an animal of any age
- Rule out intoxication (e.g. metronidazole).
- Consider infectious, inflammatory, and neoplastic disorders: Refer for further investigations if possible.
- Perform an otoscopic examination, haematology, serum biochemistry, urinalysis, body cavity screening for systemic or metastatic neoplasia, and infectious disease testing (e.g. *N. caninum* serology in dogs, *T. gondii* serology and feline coronavirus testing in cats).

4. Chronic, progressive clinical signs in a young animal

- Rule out intoxication (e.g. metronidazole).
- Consider degenerative, anomalous, infectious, inflammatory (and neoplastic) disorders: Refer for further investigations if possible.
- Perform an otoscopic examination, haematology, serum biochemistry, urinalysis, and infectious disease testing (e.g. *N. caninum* serology in dogs, *T. gondii* serology and feline coronavirus testing in cats). Search for a consistent degenerative disorder in the same breed +/− urine metabolic screening and genetic testing.

5. Chronic, progressive clinical sigs in a middle-aged or older animal

- Rule out intoxication (e.g. metronidazole).
- Consider neoplastic, inflammatory, infectious, and late-onset degenerative disorders: Refer for further investigations if possible.
- Perform an otoscopic examination, haematology, serum biochemistry, urinalysis, body cavity screening for systemic or metastatic neoplasia, and infectious disease testing (e.g. *N. caninum* serology in dogs, *T. gondii* serology and feline coronavirus testing in cats). Search for a consistent degenerative disorder in the same breed +/− urine metabolic screening and genetic testing. Consider a steroid trial before euthanasia if the clinical signs are progressive, infectious disease has been excluded, and further investigations are not possible.

6.9 Neck and/or Spinal Pain

Paul M. Freeman

Apparent pain is a very common presentation in general practice. This may be the complaint of the owner, or it may be the conclusion of the veterinary surgeon, and such cases can prove diagnostically challenging.

6.9.1 Signs of Pain

Animals may react to pain in different locations in varied ways, but there are some generalisations which can be made to assist the veterinarian when faced with such a case. Cats and dogs also react in different ways to pain; the first part of this section will be mostly concerned with canine manifestations of pain, and we will consider cats separately.

1. Neck pain

Animals with significant cervical pain classically adopt a 'head down' posture (Figure 6.9.1). They may be very reluctant to elevate the head and when tempted with a food treat, will sometimes perform a movement that will elicit an attack of pain. The adopted posture is evidently the most pain-free and is likely to be a

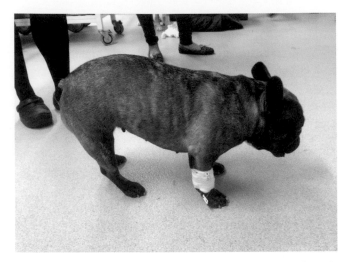

Figure 6.9.1 Low head carriage, which is commonly seen in animals with neck pain. Affected animals may be reluctant to raise their heads even when tempted with a food treat.

protective mechanism. Cervical pain may be very severe when associated with neurological disease, and it is not uncommon for dogs with cervical pain to yelp, cry, or scream intermittently, which is often very distressing to owners. If the caudal cervical region is involved, there is the possibility of a permanent or intermittent thoracic limb lameness known as 'nerve root signature' (Figure 6.9.2).

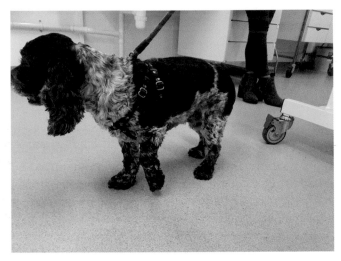

Figure 6.9.2 Nerve root signature. Animals with compression of a spinal nerve root that contributes to the major thoracic limb or pelvic limb peripheral nerves may show an intermittent or permanent non-weight-bearing lameness associated with pain. Occasionally, animals will vocalise when becoming non-weight-bearing on the affected limb. In most cases, an apparent nerve root signature indicates a lateralised problem such as an intervertebral disc extrusion affecting the C6–T2 or the L4–S3 spinal cord regions.

This is caused by mechanical or inflammatory effects on a cervical nerve root supplying the brachial plexus.

Affected animals are frequently reluctant to run, jump, or play, and may appear quite lethargic or 'depressed'. Appetite may be affected either because the animal does not feel like eating because of the pain, or more often because fully flexing the neck to eat from the ground exacerbates the pain.

2. Thoracolumbar pain

Animals with thoracolumbar pain often show a degree of kyphosis, with exaggerated flexion of the thoracolumbar spine (Figure 6.9.3). They may walk in a stiff and hunched manner, and again will be reluctant to run, jump, or play. On examination, the abdomen may feel tense due to the muscle contracture involved with the kyphotic posture, and this commonly leads to confusion and a suspicion of abdominal pain. Again, if the pain is caused by neurological disease, crying or yelping may occur, although far less commonly than with cervical pain. Shivering may occur when the pain is severe, and occasionally a tremor of the pelvic limbs may be evident when the animal is standing.

Posturing to urinate and defecate can be difficult, leading sometimes to incontinence or overfilling of the bladder, and many affected animals will choose to urinate and/or defecate whilst walking, apparently because this is more comfortable than squatting in a stationary manner.

3. Lumbosacral pain

Lumbosacral pain can be the most difficult region to localise with certainty. Animals with lumbosacral pain may walk stiffly, and again have difficulties posturing to urinate or defecate. They are most commonly reported by their owners

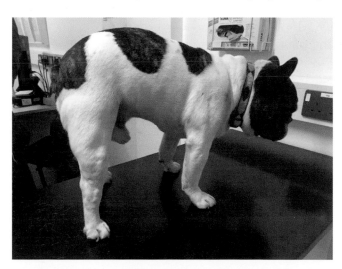

Figure 6.9.3 Kyphosis of the spine (increased dorsal flexion at the thoracolumbar region), such as in this case, is usually associated with marked thoracolumbar pain.

to be reluctant to jump up, for example into a car or onto a bed or sofa, and have difficulties climbing stairs. They may have problems sitting or lying and take excessive time to change posture. Vocalising occurs occasionally, although not commonly, and in the case of lateralised lumbosacral disease a permanent or intermittent pelvic limb lameness or nerve root signature may be seen. All of these signs may be mimicked to some extent by orthopaedic disease, such as hip dysplasia and cranial cruciate ligament disease, making this a very challenging area for diagnosis and treatment.

4. Cats in pain

Cats tend to react to pain in a different manner to dogs. Most commonly, they will become subdued, choosing to sleep much longer than normal and reject attention from their owner or other animals in the household. They may become aggressive when approached, making physical and neurological examinations very challenging. Cats rarely vocalise when in pain, but commonly become anorexic and apparently lethargic. They may show a reluctance or apparent inability to climb or jump, which can appear as weakness, and owners will often recognise changes in behaviour patterns such as choosing not to go outside, upstairs, or climb fences or trees as part of a painful syndrome. Lower back pain may make posturing to defecate or urinate painful, as for dogs, and cats may even present with an over-full bladder or constipation for this reason.

6.9.2   Physical Examination for Pain

Palpation for the presence of possible pain is an important part of the neurological examination. However, when presented with an animal with a history of suspected pain, this must be carried out with great care and sensitivity. If the clinician has a strong suspicion that pain may be present in a particular region of the spine, then it is wise to leave that region until last in the examination. By the time that many animals are presented to the veterinarian, they have become over-sensitised to their pain and this, combined with the stress and anxiety of being examined by a stranger in a strange environment, may cause them to over-react. This can make interpretation of the examination difficult. Furthermore, once an animal has been hurt by the examiner, they may react to palpation in many parts of the body where pain is not in fact located, which can lead to a very confusing examination. The basic method of palpating for pain is shown in Videos 21a and 22a of the normal neurological examination of the dog.

Where there is *not* a strong suspicion of neck pain (i.e. no head down posture, no frequent, spontaneous vocalisation), it is reasonable to work from head to tail. The author prefers to begin the examination by palpating from the atlas wings down the lateral sides of the cervical spine, followed by palpation from dorsoventrally at the level of the caudal cervical spine. This may often reveal a focal region of pain without the need to move the head and neck. However, if palpation appears unremarkable it is reasonable to flex and extend the neck, and also to turn the head and neck to the left and right, in order to assess whether any of these manoeuvres appear particularly uncomfortable. Care should be taken with full neck flexion, especially in the case of miniature and toy breeds where atlantoaxial instability (AAI) may be a differential diagnosis.

Moving on to the thoracolumbar spine, gentle pressure should be applied with a thumb and forefinger or the thumbs of both hands to the dorsal spinous processes, working cranial to caudal down to the lumbosacral region. If an area of apparent focal pain is identified (e.g. tensing of the epaxial muscles, groaning, or crying), then this area should be re-visited, this time by moving from caudal to cranial in order to see if the reaction is consistent. If no area of pain is identified, the palpation should be repeated with increasing pressure. Care must be taken to avoid compressing the abdomen during this examination, and it is a good idea to initially palpate the abdomen in order to assess how guarded the abdominal wall muscles are and whether in fact cranial abdominal pain (such as from pancreatitis) may be the cause of the animal's clinical signs.

Palpating the lumbosacral region forms a continuation of the thoracolumbar palpation as described above. However, here it is important to be sure that the pressure applied over the lumbosacral area is not creating pain through the hips or stifles. Locating the lumbosacral joint is not easy since the dorsal spines of L7 and the sacrum are rarely palpable; in most dogs, the spinous process of L7 is located in the midline just caudal to the level of the most palpable parts of the iliac wings. In some cases, it may be possible to gently elevate the animal's hindquarters while carrying out the examination in order to prevent possible misinterpretation of orthopaedic pain; however, it is still very easy to confuse lumbosacral and orthopaedic pain. It is therefore wise to palpate/manipulate the hips and stifles as a routine part of the examination in order to assess whether they could also represent a source of pain. Remember that many animals with lumbosacral disease may also have concurrent orthopaedic disease. The lordosis test involves applying pressure over the lumbosacral region whilst simultaneously extending both hips and has been recommended as a good test for identifying lumbosacral pain; however, in the author's opinion it is a very difficult test to carry out effectively, especially in larger dogs, and if the dog has hip pain this may easily create a confusing reaction.

Examining cats for pain is often unrewarding and frequently dangerous! However, there are situations where identification of a painful region may provide the clue which leads to ultimate diagnosis of the problem, and it should therefore always be attempted, particularly in cases where pain is considered possible or likely from the history. Careful and gentle palpation with minimal restraint is most likely to be rewarding and may need to be performed over a period of time. Once a cat has become hypersensitised and 'angry', the examination is likely to be unrewarding. A quiet, calm environment with minimal people and minimal restraint is most likely to yield the best results, and great patience is required to get the most from the feline neurological examination in general.

6.9.3 Pathophysiology of Pain

It is beyond the scope of this text to provide great detail on the pathophysiology of pain. However, a basic understanding is necessary in order to properly manage chronic pain. Nociceptors are the pain receptors which are free nerve endings located in high numbers in the skin, joint capsules, muscles and tendons, periosteum, and meninges. These can be variously stimulated by pressure and inflammatory mediators, causing nerve impulses to be transmitted to the dorsal horns of the spinal cord via sensory neurons. Here there are synapses relying largely on the neurotransmitters glutamate and substance P, and which also contain opioid receptors capable of modulating the transmission of impulses across these synapses. The dorsal horns project mainly to spinal cord pathways called spinothalamic tracts that carry the pain information to the thalamus and then on to the cerebral cortex. This pain information is thought to be carried in multiple tracts, bilaterally within the spinal cord, and primarily in small axon fibres which are relatively resistant to damage. Hence, the sensation of 'deep pain' is the last clinical parameter to be lost in cases of severe spinal cord damage (see later). There are also descending, modulating fibres which are capable of acting at the opioid receptors within the dorsal horns, that can be stimulated in order to downregulate and modulate the pain response.

Both the peripheral nociceptors and the central pain receptors within the cerebral cortex can undergo a process of sensitisation or 'wind-up'. This can occur either with significant damage to the CNS, such as a stroke, or may be the result of chronically painful conditions. This is a well-recognised syndrome in people, but may be more difficult to diagnose in animals. It is, however, thought to play a role in animals with chronic back or limb pain, and provides a potential target for treatment.

Because of the complex and multi-level neuropharmacology of pain, there are many different classes of drug which may be beneficial in treating pain. These range from non-steroidal anti-inflammatory drugs (NSAIDs), which target inflammatory mediators and potential sensitisation of peripheral nociceptors, through opioids, which act directly at the opioid receptors along the pain pathways, to drugs like gabapentin and amantadine, which are believed to act centrally by targeting the central sensitisation mechanisms. Ketamine and the alpha-2 agonist drugs can also act at multiple levels, with the alpha-2 drugs having a direct effect on the descending modulating pathways of pain. The table in Box 6.9.1 lists some of the more commonly used drugs that may be utilised in animals with spinal pain.

For many painful spinal conditions, it is necessary to use a multimodal approach to analgesia, and the authors will often combine an opioid with a NSAID and/or a drug such as gabapentin in conditions such as acute intervertebral disc extrusion. Paracetamol may also be safely added to this combination since its major mode of action as an analgesic is believed to be central via activation of descending serotonergic pathways.

Box 6.9.1 Analgesic Drugs and Targets

	Target	Dose rate	Side-effects and interactions
Drug – Injectable			
Methadone	Opioid receptors (full agonist)	0.1–0.4 mg/kg im or iv q 4–6 h	Respiratory depression, nausea, anorexia
Buprenorphine	Opioid receptors (partial agonist)	0.01–0.02 mg/kg im or iv q 6–8 h	May antagonise full agonists such as methadone
Ketamine	Central action via NMDA receptors in CNS	0.25–0.5 mg/kg iv followed by cri 2–5 µg/kg/min	Dysphoria, tachycardia, or cardiovascular and respiratory depression
Medetomidine	α2 adrenoreceptor agonist	10 µg/kg im or iv, followed by cri 2–5 µg/kg/h	Sedation; causes significant reduction in dose requirement of anaesthetic drugs. Bradycardia, peripheral vasoconstriction
Drug – Oral			
Tramadol	Opioid receptors, noradrenaline and 5-HT reuptake inhibition	2–5 mg/kg po q 8 h	Sedation. Care in animals taking tricyclic antidepressants (amitriptyline), monoamine oxidase inhibitors (selegiline), SSRIs, and other opioids
Gabapentin	Complex interactions in CNS to downregulate pain responses	10–20 mg/kg po q 8–12 h	Sedation and ataxia; reversible hepatotoxicity has been seen in chronic use
Amantadine	NMDA antagonism (as ketamine)	3–5 mg/kg q 24 h	None reported
Paracetamol	Anti prostaglandin, probably other mechanisms also	10 mg/kg po or iv q 12 h	Not for use in cats
NSAID	Blockage of prostaglandin synthesis	See individual data sheets	Gastrointestinal ulceration and bleeding, renal damage in hypovolaemia

6.9.4   Differential Diagnoses for Conditions Presenting Only with Pain

The diagnostic challenge of pain-only conditions is exacerbated by the fact that, by definition, there are no other significant abnormalities on the neurological examination, and the neuroanatomic localisation relies solely on identifying the origin of pain. Also, the classical features of the clinical history that we employ in order to create a differential diagnosis list for other presenting complaints may not apply as well to pain-only conditions: onset may be difficult for the owner to define, progression may or may not be clear, and is often confused by multiple visits to see multiple veterinary surgeons, with multiple attempts to control the pain with different medications. Therefore, we feel that in this situation it is important for the clinician to have a good knowledge of the specific conditions which may present with pain, and the more common signalments for these conditions.

1. Vascular

In general, vascular conditions are not painful, with the exception of the classic acute aortic thromboembolic neuromyopathy of cats.

2. Inflammatory/infectious
a. Steroid-responsive meningitis arteritis (SRMA)

Steroid-responsive meningitis arteritis (SRMA) is an autoimmune inflammatory condition of the meninges that is seen primarily in young dogs, with the first presentation usually under 3 years of age. Breeds that are over-represented for this condition include the Beagle, Boxer, Bernese Mountain Dog, Nova Scotia Duck Tolling Retriever, and Weimaraner. Affected dogs classically present with neck pain and pyrexia, although pain may be present throughout the spine and is often waxing and waning. Some affected dogs may have a chronic history, with a partial response to previously administered NSAIDs or even apparently to antibiotics. In the latter case, this is usually because the antibiotic was administered alongside an analgesic, or the condition was naturally waning at the point of treatment, which may add to confusion in diagnosis. Affected animals normally show a peripheral neutrophilia, and diagnosis requires evidence of neutrophilic inflammation in CSF. These animals do *not* have neurological deficits such as ataxia and paresis, except in rare situations where the condition is very chronic and has led to meningeal thickening.

b. Meningomyelitis of unknown origin (MUO)

A different form of autoimmune inflammation can cause focal lesions in the spinal cord and meninges that may also be painful. This is usually accompanied by neurological deficits such as paresis and ataxia. This condition may affect any age or breed of dog, as well as cats, but is more typically seen in younger and smaller dog breeds such as terriers. Systemic signs and changes in peripheral blood are inconsistent, and diagnosis relies upon identification of a typical lesion in the spinal cord on MRI, associated with a mixed, mainly mononuclear, inflammation in the CSF (see Section 6.8 'Cerebellar Dysfunction' for further discussion of this condition).

c. Discospondylitis

Bacterial (and occasionally fungal) infections of the intervertebral disc are seen sporadically, and usually present as a focal, painful region within the vertebral column with minimal or no neurological deficits. Occasionally, there is an associated disc protrusion or significant inflammation that creates a compressive myelopathy, and this may lead to signs of paresis and/or ataxia. Any age and breed of animal can be affected, but this condition appears to be most common in young to middle-aged pure breeds of dog. The most commonly affected sites are the caudal cervical, mid thoracic, thoracolumbar, and lumbosacral regions. Presumptive diagnosis may be made by survey radiography (Figure 6.9.4), although advanced imaging with culture of the infectious organism is required for definitive confirmation.

Spinal radiography in cases of discospondylitis typically reveals ventral spondylosis, erosion of vertebral endplates with loss of clear endplate structure, and lytic regions within generally sclerotic endplates. The intervertebral disc space may appear widened, although it can also be narrowed. These radiographic signs, with accompanying physical findings, may warrant a presumptive diagnosis of discospondylitis if referral for advanced imaging is not possible.

Conditions such as spinal empyema (purulent inflammation in the epidural space) and FIP in cats are rare causes of pain without neurological deficits and will not be considered further in this section. Polyarthritis and polymyositis will be discussed in Section 6.9.5 'Confounders of Spinal Pain'.

3. Traumatic

Spinal fracture and luxation will usually present with pain and often significant neurological deficits. However, trauma may occasionally result in fracture of a peripheral part of a vertebra that does not lead to instability, and these cases can present with acute and severe pain only. Most commonly, these will be cervical

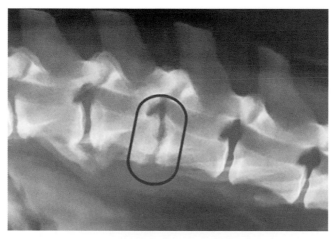

Figure 6.9.4 Discospondylitis in the lumbar spine. Bacterial infection of the intervertebral disc may be diagnosed by survey radiography when the infection has been present for at least 2–3 weeks. Changes seen in affected animals include sclerosis and irregularity of vertebral endplates at the site of the intervertebral disc infection, with lytic regions within the more sclerotic bone of the endplates. Ventral spondylosis is usually also a feature.

fractures such as those of the atlas wing, an articular facet, or even the dens of C2 (Figure 6.9.5). In most cases, a history of suspected trauma such as running into an object at speed will lead to a thorough radiographic investigation. However, some fractures (particularly when small or minimally displaced) can be difficult to identify, and CT is required for confirmation. If a spinal fracture is identified or suspected, referral for specialist advice and possible surgical treatment should always be considered.

4. Anomalous
a. Atlantoaxial instability

Some cases of AAI will present with neck pain only although in more severely affected dogs, tetraparesis and ataxia will also be seen associated with damage to the spinal cord parenchyma. Instability between the atlas (C1 vertebra) and axis (C2 vertebra) is normally a congenital problem due to malformation of the dens of the axis. In such cases, the problem is likely to present in young animals less than a year old, and miniature and toy breeds are over-represented. Diagnosis is made with survey radiography, where extended and slightly flexed lateral views should reveal a widening of the dorsal intervertebral space between C1 and C2 (Figure 6.9.6). Flexion of the neck to perform such radiography, and indeed the sedation or anaesthesia that is usually required to perform the procedure, should always be carried out with caution in any case where instability of the spine is considered a possibility. This may include cases where there is a history of known or suspected trauma, as well as in suspected cases of AAI. Clinicians should also use caution when taking radiographs under sedation or general anaesthesia in cases of suspected acute intervertebral disc extrusion, since flexion and extension of the vertebral column may potentially lead to extrusion of further nucleus

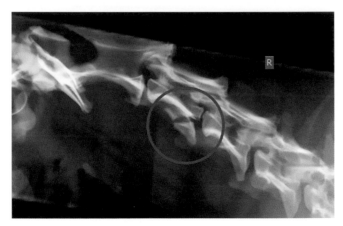

Figure 6.9.5 Vertebral body fracture at the level of C3, with mild ventral displacement but no involvement of the vertebral canal. Vertebral fractures and luxations are usually readily diagnosed by survey radiography, but orthogonal views should always be taken since minimally displaced fractures may only be apparent on a single view.

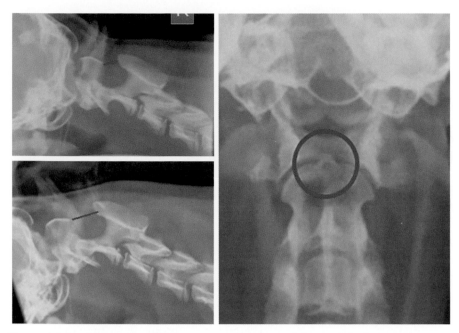

Figure 6.9.6 Atlantoaxial instability. Diagnosis may be made by carefully flexing the neck and comparing the dorsal space between C1 and C2 in neutral and flexed views. An obviously increased space, as in this case, indicates instability at the atlantoaxial joint. A ventrodorsal view may also indicate an abnormal dens, as shown. In many cases, the neutral lateral view may be enough to make the diagnosis and flexing the neck will pose a risk to the animal.

pulposus into the vertebral canal (see below). A recent study has shown that the degree of overlap of the cranial edge of the spine of the axis beyond the caudal arch of the atlas in neutral lateral views may be a safer and equally valid way to diagnose AAI in small dogs (Cummings et al. 2018).

The radiographs shown in Figure 6.9.6 illustrate the increased dorsal intervertebral space between C1 and C2 seen in dogs with confirmed AAI when the neck is flexed, compared to a normal dog where the space does not change. In the ventrodorsal radiograph the very shortened, abnormal dens is apparent.

Occasionally, AAI may be a traumatic condition, due to failure of the dorsal interspinous ligament or fracture of the dens; in such instances, even greater care should be taken when performing radiographs under sedation or anaesthesia, especially when flexing the neck, due to the possibility of spinal cord damage being exacerbated by instability at the region.

b. Chiari-like malformation/syringohydromyelia (SM)

Chiari-like malformation is defined as an overcrowding of the caudal fossa of the skull caused by malformation of the occipital bone and leading to herniation of the vermis of the cerebellum through the foramen magnum. It is often associated with other craniocervical junction abnormalities, such as atlanto-occipital overlapping and kinking of the cranial cervical spine. It is hypothesised that the changes in the flow of CSF which these abnormalities bring about are responsible for the development of syringomyelia, a condition in which CSF accumulates within the parenchyma of the spinal cord. Therefore, these two conditions often occur concurrently, although they may also occur independently to one another. Chiari-like malformation is almost ubiquitous in the Cavalier King Charles Spaniel (CKCS) breed, with clinically relevant syringomyelia seen less frequently. Syringomyelia may also be seen in association with other conditions that alter CSF flow, such as brain tumours or chronic compressive lesions of the spinal cord. There is an extensive literature concerning these conditions and the interested reader is directed to the Bibliography section at the end of this chapter for further information.

Syringomyelia is believed to be a relatively common cause of neck and spinal pain in young to middle-aged CKCS dogs, and also occurs frequently in Brussels Griffons and Chihuahuas. A recent study has shown evidence that CKCS affected with Chiari-like malformation alone may also suffer from neuropathic pain, casting doubt on the belief that syringomyelia is necessary to cause signs of pain (Rusbridge et al. 2019). However, it remains the case that both Chiari-like malformation and syringomyelia can be present asymptomatically in many dogs and other causes of acute neck pain should always be considered in susceptible breeds, such as intervertebral disc extrusion.

Syringomyelia may also cause neurological deficits, such as paresis, and a commonly associated clinical sign is phantom scratching, where the animal has bouts of sometimes frenzied scratching at the neck or flank without making contact with the skin (see Video 39). In the Chihuahua, phantom scratching appears to be the most common clinical sign, reported in 75% of affected dogs in one study (Kiviranta et al. 2017). Affected dogs will frequently scratch while walking, unlike dogs affected with skin disease. Diagnosis of Chiari-like malformation and syringomyelia may be strongly suspected from signalment and history but requires advanced imaging for confirmation (Figure 6.9.7).

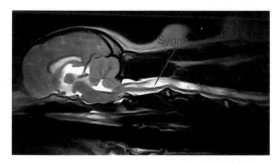

Figure 6.9.7 A T2 weighted mid-sagittal MRI of a Cavalier King Charles Spaniel showing Chiari-like malformation and syringomyelia. The syringomyelia is seen as the hyperintense (white) region on a T2 weighted scan within the parenchyma of the spinal cord.

5. Metabolic, toxic, and nutritional

These disorders rarely present as pain-only conditions.

6. Neoplastic

Most spinal tumours cause concurrent neurological deficits, and some may not be associated with pain at all. However, a vertebral tumour may occasionally present as a pain-only condition (e.g. osteosarcoma, plasma cell tumour, multiple myeloma). Survey radiography will usually identify such a lesion.

7. Degenerative

a. Intervertebral disc disease

Intervertebral disc disease covers a wide spectrum of disease, ranging from intervertebral disc degeneration without herniation, through to acute severe extrusion of non-degenerate nucleus pulposus. A more complete discussion of this disease, along with specific definitions, is given in Section 6.10 'Paresis, Paralysis, and Proprioceptive Ataxia'. However, intervertebral disc disease is a common cause of back and neck pain without neurological deficits and therefore features in the differential diagnosis list for this presentation.

Pain may be caused in a number of ways by intervertebral disc disease. It is known that degenerate discs can in themselves be a source of pain in people, so-called 'discogenic pain'. Although this is less well recognised in dogs, it seems likely that it may also occur, and should be considered in the absence of a more definitive diagnosis of back or neck pain. Better understood is the pain caused by a disc that has herniated (i.e. the disc outline extends into adjacent soft tissues, which may cause compression of spinal cord or nerve roots). Direct spinal nerve root compression may be painful, especially when associated with the inflammatory response that a herniated disc can cause. Spinal cord compression itself is not inherently painful, although accompanying stretching or inflammation of the meninges may be.

Recent work on intervertebral disc degeneration has led to some revision of our understanding of the degenerative process, and there is now believed to be much more overlap between the chondroid and fibroid degeneration than was previously thought. It remains the case that the most common form of disc herniation, the so-called Hansen type 1 intervertebral disc extrusion (where there is escape of the nucleus pulposus through the ruptured annulus fibrosus), is seen mainly in chondrodystrophic breeds such as Dachshunds, French Bulldogs, Cavalier King Charles Spaniels, Poodles, Chihuahuas, Pekingese, Pugs, Beagles, and Cocker Spaniels. The median age of presentation is 5 years although dogs as young as 1 year may be affected. Intervertebral disc extrusion is very unlikely in dogs less than a year of age. It can be seen from the previous discussion that many of the breeds affected by Hansen type 1 intervertebral disc extrusion are also commonly affected with other causes of neck pain, meaning that confirmation of diagnosis is particularly important.

Large, non-chondrodystrophic breeds, including Labrador Retrievers, German Shepherd Dogs, Dalmatians, and Dobermanns, may also be affected by Hansen type 1 intervertebral disc extrusion. However, these breeds more commonly suffer with Hansen type 2 intervertebral disc *protrusion*, where there is partial rupture and protrusion of the annulus fibrosus without escape of the nucleus pulposus. Signs typically develop more chronically with this condition and pain may be less apparent.

As previously stated, a more in-depth discussion of intervertebral disc disease will be given in Section 6.10 'Paresis, Paralysis, and Proprioceptive Ataxia', but it is important to be aware this disease is very common, affecting up to 20% of Dachshunds in their lifetime. It should therefore be at the forefront of the clinician's mind when faced with a potential painful spinal cord lesion. Cervical intervertebral disc extrusions are often significantly more painful than thoracolumbar extrusions, and frequently present with just pain and minimal or no neurological deficits. This is in contrast to thoracolumbar disease in which paresis and ataxia are more common.

Diagnosis of intervertebral disc disease may be suspected from the signalment and presenting clinical signs, and survey radiography may reveal a narrowed intervertebral disc space in the region of pain or calcified material overlying the vertebral canal. However, advanced imaging is required for confirmation, and other differential diagnoses should always be considered if this is not available.

6.9.5 Confounders of Spinal Pain

1. Immune-mediated polyarthritis

Immune-mediated polyarthritis (IMPA) may present as a painful condition, and it is a possible cause of spinal pain due to inflammation of the intervertebral joints. Affected animals are usually young, although any age can be affected. One study found that 30% of dogs with IMPA showed spinal pain, and roughly 30% of these dogs also had evidence of concurrent neutrophilic inflammation in the CSF, consistent with SRMA (Webb et al. 2002). It is therefore important to check for joint pain in any dog presented with suspected neck or back pain, with the distal joints (carpi and tarsi) most commonly affected. Synovial fluid analysis is required for diagnosis, with neutrophilic inflammation being seen in more than one joint in the absence of potential sepsis. Treatment requires immunosuppressive therapy (see below).

2. Immune-mediated polymyositis

This condition more commonly presents as generalised weakness, but significant muscular pain may be present and can mimic apparent spinal pain. Diagnosis requires evidence of significant elevations of muscle enzymes (such as creatinine kinase), although care must be taken when interpreting elevations of this enzyme since it is very labile and may be also elevated non-specifically, especially in cats. Muscle biopsy is required for confirmation of polymyositis. A specific immune-mediated myositis affecting only the muscles of mastication also occurs, called masticatory myositis, for which an antibody test is available (Type IIM antibodies). This condition usually presents as pain on opening the mouth that may occasionally be confused for neck pain. Treatment of most forms of immune-mediated myositis requires immunosuppressive doses of corticosteroid, although this may exacerbate the muscle atrophy already caused by this disease.

3. Orthopaedic disease

As already stated, orthopaedic disease may present very similarly to spinal disease, and animals that suffer from chronic osteoarthritic or degenerative conditions such as cranial cruciate ligament disease, elbow dysplasia, or hip dysplasia, may frequently show generalised pain, stiffness, and apparent 'weakness'. Such cases require careful evaluation, since many dogs presenting with genuine spinal disease, such as intervertebral disc disease and lumbosacral disease, may also have concurrent orthopaedic problems. A thorough orthopaedic examination as well as a neurological examination should be performed in all animals presenting with apparent neck or back pain, especially in cases where there are minimal or no neurological deficits. Radiographic studies must, however, be interpreted with some caution, since many animals can have clinically insignificant radiographic joint disease.

4. Neoplasia

Many forms of neoplastic disease, including osteosarcoma and even brain tumours, can present as painful animals that may be reluctant to move. Some brain tumours present with apparent neck pain and this should always be a consideration if the signalment is appropriate and the diagnosis is not immediately clear. Thorough screening for evidence of neoplasia, including thoracic radiography and abdominal ultrasound, should be performed in animals presenting with non-specific or difficult to localise pain, and any evidence of neoplastic disease investigated appropriately.

5. Abdominal pain

Abdominal pain, especially acute pancreatitis, is frequently mistaken for thoracolumbar pain and vice versa. When presented with a dog with suspected thoracolumbar pain, careful abdominal palpation should be performed in order to prevent such a mistake from being made. If there is any doubt, then a more complete abdominal diagnostic work-up, including imaging, should be considered. One recent study found an association between thoracolumbar intervertebral disc extrusion and elevations of serum canine pancreatic lipase, so it is possible that there may be an association between these two conditions (Schueler et al. 2018). However, pancreatic lipase is also an enzyme which is commonly elevated non-specifically, and so this association may be clinically insignificant. Care should be taken when making a suspected diagnosis of pancreatitis in a dog that presents with apparent abdominal pain only, particularly in a chondrodystrophic breed such as the Dachshund; in the author's experience, a significant number of dogs referred with thoracolumbar disc extrusion were initially misdiagnosed as suspected acute pancreatitis, meaning strict rest was not considered a necessary part of their treatment protocol (see Section 6.10 'Paresis, Paralysis, and Proprioceptive Ataxia').

6.9.6   Management of Pain-only Conditions

After an attempt has been made to localise the source of pain, a knowledge of the possible and likely differential diagnoses for any given presentation should allow the clinician to formulate an appropriate plan to discuss with the owner. If the animal is presenting with a first episode of pain which is mild or moderate, then in-house investigation and symptomatic treatment are usually a sensible first step. Routine haematology and biochemistry to look for evidence of neutrophilia (which might indicate SRMA, IMPA, or bacterial infection), systemic disease, or raised muscle enzymes may be indicated. Survey radiography of the painful region of the spine may provide evidence for an increased likelihood of intervertebral disc disease (narrowed intervertebral disc space, calcified material in vertebral canal), or even of discospondylitis or neoplasia.

If Hansen type 1 intervertebral disc extrusion is suspected, then the reader is referred to a more extensive discussion in Section 6.10 'Paresis, Paralysis, and Proprioceptive Ataxia'. However, the basic management strategy should include a period of confinement and appropriate analgesia.

Management strategies for other potential differential diagnoses are listed below.

1. Steroid-responsive meningitis arteritis (SRMA)

Whenever a true immune-mediated inflammatory condition of the spine is considered a significant possibility, whether it be SRMA or meningomyelitis of unknown origin (MUO), referral for specialist advice and diagnostic work-up should be offered. However, if this is not possible then what are the options for the general practitioner? Measurement of acute phase proteins such as C-reactive protein may add weight to the suspected diagnosis. This may be expected to be elevated in SRMA and not in cases with MUO, but it must always be remembered that this is a very non-specific marker of acute inflammation that can also be elevated in animals with IMPA, discospondylitis, bacterial meningitis, and neoplasia. It may be wise to perform serology for infectious diseases, such as toxoplasmosis and neosporosis, before initiating immunosuppressive therapy, although these conditions are rare compared to the prevalence of non-infectious meningitis; a recent study found results consistent with active infection in 0.25% for toxoplasmosis and 2.25% for neosporosis of dogs with suspected immune-mediated meningoencephalitis (Coelho et al. 2019).

The mainstay of treatment of SRMA (and also MUO) is prednisolone at immu-nosuppressive doses (4 mg/kg/day for 1–2 days, followed by 2 mg/kg/day for 2 weeks, then 1 mg/kg/day for 6 weeks, 0.5 mg/kg/day for 6 weeks, then 0.5 mg/kg on alternate days for 1–2 months). Pyrexia, neutrophilia, and C-reactive protein can be used for monitoring if CSF analysis is not possible, and ideally treatment should not be discontinued until all of these parameters are normal. However, it has been shown that C-reactive protein may remain elevated even after remission of disease (Lowrie et al. 2009). Relapse of SRMA is relatively com-mon and may be more likely if the disease is not treated aggressively enough or for long enough. If this occurs, prednisolone therapy should be reinstated. The disease is eventually self-limiting in most dogs by the age of 3 years, although may rarely require longer-term treatment.

2. Discospondylitis

If discospondylitis is suspected from survey radiographs (see Figure 6.9.4), an attempt should be made to culture the likely causative organism. When direct biopsy of the affected intervertebral disc is not possible, urine and blood culture should be performed. Antibiotic choice should be based on culture and sensitiv-ity results where possible, but in the absence of a positive culture empirical anti-biotic use is necessary. Because most bacterial infections of the intervertebral disc are caused by *Staphylococcus* spp., the author favours cephalexin (20 mg/kg twice daily), but potentiated-amoxycillin or clindamycin may be reasonable alternatives. Treatment should be continued for at least 3 months and well beyond the resolution of clinical signs.

3. Atlantoaxial instability (AAI)

If AAI is considered likely or is confirmed by radiography (see Figure 6.9.6), then medical and surgical management options are available. In severe cases with significant neurological deficits, specialist referral for possible surgical manage-ment is preferred. In more mild cases, conservative management with a form of external splinting and cage confinement may be sufficient to allow stabilisation of the atlantoaxial joint. In most cases of confirmed or suspected AAI, referral to a specialist for a thorough discussion of the problem and potential treatment options should be recommended.

4. Chiari-like malformation/syringomyelia

If these conditions are suspected from the clinical history and signalment, then referral to a specialist neurologist for confirmation by advanced imaging (Figure 6.9.7) and a discussion of the treatment options available is advised. Syringomyelia is a progressive condition that is likely to require lifelong treatment, although one study showed that most dogs maintain a reasonable quality of life following diagnosis (Plessas et al. 2012). If referral is not an option, then it is reasonable to offer symptomatic treatment. Analgesia and reduction in cerebrospinal fluid production are the key treatment goals. NSAIDs may be useful in early and mild cases, but often drugs more specifically acting on neuropathic pain and central wind-up may be more effective. The most commonly used medications for this role in veterinary medicine are gabapentin and amantadine, although pregabalin and topiramate may also be useful (see Box 6.9.1). Opiates such as tramadol may also be useful, although the evidence for the efficacy of tramadol in dogs is mixed. Omeprazole was proposed as a potential treatment due to experimental evidence showing that it may reduce CSF production via inhibition of proton pumping; however, a more recent paper showed no effect on CSF production following administration to Beagle dogs (Girod et al. 2016). The only drug with good evidence for a reduction in CSF production is corticosteroid, and due to its multiple other potentially beneficial effects such as inhibition of the formation of pro-inflammatory mediators and substance P, it can be a very effective drug at treating the clinical signs of syringomyelia. The author generally favours a stepwise approach to treatment of this condition, beginning with an NSAID, then adding gabapentin and perhaps also amantadine, before considering the use of prednisolone as a 'last resort'. However, at anti-inflammatory doses prednisolone can be very effective, and the dose can be titrated down to minimise side-effects in the longer term. In severely affected dogs which are poorly responsive to medical management, surgical treatment options may be available, although evidence for the long-term efficacy of these is currently lacking.

6.9.7 When Should Referral of Pain-only Spinal Disease be Actively Encouraged

Indications for referral of animals presenting with neck and/or back pain include:

- diagnosis unclear, or significantly in doubt
- initial symptomatic treatment unsuccessful
- recurring, relapsing, or chronic pain
- high suspicion of inflammatory disease, potentially requiring immunosuppressive therapy; achieving a confirmed diagnosis before embarking on prolonged immunosuppression is always preferable
- possible surgical disease (e.g. suspected AAI, history of trauma, intervertebral disc disease)
- high suspicion of syringomyelia; confirmation of diagnosis advisable since this is likely to be a progressive and lifelong disease.

6.10   Paresis, Paralysis, and Proprioceptive Ataxia

Paul M. Freeman

6.10.1   Neuroanatomic Basis of Paresis

As has already been discussed, paresis implies a reduction in voluntary motor activity, which may impair an animal's ability to weight-bear or to initiate movement. When the lower motor neurons directly innervating the skeletal muscles of the limbs are affected, the paresis is known as 'lower motor neuron paresis' and the gait is characteristically short-strided and choppy due to impaired ability to weight-bear. When the so-called upper motor neurons of the brain or spinal cord are affected, the paresis is said to be 'upper motor neuron' and the strides tend to be longer due to a reduced ability to initiate movement (see Chapter 3). Paresis in combination with proprioceptive ataxia implies brainstem or spinal cord involvement due to the effects of the lesion on the proprioceptive tracts of the spinal cord; generalised lower motor neuron paresis, such as occurs in disorders affecting the peripheral nervous system, does not usually cause ataxia because the sensory nerves and proprioceptive receptors are rarely involved. Lower motor neuron paresis is considered further in Section 6.12 'Neuromuscular Weakness'.

Paresis is generally divided into 'ambulatory' and 'non-ambulatory' as a measure of severity and for the purposes of grading spinal cord injury. The most severe injuries will cause paralysis (or plegia), which is complete absence of voluntary movement.

The following discussion will be restricted to diseases affecting the spinal cord; an approach to diseases of the brainstem, which may also result in tetraparesis and proprioceptive ataxia, has already been considered in Section 6.3 'Altered Mentation'. When faced with an animal exhibiting tetraparesis and proprioceptive ataxia, it can be assumed that the neuroanatomic localisation is cervicothoracic spinal cord if the level of mentation and cranial nerve examination are normal. The reader is also referred to Section 6.9 'Neck and/or Spinal Pain' on neck and spinal pain, since there is considerable overlap with the approach to an animal presenting with paresis and ataxia.

6.10.2   Diagnostic Approach to Paresis and Proprioceptive Ataxia

Using the approach outlined in Chapter 5, the potential differential diagnoses for a dog or cat presenting with suspected spinal cord disease may be narrowed down in the following way.

1. Clinical history

The primary considerations regarding an animal that presents for suspected spinal cord disease are the onset and progression of the clinical signs, the presence or absence of pain, and the degree of asymmetry. A recent study evaluated the usefulness of this approach and concluded that the only spinal disorders presenting as a peracute, improving, non-painful, and lateralising myelopathy are fibrocartilaginous embolism (FCE) and acute non-compressive nucleus pulposus extrusion, so this is clearly very valuable information (Cardy et al. 2015). The same study concluded that most cases of type 1 intervertebral disc herniation present as an acute onset of painful, often progressive, and symmetrical clinical signs.

a. Onset of clinical signs

i. Peracute onset

• *Fibrocartilaginous embolism (FCE)*
  FCE is a condition in which a small piece or pieces of fibrocartilage, which are thought to arise from an intervertebral disc, embolise into an arteriole(s) supplying a focal region of the spinal cord. This causes ischaemic damage to the parenchyma of the spinal cord and often leads to asymmetrical signs due to the nature of the blood supply to the spinal cord. The precise route by which this material gains entry to the vascular system is unknown but may involve invasion of a degenerate intervertebral disc with blood vessels from the adjacent vertebral endplate. Most affected dogs are middle-aged or older, large and giant breeds, and occasionally there is a history of onset during exercise. However, there is frequently no association with trauma and affected dogs are found at home by their owners having suffered an acute onset of paresis or plegia. The dog may yelp at the time of onset and there may be mild pain on palpation over the affected region of the spine which only lasts for a few hours, so that by the time affected dogs are seen by a veterinary surgeon there is usually no apparent spinal pain (see below).

• *Acute hydrated nucleus pulposus extrusion (compressive or non-compressive), or 'traumatic disc extrusion'*
  These terms (along with others) are used to describe the peracute extrusion of non- or partially degenerate, gelatinous nucleus pulposus material from an apparently healthy intervertebral disc. This condition is commonly referred to as acute non-compressive nucleus pulposus extrusion or ANNPE, or, if spinal cord compression is seen, hydrated nucleus pulposus extrusion or HNPE. This is presumed to be associated with forceful compression of the disc during some kind of trauma. Such an extrusion may be associated with external trauma, such as a road traffic accident, but is also seen in association with vigorous exercise such as jumping and ball chasing. Affected dogs are often heard to cry or yelp in pain at the time of a sudden onset of paresis or plegia.

As for FCE, the neurological deficits are often asymmetrical, meaning that these two conditions are very difficult to distinguish clinically. Pain on palpation may be present for up to 24 hours after the onset of signs, but again may be absent by the time animals are presented. Neurological deficits can be severe, with some animals presenting with tetra- or paraplegia. Staffordshire Bull Terriers may be over-represented. Most often, the extruded nuclear material is minimally or non-compressive and the spinal cord damage is a result of contusion; compressive lesions have also been described, although a recent study showed no difference in outcome between these treated surgically and non-surgically (Nessler et al. 2018).

- *Vertebral fracture/luxation*

  This diagnosis would normally be associated with a known trauma and would therefore be suspected. However, a fracture of an articular process or the atlas wing for example may occur without an obvious (to the owner at least) trauma and can be difficult to diagnose with survey radiography. Neurological deficits are related to the level and degree of trauma and, in some situations, fractures may cause pain only with no apparent deficits (see Section 6.9 'Neck and/or Spinal Pain').

ii. Acute onset over minutes to hours

- *Hansen type 1 intervertebral disc extrusion*

  See below.

- *Meningomyelitis of unknown origin (MUO)*

  MUO affecting the brain has already been discussed in Section 6.8 'Cerebellar Dysfunction'. However, autoimmune inflammation may also affect the spinal cord, leading to focal or multifocal lesions that can present as an acute or subacute onset of paresis and proprioceptive ataxia. These lesions may be variably painful and can also cause a more chronic and insidious progression of signs. Neurological deficits are usually progressive, with disease progression sometimes being quite rapid. Diagnosis requires the identification of characteristic T2-weighted hyperintense lesions within the parenchyma of the spinal cord on MRI, most often associated with a mixed, mononuclear inflammatory CSF sample. Treatment requires immunosuppression, with corticosteroids being the most widely used and often effective treatment. Prognosis, as for MUO affecting the brain, is guarded.

- *Infectious disease*

  Bacterial infection causing accumulation of purulent exudate within the epidural space (empyema) is an uncommon cause of acute spinal cord disease. Such infections are frequently associated with systemic signs such as pyrexia and may be extremely painful. They usually lead to a rapid progression of neurological signs within a short period of time (hours to days). Many cases are associated with an infectious focus somewhere in the body, such as a foreign body, urinary tract infection (UTI), or skin disease, although they are occasionally spontaneous. Diagnosis may be suspected from clinical history and physical examination but requires advanced imaging +/− sampling or surgical exploration for confirmation. Treatment may be medical or surgical, although if there is a rapid deterioration and significant pain then surgery may provide more rapid resolution of clinical signs.

Toxoplasmosis and neosporosis can in theory cause focal cystic lesions affecting the spinal cord. However, these infections are extremely rare when compared to non-infectious inflammatory disease as described above.

iii. Subacute onset over a few days

Conditions with a possible subacute onset of clinical signs include meningoencephalomyelitis of unknown origin and infectious disease (as discussed above), Hansen type 1 intervertebral disc extrusion (see below), and neoplasia.

iv. Chronic onset over several days to several weeks

- *Hansen type 2 intervertebral disc protrusion*
  See below.
- *Syringomyelia*
  See Section 6.9 'Neck and/or Spinal Pain'.
- *Degenerative myelopathy*

There are a number of chronic, progressive neurodegenerative conditions that may affect the spinal cord of dogs and cats. These are generally rare but the most well known and common is degenerative myelopathy in dogs. This chronic, progressive neurodegenerative disease is seen in many large breeds of dog, most notably the German Shepherd Dog. It is also known to affect the Corgi, Chesapeake Bay Retriever, Siberian Husky, Boxer, Bernese Mountain Dog, Rhodesian Ridgeback, Golden Retriever, Pug, and Standard Poodle, amongst others. Affected dogs are typically middle-aged or older (>8 years), but it may be seen in dogs as young as 5 years old. In the Corgi, especially Cardigan Corgis, disease onset is often much later.

Degenerative myelopathy is caused by a genetic mutation affecting the superoxide dismutase (SOD) enzyme system responsible for destroying free radicals within the body. This leads to degeneration of white matter tracts in the spinal cord, predominantly in the thoracic region. This causes a chronic, progressive pelvic limb paresis and ataxia, with classical signs of toe-dragging, scuffed nails, and significant ataxia. The condition is not painful, but over time may progress to urinary and faecal incontinence, thoracic limb involvement, and complete paraplegia. Diagnosis is by exclusion of other conditions that may also present as a chronic, progressive T3–L3 myelopathy, such as Hansen type 2 intervertebral disc protrusion and neoplasia. There is currently no treatment. A genetic test is available for identification of the SOD-1A mutation associated with the disease in the German Shepherd Dog and probably most affected breeds, although an additional mutation SOD-1B has been identified specifically in the Bernese Mountain Dog. Affected dogs are usually homozygous for the mutation, with heterozygous dogs being carriers of the disease but rarely showing clinical disease. It is important to remember that a positive genetic test result does *not* mean that an affected animal has degenerative myelopathy, only that it is at an increased risk of acquiring the condition at some point in its lifetime. The results must therefore always be combined with other factors when forming a diagnosis, such as the signalment, clinical history, and exclusion of other possible differential diagnoses by advanced imaging.

- *Arachnoid space disease*

  A chronic, progressive myelopathy may be seen in association with a focal accumulation of CSF in the subarachnoid space, usually dorsal to the spinal cord in either the cervical or thoracic regions. Such 'arachnoid diverticuli' are seen mainly in young Rottweilers in the cervical region, and older Pugs in the mid-thoracic spine. The aetiology is uncertain in many cases but is suspected to be related to chronic instability secondary to hypoplasia of the articular facets in the thoracolumbar region of older Pugs. Many affected Pugs show signs of faecal incontinence as well as paraparesis and proprioceptive ataxia. The condition is usually non-painful, chronic, and progressive. Diagnosis requires advanced imaging, and treatment usually involves some form of surgical drainage of the diverticulum +/− stabilisation.

- *Cervical spondylomyelopathy (osseous- and disc-associated 'wobbler syndrome')*

  'Wobbler syndrome' is caused by cervical spinal cord compression, either by bony structures or soft tissues. Young giant breed dogs, such as the Great Dane, Bernese Mountain Dog, and Rhodesian Ridgeback, may be affected by osseous wobbler syndrome, in which the cervical spinal cord is compressed at multiple levels by bony enlargement of articular processes or the vertebral arch causing constriction of the vertebral canal. Affected dogs are typically 2–3 years old, but may present at less than 1 year of age, and show a progressive tetraparesis which may be moderately painful. Diagnosis may be suspected from survey radiographs but requires advanced imaging for confirmation. Treatment usually requires surgical removal of compressive bone, although many cases will stabilise or can be managed medically, and a recent case report described spontaneous resolution of signs in a growing Mastiff dog (Doran et al. 2019).

  Disc-associated wobbler syndrome is more common and is seen in the Dobermann and other large breeds of dog such as the Labrador Retriever and Dalmatian. Clinical signs of tetraparesis develop in middle-aged and older dogs and may be progressive, with variable pain. The pelvic limbs are often more severely affected than the thoracic limbs. The disc-associated lesions responsible for the clinical signs are more common in the caudal cervical spine, typically at the C5–C6 and C6–C7 levels. These range from a simple intervertebral disc protrusion to more complex compressive lesions involving the intervertebral disc and associated soft tissues, such as the intervertebral ligaments and facet joint capsules. The location of the spinal cord lesions within the C6–T2 intumescence can lead to the typical 'two-engine' gait, with short, choppy thoracic limb strides and long, ataxic pelvic limb strides (see Chapter 4). Diagnosis again requires advanced imaging to demonstrate the site and nature of the spinal cord compression. Occasionally, dogs may suffer acute deterioration to severe, non-ambulatory tetraparesis or -plegia, potentially associated with trauma. Treatment may be surgical or medical (see below). Many dogs will respond well to initial treatment with anti-inflammatory doses of prednisolone, although the long-term prognosis may be better with surgical treatment.

- *Degenerative lumbosacral stenosis*
  Dogs affected by lumbosacral disease rarely show significant ataxia, and frequently only have mild to moderate paraparesis. Similar to the disc-associated wobbler syndrome described above, degenerative lumbosacral stenosis is a complex condition that results in compression of the cauda equina at the level of L7–S1 by a combination of intervertebral disc and/or associated bony and soft tissue structures. It may result in lateralising signs, such as pelvic limb lameness associated with compression of the L7 nerve roots as they exit the vertebral canal at this level. It can also present as bilateral lameness, paraparesis, lower back pain, tail, bladder, or even anal sphincter weakness. A common presenting sign of lumbosacral stenosis is a dog that has become reluctant to jump into the car or onto the sofa or is reluctant to go up steps and stairs. Diagnosis requires confirmation of cauda equina compression using MRI or CT and exclusion of other causes for the presenting clinical signs. Treatment may be medical or surgical and, as for wobbler syndrome, many different surgical techniques have been described. Medical treatment is successful in a number of dogs, and epidural injection of methylprednisolone acetate has also been reported to be effective in a high percentage of dogs.

b. Progression of clinical signs

i. Improving signs

- FCE, acute non-compressive nucleus pulposus extrusion

These two conditions may both show quite rapid improvement, sometimes within 48 hours. However, more severely affected dogs will take several weeks to improve, and some cases fail to improve at all, particularly if there is an absence of nociception (deep pain perception) in the affected limbs or if the lesion involves the spinal cord grey matter in the C6–T2 or L4–S3 spinal cord regions.

ii. Static signs
• Trauma, Hansen type 1 intervertebral disc extrusion

iii. Deteriorating signs
• Meningomyelitis of unknown origin, infectious disease, syringomyelia, arachnoid space disorder, cervical spondylomyelopathy, neoplasia, Hansen types 1 and 2 intervertebral disc herniation, degenerative myelopathy

The speed of deterioration for these conditions can be very variable; some conditions, such as syringomyelia, arachnoid space disorders, and degenerative myelopathy, take a slow, chronic, progressive course over months. In contrast, neoplastic conditions affecting the spinal cord can have a very rapid progression but may also progress more slowly as would be perhaps more expected for neoplasia. Hansen type 2 intervertebral disc protrusions usually progress slowly over weeks to months but can also show an acute deterioration. Hansen type 1 intervertebral disc extrusions normally progress more quickly, and this disease may take a very variable course; some cases improve following an acute onset, others progress over hours to days, and yet others have a static or even apparently waxing and waning time course (see below).

c. The presence/absence of pain

i. Non-painful pain conditions
FCE, acute non-compressive nucleus pulposus extrusion (after initial 24 hours), many anomalous diseases (such as arachnoid space disorders), most intramedullary neoplasia, neurodegenerative disorders (e.g. degenerative myelopathy).

ii. Painful conditions
Inflammatory/infectious disorders are frequently painful, including meningomyelitis of unknown origin. Some protozoal or viral infections, such as toxoplasmosis and FIP, may present without apparent pain but most bacterial disease is very painful. Discospondylitis and epidural empyema may be two of the most painful conditions seen in small animal practice. Traumatic vertebral fractures are usually very painful due to compression and inflammation of associated nerve roots and meninges. Anomalous disorders such as Chiari-like malformation and syringomyelia, as well as AAI, may be significantly painful (see Section 6.9 'Neck and/or Spinal Pain'). Neoplastic disease affecting the vertebral column and spinal cord is often painful, especially vertebral body osteosarcoma. Most cases of Hansen type 1 and type 2 intervertebral disc herniation are associated with a degree of apparent pain on examination, with this being particularly true for type 1 disc extrusions.

d. Symmetry of neurological deficits

i. Asymmetrical conditions

FCE, acute non-compressive nucleus pulposus extrusion, (Hansen type 1 intervertebral disc disease, neoplasia, degenerative myelopathy).

ii. Symmetrical conditions

Most intervertebral disc herniations (especially Hansen type 2 disc protrusions), inflammatory/infectious disease, anomalous disorders, degenerative myelopathy.

2. Signalment

There may be clues to the most likely differential diagnoses through a knowledge of breed predispositions (see Chapter 2), and although these can rarely, if ever, be taken as absolutes, they can help the clinician to make informed choices and provide reasonable advice in situations where specialist referral for diagnosis is not an option. A few of the known breed predispositions include the following.

* *Fibrocartilaginous embolism and acute non-compressive nucleus pulposus extrusion*
  One study found that Staffordshire Bull Terriers and Border Collies were over-represented (Fenn et al. 2016), and this is also the author's experience. Furthermore, 70–80% of all cases of FCE occur in middle-aged and older, large and giant breed dogs.
* *Hansen type 1 intervertebral disc extrusion*
  At least 75% of cases occur in chondrodystrophic breeds of dog, with the Dachshund, French Bulldog, and Cocker Spaniel being over-represented.
* *Degenerative myelopathy*
  The German Shepherd Dog and Pembroke Welsh Corgi are predisposed, but this disease also occurs in many other breeds of dog (see above).
* *Cervical spondylomyelopathy*
  Young Great Danes are predisposed to the osseous form, where the onset of clinical signs is usually in juvenile growing dogs. The Dobermann is the breed most commonly affected by the disc-associated form, but the disease may also be seen in other breeds, including the Dalmatian and the Labrador Retriever. Affected dogs are usually middle-aged or older.
* *Atlantoaxial instability*
  Chihuahuas, Yorkshire Terriers, and other toy breeds are predisposed to this condition, with signs usually becoming apparent in young dogs.
* *Arachnoid space disorders*
  Thoracolumbar arachnoid diverticuli are seen mainly in Pugs and French Bulldogs, often associated with vertebral abnormalities. A recent study found male dogs are significantly over-represented (Mauler et al. 2014). Pugs also

suffer from a fibrotic constrictive myelopathy in this region. Larger breeds, especially the Rottweiler, are affected by cervical arachnoid diverticulum. There is no significant age predisposition, with the study mentioned above finding a median affected age of 3 years.

3. Neurological examination

Mentation: Expected to be normal unless affected by severe pain or shock in trauma cases.

Gait and posture: Tetra-, hemi-, or paraparesis with concurrent proprioceptive ataxia. A low head carriage may be seen in painful cervical lesions and kyphosis in painful thoracolumbar lesions. Kyphosis and/or scoliosis may also be associated with vertebral malformations and severe cases of syringomyelia. Schiff–Sherrington posture may be present in cases of acute, severe thoracolumbar spinal cord injury, with rigidly extended thoracic limbs and paralysed pelvic limbs (see Figure 6.10.1, Video 23, and Chapters 3 and 4).

Postural reactions: Abnormalities of either one, two, three, or four limbs, depending on the lesion location. In cervical lesions, all limbs may be expected to be abnormal, but if the lesion is markedly lateralised then there may be a hemiparesis and postural reaction deficits on only the affected side. With thoracolumbar lesions, just the pelvic limbs should be affected, and in a very lateralised lesion just a single pelvic limb may have postural reaction deficits.

Spinal reflexes: May be normal in all limbs for lesions affecting the C1–C5 spinal cord segments. If the lesion affects the C6–T2 spinal cord segments, spinal reflexes may be reduced in the thoracic limbs, and if the lesion affects the L4–S3 spinal cord segments, the spinal reflexes in the pelvic limbs may be reduced (see Chapter 4). However, the relative strength of the withdrawal reflexes can be

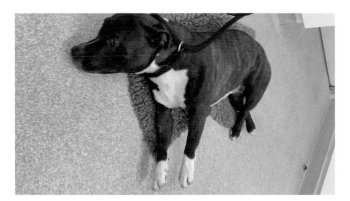

Figure 6.10.1 Schiff–Sherrington posture in a dog with an acute, severe thoracolumbar spinal cord injury. The rigid extension of the thoracic limbs is caused by a loss of ascending inhibitory influence on the thoracic limb extensor muscles from interneurons in the lumbar spinal cord known as Border cells. Voluntary limb function and postural reactions in the thoracic limbs are normal in such cases, and this presentation does not affect the prognosis for recovery.

difficult to determine, even for a specialist neurologist, and is open to a degree of subjectivity which can make neuroanatomic localisation difficult.

In acute, severe thoracolumbar spinal cord lesions, the spinal reflexes may be reduced in one or both pelvic limbs for a variable period of time by a phenomenon known as spinal shock (see Chapters 4 and 7.3). The correct neuroanatomic localisation in these cases is usually possible by using the cutaneous trunci reflex, which is frequently interrupted close to the level of the lesion.

Cranial nerve examination: Expected to be normal. Horner syndrome may be seen in some cases of cervical spinal disease, especially with lesions affecting the brachial plexus outflow.

Palpation: Careful palpation for pain may help with the neuroanatomic localisation as well as the list of differential diagnoses (see above).

4. Neuroanatomic localisation

Following the neurological examination, it should be possible to localise the spinal cord lesion in an animal presenting with paresis and ataxia to one of four regions within the spinal cord: C1–C5, C6–T2, T3–L3, L4–S3 (see Chapter 4).

The neuroanatomic localisation does not necessarily aid construction of a differential diagnosis list, except in cases of certain anatomically restricted diseases, but may focus diagnostic evaluation. There are, however, certain causes of paresis and proprioceptive ataxia for which a specific localisation would be expected, such as AAI (C1–C5), disc-associated wobbler syndrome (C6–T2), and degenerative myelopathy (T3–L3). An alternative neuroanatomic localisation would make these particular diseases unlikely.

6.10.3 Formulating a Plan

Once a reasonable differential diagnosis list has been produced by adopting the approach outlined above, the clinician must decide how best to approach the case (i.e. whether to initiate further investigations or seek specialist assistance via referral). As before, the purpose of this text is to provide maximum assistance when referral is not an option, but also to give guidance as to when referral is likely to be most urgent.

Cases can be differentiated in a number of ways, with onset, progression, and the presence/absence of pain perhaps being most useful when it comes to establishing potential differential diagnoses and considering an appropriate course of action.

1. Peracute onset of clinical signs
a. Painful conditions

Trauma is the most likely cause, so consider immediate referral if possible, especially if neurological deficits are severe. In cases of spinal cord trauma with an absence of deep pain perception, the prognosis is likely to be grave and recovery very unlikely, so euthanasia should always be discussed with owners. Cervical lesions that are severe enough to cause loss of deep pain perception usually result in death through respiratory failure. Be aware of the possibility for spinal instability, provide support if possible, and take great care with anaesthesia and sedation. If referral is not an option and deep pain perception is preserved, consider survey radiographs of the affected region. Cage confinement may lead to eventual recovery if the spinal cord damage is not too severe and the injury is stable or can be supported by an external splint or cast, especially in the case of cervical or low lumbar injuries.

b. Non-painful conditions

FCE and ANNPE are most likely, especially if the neurological deficits show some asymmetry and the signs are static or improving. Supportive care should be instigated as appropriate for acute spinal cord injury, including intravenous fluid therapy, maintenance of normal systemic mean arterial pressure, nursing care, and bladder management if required (see Chapter 7). Cases carry a favourable prognosis and the majority of dogs with intact nociception will recover the ability to walk with nursing care alone. Referral for advanced imaging is always appropriate but is not necessary to distinguish between these two conditions since their basic management is the same (see below). Although some cases of traumatic, non-degenerate disc extrusion may lead to a compressive spinal cord lesion (so-called compressive HNPE), a recent study showed that outcomes with surgical and medical management may be very similar (Nessler et al. 2018).

2. Acute or subacute onset of clinical signs

a. Painful conditions

Inflammatory disease, either infectious or non-infectious, and intervertebral disc extrusion are the most likely differential diagnoses in this category. The decision whether to investigate, treat, or refer (if possible) should be governed by the neurological status at presentation and the speed of progression. Any animal that is showing a rapid deterioration or is unable to walk at the time of presentation is a candidate for referral for specialist assessment. Inflammatory and infectious diseases can progress rapidly if appropriate treatment is not initiated, and some cases of intervertebral disc extrusion may progress to loss of deep pain perception, in which case the prognosis for recovery is greatly reduced. If the animal is able to walk, it is reasonable in most cases to consider investigations in-house, which may include haematology and serum biochemistry, infectious disease testing +/– survey radiography of the affected area. Analgesic therapy should be given, but corticosteroids should be avoided due to their ability to mask clinical signs, exacerbate infections, and make potential future diagnosis more difficult. If referral is not an option, then the clinician must make decisions based on the most likely suspected diagnosis. A more detailed description of the approach to intervertebral disc disease is given in Section 6.10.4 'Intervertebral Disc Disease'.

b. Non-painful conditions

There are few non-painful conditions that will show a genuinely acute onset of signs, with the exception of acute non-compressive nucleus pulposus extrusion and FCE, as already discussed. Some intramedullary neoplasms may be non-painful and occasionally present in an acute or subacute manner. Some cases of arachnoid space disorder may also present relatively acutely and with little pain, but this is unusual.

Tetanus is a condition that is caused by infection with spores of the bacterium *C. tetani*, which release a neurotoxin that affects inhibitory interneurons to the extensor muscles of the limbs. This leads to a generalised spastic paresis/paralysis which may initially present as an acutely tetraparetic animal. Other signs may include facial muscle contraction ('risus sardonicus' – Figure 6.10.2) and an elevated or semi-elevated tail. Occasionally tetanus may be focal, with the clinical signs restricted to a single limb. It is a rare condition in dogs and cats, with a potentially guarded prognosis in generalised cases due to the degree of nursing care required until spontaneous recovery can occur. Referral for specialist advice and intensive care is recommended in suspected cases, as intensive nursing will improve the prognosis and may be required for a prolonged period of time. For further information the reader is referred to the many other texts on specific neurological diseases.

3. Chronic onset of clinical signs

a. Painful conditions

This group consists mainly of Hansen type 2 intervertebral disc protrusion (and occasional cases of Hansen type 1 disc extrusion), spinal cord neoplasia, and

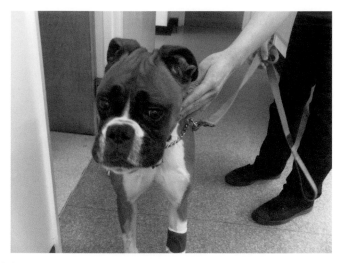

Figure 6.10.2 Risus sardonicus in a dog. This facial expression is typically seen in cases with tetanus due to spasticity of the muscles of facial expression.

certain anomalous diseases, such as syringomyelia (see Section 6.9 'Neck and/or Spinal Pain'). Cervical spondylomyelopathy and degenerative lumbosacral stenosis are often associated with apparent pain on examination, although with many of these more chronic conditions the degree of pain is variable. Chronic conditions, by their nature, tend to present in a less severely affected way and because they are generally slowly progressive, the clinician usually has more time to consider options and even perform investigations or trial treatment options. Indications for referral include rapidly deteriorating animals (which may well have a neoplastic disease), and animals where the pain cannot be controlled or is recurrent. Such animals may be suffering with intervertebral disc disease, and chronic recurrent pain may justify surgical management.

b. Non-painful conditions

The most likely presentations in this category would be neurodegenerative diseases (such as degenerative myelopathy), certain intramedullary neoplasms, and some anomalous conditions (such as arachnoid diverticulum and arachnoid fibrosis). The signalment should help with deciding which condition is more or less likely, and again the clinician usually has time to consider further investigation or referral. Submitting blood for genetic testing for the SOD-1 mutation known to predispose to degenerative myelopathy may be worthwhile if signalment and neuroanatomical localisation and signs are consistent. Radiographs may reveal vertebral column abnormalities, particularly in Pugs, which may be associated with arachnoid space disorders, or may even suggest severe kyphosis, which can be the cause of the paresis and ataxia.

One condition that may present as chronic paraparesis, often with a waxing and waning course, is *aortic thromboembolic disease in dogs*. Unlike in cats, where the classical presentation is acute, painful, severe, and easily recognised, the thromboembolic disease of dogs is commonly partial, leading to a presentation of exercise intolerance and pelvic limb weakness (see Chapter 3 and Videos 24 and 40). This presentation may therefore be confused for a thoracolumbar myelopathy or myasthenia gravis. Diagnosis is suggested by the presence of poor femoral pulses on general physical examination but requires imaging confirmation of a thromboembolism in the distal aorta. Treatment is aimed at preventing further enlargement of the thrombus and reversing, if possible, any underlying predisposing medical conditions, such as protein-losing nephropathy and loss of anti-thrombotic factors through damaged renal tubules.

6.10.4 Intervertebral Disc Disease

Intervertebral disc disease in one form or another is probably the most common neurological condition that the general practitioner will face, with one epidemiological study reporting that around 2% of dogs, and as many as 20% of Dachshunds, are affected by intervertebral disc disease during their lifetime (Bergknut et al. 2012).

The intervertebral disc consists of an outer, fibrous annulus fibrosus and an inner, initially gelatinous nucleus pulposus. The disc undergoes a process of degeneration in all dogs, with the chondrodystrophic breeds tending to show a more rapid degeneration, whilst in the larger, non-chondrodystrophic breeds degeneration is usually a slower process. There are also differences in the nature of the degenerative process between breeds of dog, as described initially by Hansen. These differences are proposed as the reason why chondrodystrophic breeds tend to suffer more disc *extrusion* (Hansen type 1 disc disease), where the nucleus pulposus escapes through a tear in the annulus fibrosus. Non-chondrodystrophic breeds are more likely to suffer a disc *protrusion* (Hansen type 2 disc disease), where the annulus remains intact but thickens and bulges in various ways (Figure 6.10.3).

The differences in degeneration between chondrodystrophic and non-chondrodystrophic breeds are now known to overlap far more than was originally believed, and this probably explains why a significant number of Hansen type 1 extrusions may also occur in non-chondrodystrophic breeds, such as Labrador Retrievers and German Shepherd Dogs. Recent work has also led to the identification of a genetic mutation thought to be responsible for the chondrodystrophic degenerative process, as well as intervertebral disc disease itself (Brown et al. 2017), and this may lead to more effective treatments and breeding strategies in the future.

Some authors favour the term intervertebral disc *herniation* to encompass all the different types of intervertebral disc disease in which displacement of the disc occurs in some way. The term intervertebral disc *disease* may include also the degenerative process itself rather than true herniation. It is well known that a degenerate, but non-herniated, disc, is capable of causing pain in human patients. This should potentially be considered as a possibility in animals,

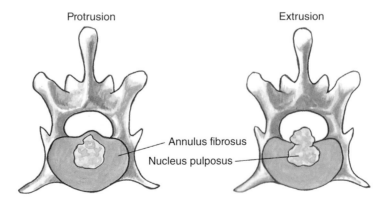

Figure 6.10.3 The two main types of intervertebral disc herniation. Hansen type 1 disc extrusion occurs when degenerate nucleus pulposus material herniates through a ruptured annulus fibrosus; Hansen type 2 disc protrusion occurs when the degenerate annulus bulges into the vertebral canal without being ruptured.

although it would be much more difficult to prove. For the purposes of this discussion, the term intervertebral disc *herniation* will be used, being defined as localised displacement of the intervertebral disc beyond the boundaries of the intervertebral disc space. This displacement may be contiguous with the remainder of the disc or may also include material which is separated from the disc and lying some distance away from the affected intervertebral disc space. Where discussion is confined to the Hansen type 1 extrusion of degenerate (and often calcified) nucleus pulposus through a ruptured annulus fibrosus, the term intervertebral disc *extrusion* will be used. Likewise, when discussing the Hansen type 2 protrusion of a degenerate but intact annulus fibrosus, with no escape of nucleus pulposus, the term intervertebral disc *protrusion* will be used. When the term, intervertebral disc *herniation* is used it refers to the generic displacement of disc material, and this may encompass both extrusion and protrusion, as well as escape of non-degenerate nuclear material as in the acute non-degenerate nucleus pulposus extrusion.

1. Hansen type 1 intervertebral disc extrusion

History: Usually acute or subacute, painful, frequently progressive, and often more or less symmetrical.

Signalment: Mainly chondrodystrophic breeds, especially the Dachshund, French Bulldog, Beagle, Cocker Spaniel, Pekingese, but can occur in any breed. Mean age at presentation 5 years but can occur in any dog over 1 year old.

Presenting signs: Can be very variable, ranging from back pain alone through to complete tetra- or paraplegia with absent deep pain perception. Tetraplegia with loss of deep pain perception is uncommon, as already stated, due to the vital cardiorespiratory functions that can be affected by such a severe lesion in the cervical spinal cord. A very common presentation is for an animal to show a few days of apparent pain or lethargy, which may easily be mistaken for abdominal pain, followed by a rapid progression to paraparesis or even paraplegia.

The location of Hansen type 1 intervertebral disc extrusions may be cervical or thoracolumbar, with the most common disc spaces affected in the cervical region being C2–C3 in small breeds and C6–C7 in large breeds, whilst in the thoracolumbar region around 90% of extrusions occur between T11 and L3. Cervical intervertebral disc extrusions commonly present with severe pain (e.g. vocalisation) and minimal neurological deficits, whereas thoracolumbar extrusions more often present with varying degrees of neurological deficit and apparently less severe pain.

Diagnosis: May be presumptive based on the appropriate history and signalment and neurological examination findings pointing to a focal myelopathy in an appropriate location. Survey radiography may provide further evidence if a narrowed intervertebral disc space is noted in the suspected region, or calcified material is seen within the vertebral canal or intervertebral foramen. Survey radiographs must be of sufficient quality for these findings to be reliable, with centering over the suspected disc space and good collimation; a disc space narrowing is unreliable if it is seen on the edge of the field of view, and it should be possible to identify wider spaces on each side of the affected space if the narrowing is genuine. It should also be remembered that T10–T11 frequently appears narrowed in cats and dogs, and is uncommonly the location of an extrusion.

Confirmation of diagnosis requires advanced imaging; myelography is a relatively reliable technique but has largely been superseded by three-dimensional imaging such as CT and MRI. These modalities are increasingly available and, although still relatively expensive in veterinary medicine, they provide essential diagnostic information when surgical treatment is being considered or there is significant doubt surrounding the diagnosis. CT is more rapid and usually reliable in cases of intervertebral disc extrusion, but MRI is superior at eliminating the possibility of other less common differential diagnoses such as neoplasia and inflammatory disease.

Treatment options: Conservative or surgical for both cervical and thoracolumbar extrusions. Conservative management entails a period of strict rest and confinement, together with analgesia. It may be necessary, especially with cervical disease, to use multimodal analgesic drugs and the author commonly prescribes a combination of a NSAID, paracetamol (10 mg/kg per os twice daily), and gabapentin (10 mg/kg per os twice or three times daily). Controlling the pain is very important for the owner and for successful resolution of signs. Corticosteroids are best avoided, except in situations where referral is definitely not an option and the pain has been prolonged, unremitting, and poorly controlled with other medications. Cage confinement is considered essential to prevent further nucleus pulposus from extruding and to potentially allow healing of the ruptured annulus fibrosus. The length of time that cage rest should be recommended is not known, with 2–4 weeks being commonly proposed. However, one study found no association between the length of cage rest and a successful outcome (Levine et al. 2007). The author usually recommends an initial week of very strict cage confinement, followed by a further 3 weeks of gradual relaxation of the confinement.

The decision as to whether and when to refer for possible surgical treatment is probably one of the biggest concerns for a general practitioner, therefore a set of broad guidelines is given below.

a. Suspected cervical intervertebral disc extrusion

Neck pain only: Medical management. Consider referral if pain is not controlled within 48 hours or there are signs of progression to paresis and ataxia.

Pain and ambulatory tetraparesis: Medical management is reasonable initially. If neurological deterioration occurs then consider referral, but if the clinical signs are stable and/or improving then medical management may be successful.

Pain and non-ambulatory tetraparesis: Refer for potential surgical management if this is an option. If not, medical management may still be successful.

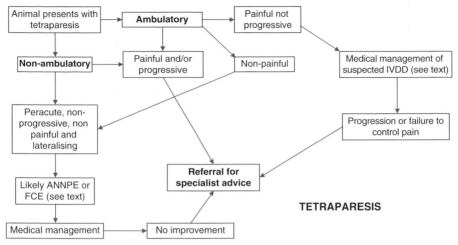

Approach to cases of tetraparesis in practice.

b. Suspected thoracolumbar intervertebral disc extrusion

Back pain only: Medical management. Owners should be instructed to pay careful attention to cage confinement, and to report immediately any signs of neurological deterioration. They should be warned that after appropriate analgesia their pet may appear recovered, but that the cage confinement is still essential for prevention of deterioration or recurrence.

In all cases where a suspected thoracolumbar intervertebral disc extrusion is managed conservatively, it is important for the veterinarian to discuss with the pet owner that acute deterioration to paraplegia with absent deep pain perception can occasionally occur, and that this would reduce the prognosis for recovery (see below). The veterinarian must necessarily protect him or herself from any possible accusation that a future deterioration may have occurred due to incorrect or false advice or information being provided. Any owner who is uncomfortable with this should be offered early referral for specialist advice.

Pain and ambulatory paresis: Medical management is appropriate, with the provisos stated above. Many dogs will recover (recovery rates of 80% are commonly reported), although recurrence rates may be higher with surgical treatment. However, the risks and costs of surgical treatment should also be discussed, since many owners will be unable to afford a second surgical treatment if there is recurrence after an initial surgery, and recurrence rates after surgical treatment if multiple site fenestration is not employed may be as high as 15–20%. For this reason, it may be in the owner's best interest to employ medical management in such situations, 'saving' any available funds/ insurance for a situation where there is better evidence for the superiority of surgical treatment.

Non-ambulatory paresis or paraplegia: Refer for specialist advice and potential surgical management if possible. If this is not an option, then medical management may still be successful in as many as 80% of cases where deep pain perception is retained, although recovery may be prolonged and incomplete.

Paraplegia with loss of deep pain perception. The loss of the ability to feel a painful stimulus applied to the deep structures of the foot/toes of the pelvic limb is a sign of severe spinal cord injury (see Chapter 3). It is the only factor which has been consistently shown to be linked to prognosis in cases of thoracolumbar interverte-bral disc extrusion. For dogs that lose deep pain perception, recovery rates are reduced from around 90% to just over 50% in dogs that are treated surgically. The recovery rate for dogs treated medically is thought to be considerably lower than this, although the true rate may be higher since there is very little information regarding the medical management of dogs with absent deep pain perception. In any event, recovery is likely to be prolonged and potentially expensive due to the nursing requirements and associated urinary incontinence which is usually seen. Referral of dogs that lose pelvic limb deep pain perception should be arranged as quickly as possible, although a recent study concluded that speed of surgical treat-ment is not associated with outcome (Jeffery et al. 2016), and most neurosurgeons are now happy to delay surgery until such time as an animal is stable. The chances of successful outcome, potential costs involved, and length of time expected for recovery (recovery to ambulation and regaining ability to urinate may be pro-longed and usually between 2 and 8 weeks) should be discussed prior to referral, since some owners may unfortunately elect to euthanise their pet at this point.

Medical management in paraplegic dogs

As already stated, rest is important, although in dogs which are plegic this is not usu-ally a problem! It is important to ensure that care is taken when handling affected dogs so as to minimise the risks of causing extrusion of further nucleus pulposus material into the vertebral canal, although the real risks of this are unknown.

i. Bladder management

Most dogs rendered paraplegic by a thoracolumbar intervertebral disc extrusion will suffer a period of urinary incontinence associated with loss of the upper motor neuron control of micturition (see Chapter 3). This presents as a dog that is unable to empty the bladder, but with a spastic external urethral sphincter so that the bladder becomes over-full with urine until the pressure inside is great enough to force open the sphincter. This is known as urinary retention and overflow. It is common for veterinarians and nurses who are inexperienced at dealing with such dogs to mistakenly assume that such urine overflow repre-sents conscious urination by the dog. This may be a dangerous mistake, since if the bladder is allowed to remain in an over-full state with the detrusor muscle stretched for more than just a couple of days, permanent detrusor damage can result. This can lead to the very unfortunate situation where a dog recovers the ability to walk but remains permanently urinary incontinent.

Any dog that is paraplegic or non-ambulatory paraparetic should have regular (at least three times a day) bladder checks. Palpation of the caudal abdomen may be sufficient to determine the level of filling of the bladder, but this also requires a level of experience in order to be reliable. Where there is any doubt, ultrasound scanning of the abdomen may give a more reliable picture of the true state of bladder filling. When a dog has potentially passed some urine, and either the passing was unobserved (e.g. found on the dog's bed) or there is some doubt as to whether the urination was conscious and voluntary or unconscious overflow, then the bladder must be checked in some way as soon as possible afterwards. If the urination was involuntary overflow, then the bladder is likely to be full or overfull when checked. If, on the other hand, it was a genuine conscious act of bladder emptying, then the bladder should be small or close to empty when checked.

If there is a concern that the patient is not able to pass urine voluntarily, then a plan must be put in place to manage bladder emptying. There are three options which are available to ensure that the bladder is prevented from becoming overfull, and each has different pros and cons. The clinician may need to be able to adapt and switch between options depending on how the case is progressing.

Bladder management options in spinal cord disease

Manual expression: Regular manual bladder expression via caudal abdominal palpation is possible in many cases. The technique is not easy, and it can be difficult even for an experienced clinician to ensure that the bladder is properly emptied. As mentioned above, the use of an ultrasound scanner to check bladder filling after manual expression is a reliable way of monitoring the effectiveness of emptying. Where this is not possible, passing a rigid urinary catheter after manual expression allows the clinician to check their technique. Advantages of manual expression include reduced cost and level of nursing care, and the possibility for owners to be trained to express their own animal's bladder. Disadvantages revolve around the potential for inadequate emptying, and the fact that the technique may cause discomfort to the patient, making other nursing procedures and physiotherapy more difficult.

Intermittent rigid catheterisation: Passing of a rigid catheter at regular intervals is possible, especially in male dogs. This needs to be performed three times daily in order to ensure the bladder does not become over-full, and therefore can become expensive if it needs to be continued for a prolonged period. It can also lead to inflammation of the urethra, as well as being technically challenging in females.

Indwelling urinary catheter: Placement of a permanent indwelling soft urinary catheter allows continuous bladder drainage with minimal handling of the patient. It also allows for close monitoring of urine output, and is the only way of ensuring the bladder is kept properly emptied, which can be important, especially in cases where it may have been over-full for 24 hours or more. Catheter management is important, and aseptic precautions should be taken when placing and handling catheters. The use of closed collection systems is preferred for both hygiene reasons and to allow proper monitoring of urine production. If urine output appears to fall, the catheter should always be checked to ensure it has not become kinked or blocked. A Buster collar or similar needs to be worn to prevent the patient licking, chewing, or pulling the catheter out. Disadvantages include added cost and the increased difficulty of moving affected patients with attached urinary collection bag. However, the author's preference is to place an indwelling catheter in most cases that present paraplegic, at least to allow easy bladder management in the first few days.

With all of the above techniques, urinary tract infection (UTI) is common. Several studies have shown that UTI is a common complication in dogs suffering with severe paraparesis and paraplegia associated with spinal cord injury, and so careful aseptic technique and ensuring that bladders are properly emptied is important. The use of prophylactic antibiotics has not been shown to be effective and is not advised during a period of indwelling catheterisation due to the risk of development of antimicrobial-resistant bacteria. However, a short period of prophylactic antibiosis following catheter removal may reduce the incidence of clinical UTI (Marschall et al. 2013) and may be considered. Specific antibacterial treatment should generally be reserved for patients with clinical signs of UTI, preferably following urine bacterial culture and antibiotic sensitivity testing from a cystocentesis sample. If a clinical UTI occurs, it is advisable to remove an indwelling catheter and use an alternative method of bladder management. However, it is important to be aware that the risk of UTI is not significantly different with any of the above methods, since there is a risk from leaving residual urine in the bladder as is likely with manual expression, as well as through the use of catheters.

ii. Physiotherapy and rehabilitation

Active rehabilitation employing physiotherapy techniques and potentially hydrotherapy is considered an important part of recovery from acute spinal cord injury whether from intervertebral disc disease or other causes of myelopathy such as FCE. Care must be taken when dealing with patients suffering with acute Hansen type 1 intervertebral disc extrusion, since there is always a possibility of further nucleus pulposus material extruding into the vertebral canal during recovery, especially in patients managed medically rather than surgically. Furthermore, the evidence for the effectiveness of physical therapy in neurologic patients is somewhat limited, with one recent study finding no benefit (Olby et al. 2019). In the author's experience, passive range of motion exercises and limited physiotherapy may be beneficial in avoiding joint stiffness especially in long-term paraplegic patients, and should be performed in a careful way on acutely paraplegic and non-ambulatory paraparetic patients when possible. Once such animals recover ambulation, the emphasis should be more on exercises aimed at improving coordination and proprioception, and the assistance or involvement of a properly trained animal physiotherapist or rehabilitation practitioner is advisable. For spinal cord conditions other than intervertebral disc disease, again the evidence for the effectiveness of physical therapy is varied, but one study showed an increased life expectancy for dogs suffering from degenerative myelopathy (Kathmann et al. 2006). The other benefits of employing rehabilitation techniques include improved well-being for the patient and greater owner participation in their animal's recovery, which for some owners can be a significant factor.

Alternative therapies, such as the use of laser therapy, have so far not been shown to be of benefit in the recovery of dogs with intervertebral disc disease (Bennaim et al. 2017). Acupuncture has, however, apparently improved recovery rates in severely affected dogs and reduced the degree of pain associated with intervertebral disc disease. This therapy is therefore worth considering, especially in situations when the traditional approach of MRI and decompressive surgery is not an option (Joaquim et al. 2010).

2. Hansen type 2 intervertebral disc protrusion

History: Chronic, progressive, sometimes painful, usually symmetrical.

Signalment: Large breed, non-chondrodystrophic dogs, especially German Shepherd Dogs, Labrador Retrievers, Dalmatians, Dobermanns. Usually older (>5 years).

Presenting signs: Progressive tetra- or paraparesis with proprioceptive ataxia and variable neck or back pain.

Diagnosis: As for type 1 disc extrusions above.

Treatment: Medical or surgical management may be employed. In a recent study, surgical treatment was found to be more effective than medical management for thoracolumbar disc protrusions (Crawford and De Decker 2017), and referral should therefore always be discussed with the owner. However, many affected dogs are older at the time of diagnosis and owners may be reluctant to pursue surgical treatments which can, in the case of chronic thoracolumbar disc protrusions, have significant morbidity. Medical management is therefore common in these cases. In this situation, controlled exercise and the judicious use of anti-inflammatory doses of corticosteroids may give superior results to NSAIDs, at least in the short-term.

A tapering dose of prednisolone has also been recommended for the medical management of disc-associated cervical spondylomyelopathy (0.5 mg/kg twice daily for 7 days, 0.5 mg/kg once daily for 7 days, 0.5 mg/kg on alternate days). This condition is seen especially in the Dobermann, where chronic intervertebral disc protrusion in the caudal cervical region leads to progressive signs of tetraparesis +/− neck pain. This is a specific variant of Hansen type 2 intervertebral disc protrusion that may also involve other sources of spinal cord compression, both bony and soft tissue, as well as instability at the intervertebral joint. Corticosteroids are likely to be efficacious through reduction of vasogenic spinal cord oedema associated with chronic spinal cord compression in these cases, and it is the author's experience that this is often also the case for thoracolumbar disc protrusions. This is in contrast to acute intervertebral disc extrusions, in which the nature of the spinal cord injury differs, and corticosteroids play little role in the management. For disc-associated cervical spondylomyelopathy, controversy remains as to which treatment modality is superior, and many different surgical approaches have been described.

Prognosis in all cases of Hansen type 2 intervertebral disc protrusion remains guarded, with most cases showing progression when managed medically, and outcomes with surgical management are less predictable than for type 1 disc extrusions.

3. Acute non-compressive (or moderately compressive) nucleus pulposus extrusion (ANNPE)

History: Peracute, non-progressive, initially painful but rapidly becoming non-painful, usually asymmetrical.

Signalment: Any age and breed may be affected. Border Collies over-represented.

Presentation: Peracute onset of moderate to severe neurological deficits, often asymmetrical, non-painful within 24 hours of onset, and frequently improving at a variable rate.

Diagnosis: May be presumptive based on the factors above, with FCE being the primary differential diagnosis. Confirmation requires MRI.

Treatment: Medical management carries a favourable prognosis, with most animals that retain deep pain perception recovering ambulation, usually within 2–4 weeks. Analgesia is not usually required, and cage confinement is not necessary. Physiotherapy and rehabilitation techniques from an early stage will potentially assist in the recovery. Initial management of suspected spinal cord contusion by maintaining adequate mean arterial pressure and oxygenation may be beneficial. Management of FCE is similar and therefore differentiation of these two conditions is not essential to ensure a favourable prognosis.

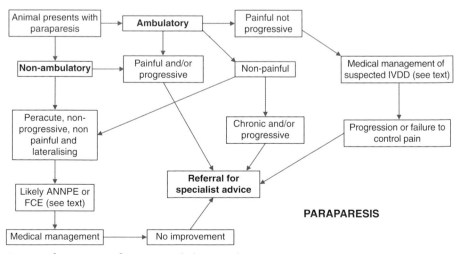

Approach to cases of paraparesis in practice.

6.11   Monoparesis and Lameness

Paul M. Freeman

Many of the conditions that are discussed in Section 6.10 'Paresis, Paralysis, and Proprioceptive Ataxia' as possible causes of paresis and ataxia can also present as a monoparesis or apparent lameness, and these conditions can be difficult to distinguish from orthopaedic disease (e.g. elbow dysplasia, cranial cruciate ligament disease, hip osteoarthritis, septic arthritis, osteosarcoma). The following section is a guide to the recognition, differential diagnosis, and approach to monoparesis in cats and dogs.

6.11.1   Recognition of Potential Neurogenic Lameness

There are a number of potential clues to assist with the recognition of neurogenic lameness as opposed to orthopaedic lameness.

Muscle atrophy: Neurogenic muscle atrophy is usually much more rapid and severe than the atrophy of disuse which is commonly associated with orthopaedic disease. However, if an animal presents with a chronic history of gait abnormality the distinction can be more difficult, because significant disuse muscle atrophy may have already occurred (e.g. secondary to chronic cranial cruciate ligament insufficiency). In general, whenever an animal is presented with a lameness that is accompanied by severe muscle atrophy affecting all or part of the limb, a neurogenic cause should be considered.

Paresis and postural reactions: A reduction in the *ability* to weight-bear (lower motor neuron paresis) or a reduced ability to initiate movement (upper motor neuron paresis) are features of neurogenic lameness, termed 'monoparesis' when they affect a single limb. An animal may drag the toes of the affected limb leading to abnormal wearing of the nails. Postural reaction deficits (paw replacement and/or hopping) may also be present, particularly in cases of upper motor neuron monoparesis. In contrast, orthopaedic lameness results from a *reluctance* to weight-bear on the affected limb and the postural reactions should be normal. However, caution should be exercised when diagnosing a neurogenic lameness based on reduced postural reactions alone, since painful orthopaedic conditions (such as osteosarcoma) may lead to apparent deficits of weight-bearing, paw replacement, and hopping, and may cause toe dragging during ambulation secondary to pain and reluctance to move the limb.

Reduced spinal reflexes: The flexor withdrawal reflex, as well as other spinal reflexes such as the patellar reflex and extensor carpi radialis reflex, may be significantly reduced in cases with neurogenic lameness and lower motor neuron monoparesis. Again, the clinician should be careful not to over-interpret such signs since an animal with a painful orthopaedic problem may be reluctant to withdraw the affected limb, and the patella reflex is commonly absent in some older dogs and dogs which have significant stifle pathology (see Chapter 3).

Reduced sensation: Significant nerve damage may lead to loss of sensation in the skin supplied by the affected nerve (e.g. following traumatic avulsion of the roots of the brachial plexus). A knowledge of the so-called autonomous zones (the areas of skin supplied by an individual nerve, see Figure 1.3) may allow accurate localisation of a specific nerve injury but is not generally required for diagnosis and management of the majority of cases in general practice.

Pain: Many cases of neurogenic lameness may be accompanied by significant pain; a neurogenic cause should be considered in any animal presenting with a severely painful lameness that is resulting in spontaneous vocalisation.

6.11.2   Differential Diagnosis for Monoparesis

1. Vascular conditions

Fibrocartilaginous embolism (FCE) may cause an acute mono- or hemiparesis dependent on the site and extent of the lesion. In this condition, small fragments of fibrocartilaginous material from an intervertebral disc embolise into small spinal arterioles leading to a peracute ischaemic myelopathy. If the area of spinal cord ischaemia is sufficiently lateralised then a monoparesis may result, which can be severe enough to result in monoplegia. It is rare for a single thoracic limb to be involved without a corresponding upper motor neuron paresis of the ipsilateral pelvic limb, but if lesions occur caudal to the C6–T2 spinal cord segments then monoparesis of a pelvic limb may be seen (see Video 41). This will be an upper motor neuron monoparesis if the lesion is cranial to the L3 spinal cord segment, or a lower motor neuron paresis if the lesion occurs within the L4–S3 spinal cord segments. As discussed in Chapters 3 and 4, upper motor neuron paresis will be accompanied by intact spinal reflexes, whilst lower motor neuron paresis typically leads to reduced or absent local spinal reflexes. Dependent on the location of the lesion, there may also be an interrupted cutaneous trunci reflex just caudal to the site of the lesion. Diagnosis requires referral for MRI, but a presumptive diagnosis may often be made based on the clinical history, neurological examination, and signalment. The prognosis is generally good in cases of monoparesis, although may be guarded for recovery of limb function if there is severe lower motor neuron monoparesis/monoplegia. Management of these cases is medical and involves physiotherapy and rehabilitation (see Section 6.10 'Paresis, Paralysis, and Proprioceptive Ataxia').

Aortic thromboembolism, as discussed in Section 6.10 'Paresis, Paralysis, and Proprioceptive Ataxia', may present as a monoparesis or unilateral 'lameness'. In cats, a single thoracic limb may be involved, and the prognosis is generally guarded. In dogs, rare cases may involve just one pelvic limb.

2. Inflammatory conditions

Meningomyelitis of unknown origin (MUO) (see Section 6.10 'Paresis, Paralysis, and Proprioceptive Ataxia') may rarely present as a monoparesis secondary to the presence of a focal, asymmetric lesion within the spinal cord; however, this is very uncommon.

Idiopathic or immune-mediated neuritis: Occasionally, an autoimmune inflammatory response is triggered in an individual peripheral nerve or nerve root, usually at the level of the spinal cord, that results in lameness and/or monoparesis if the affected nerve is responsible for innervating the muscles of a single limb (e.g. C6–T2 or L4–S2 nerve roots). Reports and information regarding this condition are limited, but significant nerve root enlargement can occur, mimicking neoplastic disease.

3. Trauma

Trauma is a relatively common cause of peripheral nerve injury and may also accompany orthopaedic injury (e.g. pelvic fractures following road traffic accidents). The clinical history should facilitate diagnosis, and radiographic evidence of a fracture in a region of bone that lies close to a peripheral nerve or nerve root (e.g. the iliac shaft or distal humerus) along with accompanying neurological deficits should always raise suspicion for concurrent neurological injury. Traumatic nerve injury may range from neuropraxia, which includes nerve injuries such as stretching, compression, or blunt trauma where the axons remain intact, through to axonotmesis, which is defined as complete physical disruption of the axons in a nerve. When nerve injury is suspected, the loss of deep pain perception in regions of the limb supplied by the nerve carries a guarded prognosis for recovery of function and implies likely axonotmesis. However, care must be taken in interpreting loss of deep pain perception in animals suffering from shock, and it is sensible to delay such testing until systemic stabilisation is complete. Significant pain may be present if there is entrapment of a peripheral nerve or nerve root within a fracture site, and in animals that present with pelvic injuries where the pain is difficult or impossible to control, consideration should always be given to the possibility of nerve entrapment; referral for specialist assessment should be considered at an early stage in these cases.

Brachial plexus avulsion is a specific condition in which the nerve roots of the brachial plexus are avulsed from the cervicothoracic spinal cord by significant trauma, often involving excessive abduction of a thoracic limb. The limb is typically flaccid and paralysed, with an absent flexor withdrawal reflex, absent postural reactions, and rapid denervation muscle atrophy. Loss of the ipsilateral cutaneous trunci reflex and/or the presence of Horner syndrome may also be seen. In severe cases, with complete loss of motor and sensory function, the prognosis is guarded. If some degree of function is retained (particularly radial nerve function and the ability to extend the elbow to bear weight), then many animals will recover to at least some extent. However, this recovery may be very protracted and limb amputation should still be considered, particularly if there is self-trauma or recurrent damage to the affected distal limb.

Radial nerve paralysis (or paresis) is a specific nerve injury affecting the radial nerve that is thought to be caused by blunt trauma where this nerve is closely associated with the distal portion of the humerus. It is therefore also occasionally associated with humeral fractures. Again, prognosis is related to extent of nerve damage, and complete loss of motor and sensory function implies a guarded prognosis.

4. Neoplastic conditions

Peripheral nerve neoplasia is a relatively common cause of monoparesis or neurogenic lameness.

Peripheral nerve tumours may affect a single peripheral nerve (usually proximally) and commonly cause a chronic, progressive lameness that may be poorly responsive to analgesics and anti-inflammatory drugs. These cases are frequently accompanied by significant muscle atrophy in the affected limb. Hemiparesis (lower motor neuron paresis of a thoracic limb and upper motor neuron paresis of the ipsilateral pelvic limb) may be seen secondary to spinal cord compression if a tumour of the C6–T2 nerve roots invades into the vertebral canal via the intervertebral foramen. Diagnosis requires MRI in most cases, and treatment may be palliative or surgical. The prognosis is generally guarded, with most studies showing median survival times of less than 1 year following surgical excision and limb amputation. However, a recent study where compartmental excision and limb-sparing was performed reported a median survival time of 1303 days (Stee et al. 2017).

Lymphoma should always be considered as a differential diagnosis in cases with peripheral nerve or nerve root enlargement, and evaluation for signs of systemic involvement or other locations of lymphoma may prevent inappropriate treatments or unnecessary referral.

5. Degenerative conditions

Intervertebral disc disease (see Section 6.10 'Paresis, Paralysis, and Proprioceptive Ataxia'). Hansen type 1 intervertebral disc extrusions may occasionally present as a monoparesis/lameness if the extruded disc material herniates laterally into the intervertebral foramen in the region of the brachial plexus or lumbosacral plexus nerve roots. Lameness may be moderate to severe and painful, with permanent or intermittent episodes of non-weight-bearing ('nerve root signature'). Even with advanced imaging, diagnosis can be difficult and surgical treatment may be technically demanding, dependent upon the location of the extruded material. Medical management may be successful and is generally reasonable in the first instance, although persistent pain is an indication for surgical treatment. However, resolution of lameness can be protracted over weeks or months whichever treatment method is employed. Hansen type 2 intervertebral disc protrusions may also present as monoparesis/lameness if an annular protrusion is lateralised and compresses a peripheral nerve root at the level of the intervertebral foramen.

Degenerative lumbosacral stenosis is a syndrome where the vertebral canal at the level of the lumbosacral junction is narrowed by various bony and/or soft tissue structures, commonly including the L7–S1 intervertebral disc. It occurs in middle-aged and older large breed dogs, notably the German Shepherd Dog, but many breeds may be affected. Clinical signs commonly include lower back pain and reluctance to climb stairs or jump up (see Section 6.9 'Neck and/or Spinal Pain') but may also involve some degree of tail paresis or even urinary or faecal incontinence. If the L7–S1 intervertebral foramen is narrowed on one side, leading to compression of the L7 nerve root, then this condition may involve a pelvic limb lameness or monoparesis. Definitive diagnosis requires advanced imaging and treatment may be medical or surgical. Epidural injection of methylprednisolone acetate can provide pain relief and reduction of inflammation, with one study reporting good results with this treatment (Janssens et al. 2009). Diagnosis should preferably be confirmed prior to using corticosteroid treatment since a possible differential diagnosis may be bacterial discospondylitis, in which the use of corticosteroids would be contraindicated.

6.11.3 Approach to Monoparesis

When faced with a case of monoparesis, a knowledge of the conditions that may present with this clinical sign, and their differences in expected clinical history and signalment, should allow the clinician to limit the possible differential diagnoses to a small number. Unfortunately, advanced imaging +/− specialist electrodiagnostic evaluation is usually required for confirmation of the diagnosis. Therefore, referral for specialist advice and investigation should always be considered if an orthopaedic cause of lameness has been ruled out. Referral is seldom an emergency in these situations, except in cases of potential nerve injury following trauma where surgical intervention to stabilise fractures may be urgently required to prevent permanent nerve damage. In other peracute presentations, such as FCE and brachial plexus avulsion, referral may help to confirm the diagnosis and offer guidance in terms of prognosis but will rarely affect the outcome.

In subacute and chronic cases, referral should be considered whenever the diagnosis remains unclear. Survey radiographs to look for evidence of orthopaedic disease may be considered, as well as spinal radiographs looking for evidence of neoplasia, degenerative lumbosacral stenosis, or intervertebral disc disease when appropriate. Screening for metastatic and primary disease should be considered if neoplasia appears likely (e.g. lymphoma), although peripheral nerve tumours are rarely metastatic.

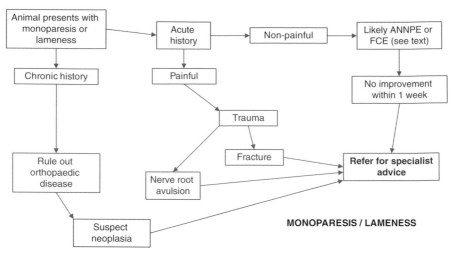

Approach to monoparesis/lameness in practice.

6.12   Neuromuscular Weakness

Edward Ives

Neuromuscular disease is the broad term used to describe disorders affecting one (or more) of the following neuroanatomic structures:

- the peripheral motor and/or sensory nerves residing outside the central nervous system (CNS)
- the neuromuscular junction (NMJ) that provides the connection between the peripheral motor nerves and the skeletal muscles they innervate
- the skeletal muscles themselves.

Neuromuscular disorders can therefore be divided into the following categories:

- peripheral neuropathies
- junctionopathies
- myopathies.

Before considering these individual categories, the most important step is recognising that the neuromuscular system is affected in the first place. This may sound obvious; however, disorders affecting other body systems can mimic neuromuscular weakness, and neuromuscular disorders can appear clinically similar to disorders affecting the CNS. The neurological examination should therefore be repeated and reconsidered until you are as confident as you can be that a neuromuscular disorder is responsible for the presenting complaint and clinical signs (Glass and Kent 2002). This will allow you to formulate a list of the most likely causes, from which a logical and efficient set of diagnostic investigations can be planned.

Tips for recognising neuromuscular disease and differentiating these disorders from lesions affecting the brain or spinal cord are listed below. The typical clinical signs associated with neuromuscular disease and the clinical distinction between peripheral neuropathies, myopathies, and junctionopathies is further discussed in Chapter 4.

1. **Stride length, joint posture, and muscle tone**

    The peripheral motor nerves, NMJ, and skeletal muscles form the final common pathway for motor function. Disorders affecting these structures result in an inability to maintain normal muscle strength and tone. A reduction in extensor muscle tone will influence the ability to support body weight against the force of gravity. This will be clinically-apparent as reduced joint extension and a short-strided gait as the animal rapidly shifts its weight from limb to limb to avoid collapse. The limbs may appear flaccid when the animal is in lateral recumbency and the flexor withdrawal reflexes may be reduced in all limbs (see Videos 31 and 42). This generalised reduction in muscle tone and the recognition of weak withdrawal reflexes in all limbs can be used to differentiate neuromuscular weakness as the cause for non-ambulatory tetraparesis from a cervical spinal cord lesion, in which the trunk tone, pelvic limb muscle tone, and pelvic limb withdrawal reflexes would be expected to be normal.

2. **Is the animal ataxic or just weak? Is the proprioception normal?**

    The NMJ and skeletal muscles are only involved in motor function and play no role in sensory modalities, such as proprioception or the coordination of movement. The clinical signs of the most common peripheral neuropathies primarily reflect peripheral motor nerve involvement, with relative sparing of sensory function. Therefore, as long as there is sufficient muscle strength to perform some degree of voluntary movement, animals with neuromuscular disease will frequently have normal proprioception and will not be ataxic, even if they are too weak to support their weight (see Video 31). In contrast, lesions affecting the spinal cord will equally affect the ascending sensory (proprioceptive) tracts and descending motor fibres, resulting in a combination of ataxia, paresis, and proprioceptive deficits in the affected limbs. This relative sparing of sensory function and proprioception in neuromuscular disease can be very useful to differentiate it from spinal disorders as a cause for an abnormal gait in all limbs (tetraparesis).

3. **Are the neurological deficits symmetric or asymmetric?**

    The majority of neuromuscular disorders, particularly myopathies and junctionopathies, present with generalised and symmetric clinical signs involving all limbs (i.e. tetraparesis). These clinical signs may be initially most apparent in the pelvic limbs, or less commonly in the thoracic limbs, but will usually progress to involve all limbs over a relatively short period of time. In contrast, spinal cord and brain lesions can result in markedly asymmetric/lateralised clinical signs dependent on the lesion location and extent (i.e. hemiparesis). An exception to this rule is monoparesis secondary to involvement of a one or more peripheral nerves innervating a single limb (see Section 6.11 'Monoparesis and Lameness'). Neurological deficits involving individual cranial nerves and the condition of isolated masticatory myositis are discussed in Section 6.6 'Cranial Nerve Dysfunction'. This section will focus on the presentation and clinical approach to generalised neuromuscular weakness.

4. **Are the clinical signs exacerbated by exercise?**
The reduction in muscle strength and tone resulting from neuromuscular disease may be more apparent in the face of increased demand during exercise, particularly for junctionopathies and myopathies. Therefore, the clinical signs may be exacerbated by exercise and some animals will have a clinical history of exercise intolerance. In contrast, the severity of the neurological deficits associated with spinal cord lesions is usually independent of exercise unless there is significant discomfort or vertebral instability.

5. **Are there any cranial nerve deficits?**
The function of skeletal muscles throughout the body, including those innervated by the cranial nerves, may be affected by neuromuscular disease. Therefore, a condition affecting the neuromuscular system should always be considered in animals that present with appendicular muscle weakness and concurrent cranial nerve deficits (e.g. facial paresis, dropped jaw, pharyngeal dysphagia, or megaoesophagus). These cranial nerve deficits will usually be bilateral and, in contrast to brainstem lesions resulting in cranial nerve dysfunction, the level of mentation will be normal.

6.12.1 Differential Diagnoses for Generalised Neuromuscular Weakness

If neuromuscular weakness is suspected on the basis of the neurological examination, then the next step is to decide whether this represents a clinical sign of systemic disease or a primary neuromuscular disorder.

1. A systemic disease that is affecting delivery of oxygen and nutrients to the peripheral nerves and muscles resulting in 'secondary' neuromuscular weakness
   Examples of conditions that can present with clinical signs of generalised weakness, and thus mimic primary neuromuscular disease, include:
   • cardiorespiratory disease (reduced cardiac output or blood oxygenation)
   • anaemia or polycythaemia
   • thromboembolic disease obstructing delivery of blood to nerves/muscles
   • hypoglycaemia

- sepsis
- shock
- hyperthermia
- pheochromocytoma
- diabetic ketoacidosis
- electrolyte abnormalities.

These disorders can often be excluded on the basis of a thorough general physical examination, blood pressure testing, haematology, serum biochemistry, and urinalysis. Mimics of neuromuscular weakness should also be excluded at this time, such as abdominal pain or generalised orthopaedic conditions that are resulting in a reluctance to walk rather than an inability to support weight.

2. A primary neuromuscular disorder affecting the peripheral nerves, NMJ, or skeletal muscles

A list of differential diagnoses for primary neuromuscular disease is given below, separated into those for generalised peripheral neuropathies, junctionopathies, and myopathies. An asterisk (*) has been used to highlight the most common conditions that may be observed in general practice. The reader is referred to the Bibliography for further information regarding the diagnosis and treatment of these individual conditions.

a. Generalised peripheral neuropathies:
- Inflammatory – chronic inflammatory demyelinating polyneuropathy
- Infectious – *N. caninum, T. gondii*
- Toxic – vincristine, cisplatin, organophosphates (cats)
- Metabolic – hypothyroidism, diabetes mellitus*, hypoglycaemia, hyperlipidaemia
- Idiopathic – acute canine polyradiculoneuritis* (Box 6.12.1), motor polyneuropathy in young cats* (Box 6.12.2), distal denervating disease
- Neoplastic – insulinoma, paraneoplastic polyneuropathy, lymphoma
- Degenerative – motor neuron diseases, laryngeal-paralysis polyneuropathy*, sensory neuropathy, other inherited breed-specific neuropathies.

b. Myopathies:
- Inflammatory – idiopathic polymyositis* (Box 6.12.3)
- Infectious – *N. caninum*, *T. gondii, Ehrlichia canis, Leptospirosis spp., Leishmania infantum*
- Toxic – adverse drug reaction, snake bite envenomation
- Metabolic – hypothyroidism (dogs)*, hyperthyroidism (cats), hypoadrenocorticism*, hyperadrenocorticism*, chronic corticosteroid therapy*, hypokalaemic myopathy*
- Neoplastic – paraneoplastic polymyopathy, lymphoma
- Degenerative – muscular dystrophies, centronuclear myopathy, congenital myotonia, other inherited breed-specific myopathies

Box 6.12.1 Acute Canine Polyradiculoneuritis

Pathogenesis: Uncertain but suspected to represent an immune-mediated disorder targeted against peripheral myelin and/or axons (Rupp et al. 2013).

Typical presentation: Acute onset, rapidly-progressive, flaccid tetraparesis, frequently starting in the pelvic limbs and progressing to involve the thoracic limbs (see Video 42). Typically progresses over 5–10 days to non-ambulatory tetraparesis or tetraplegia. Proprioception remains normal in those animals with sufficient strength to correct for changes in limb position. Weak withdrawal reflexes and reduced muscle tone in all limbs. The cranial nerves and tail function are usually spared, but an altered pitch and strength of bark (dysphonia) is common in affected dogs. Oesophageal function, urinary and faecal continence are normal. Jack Russell Terriers and West Highland White Terriers had greater odds of developing acute canine polyradiculoneuritis compared to a baseline group of dogs in one study (Laws et al. 2017).

Diagnosis: Typical clinical presentation (likely to represent the most common cause of non-ambulatory, flaccid tetraparesis in the UK), exclusion of other causes of polyneuropathy (e.g. endocrine disease, neoplasia, *N. caninum, T. gondii*), electrodiagnostics, muscle/nerve biopsy.

Treatment: Spontaneous resolution with supportive care – frequent turning, assisted feeding, intensive physiotherapy. Corticosteroids do not appear effective, can exacerbate muscle weakness, and predispose to complications (e.g. urinary tract infections). Human intravenous immunoglobulin may reduce the time to recovery (Hirschvogel et al. 2012).

Prognosis: Usually good. Variable length of recovery from 2 weeks to over 6 months. Relapses may occur if exposed to same trigger, which is usually unknown (Laws et al. 2017).

Box 6.12.2 Motor Polyneuropathy in Young Cats

Pathogenesis: Currently unknown and likely to be heterogeneous dependent on the breed and individual.

Typical presentation: Acute onset, relapsing or progressive tetraparesis characterised by reduced muscle tone in the affected limbs, weak withdrawal reflexes, and wide scapula excursions if able to walk (see Video 43). The cranial nerves are frequently spared but facial paresis and dysphonia can be observed. A waxing/waning or relapsing clinical course is common. Affected cats are typically less than 1 year of age at the onset of the first clinical manifestations (Aleman et al. 2014). Any breed can be affected but a specific form of recurrent polyneuropathy has been reported in Bengal cats (Bensfield et al. 2011).

Diagnosis: Typical clinical presentation, exclusion of other causes of polyneuropathy, electrodiagnostics, muscle/nerve biopsy.

Treatment: The optimal treatment is currently unknown and is likely to vary between cases. Some cats show a spontaneous resolution of clinical signs without treatment, whilst others appear to respond to prednisolone (tapering from 1 mg/kg per os twice daily).

Prognosis: Generally good but relapses appear common and some cats may show progressive clinical signs in spite of attempted treatment.

Box 6.12.3 Idiopathic Polymyositis

Pathogenesis: Unknown but suspected to represent an autoimmune disorder targeted against certain sarcolemmal antigens (Evans et al. 2004; Podell 2002).

Typical presentation: Most common in middle-aged, large breed dogs (e.g. Boxers, Newfoundlands, Labrador Retrievers). Generalised weakness, stiff/stilted gait in all limbs, lethargy, exercise intolerance, muscle atrophy, weight loss +/− discomfort on muscle palpation, dysphagia, and regurgitation. Proprioception is normal in all limbs and withdrawal reflexes are usually adequate. A specific disorder in the Hungarian Vizsla breed is characterised by dysphagia and masticatory muscle atrophy (Tauro et al. 2015).

Diagnosis: Clinical presentation, elevated serum muscle enzymes, exclusion of other causes of polymyopathy (e.g. endocrine disease, neoplasia, *N. caninum, T. gondii*), electrodiagnostics, muscle biopsy.

Treatment: Immunosuppressive doses of prednisolone (1 mg/kg per os twice daily for 2–4 weeks, tapering to the lowest effective dose). Adjunctive immunosuppressive agents, such as cyclosporine or azathioprine, can be used in dogs that do not adequately respond to prednisolone alone. These can also be useful as steroid-sparing agents, particularly in large dogs that may not tolerate high oral doses of prednisolone.

Prognosis: Generally good but relapses can occur as treatment is withdrawn.

---

c. Junctionopathies:
- Inflammatory – acquired myasthenia gravis* (Box 6.12.4)
- Toxic botulism, tick paralysis, organophosphates, snake bite, Black Widow spider envenomation
- Anomalous – congenital myasthenia gravis.

6.12.2 Clinical Approach to Generalised Neuromuscular Weakness

1. Confirm the presence of a neuromuscular disorder

- Clinical history and presenting complaint
- General physical examination
- Neurological examination

As discussed in Chapter 4, the clinical history and neurological examination findings should first be used to localise the lesion to the neuromuscular system. Important information to gather from the clinical history should include concurrent clinical signs (e.g. weight loss, regurgitation), current and previous medical conditions, medications that the animal is receiving, travel history, and exposure to toxins. Differentiating between a peripheral neuropa-

---

Box 6.12.4 Acquired Myasthenia Gravis

Pathogenesis: Autoimmune disease resulting from the production of autoantibodies against the nicotinic acetylcholine receptor. Blockade and accelerated degradation of these bound receptors affects normal neuromuscular transmission, resulting in skeletal muscle weakness, particularly at times of increased demand (e.g. exercise). A concurrent thymoma has been reported in around 3% of affected dogs and 15–52% of affected cats (Hague et al. 2015; Shelton 2002; Shelton et al. 1997).

Typical presentation: Reported bimodal age at onset (e.g. 3–4 years old and 10–12 years old). Rare in cats compared to dogs but Abyssinian and Somali cats are over-represented (Hague et al. 2015). Neurological examination may be normal at rest. The focal form frequently affects the oesophagus, larynx, pharynx, and/or facial muscles resulting in clinical signs of regurgitation, dysphagia, dysphonia, and weak palpebral reflexes. The generalised form results in exercise-induced/exacerbated muscle weakness presenting as exercise-intolerance, progressive stiffness when walking (particularly affecting the pelvic limbs), and frequent sitting/lying down at exercise (see Video 44). These signs are commonly accompanied by excessive drooling, megaoesophagus, and regurgitation in dogs. A less common, acute, and severe fulminant form results in recumbency, regurgitation +/− respiratory difficulty in affected animals (Dewey et al. 1997; King and Vite 1998).

Diagnosis: Clinical presentation, rule out other causes of neuromuscular weakness, conscious thoracic radiography (to assess for the presence of a thymoma, megaoesophagus, and aspiration pneumonia), nicotinic acetylcholine receptor antibody testing, edrophonium-response test, repetitive nerve stimulation.

Treatment: Supportive care and nutrition for an animal with megaoesophagus +/− omeprazole to manage oesophagitis and to increase the pH of gastric content that may be aspirated (see Section 6.6.3 'Vagus Nerve') (Khorzad et al. 2011). Anticholinesterase therapy to increase the amount of acetylcholine available at the NMJ to bind to the remaining receptors (pyridostigmine bromide 0.5–3.0 mg/kg (dogs) or 0.25 mg/kg (cats) per os every 8–12 hours). Immunosuppressive medications can be used in animals that do not respond to supportive care and pyridostigmine therapy, but this should be carefully monitored. This is because of the high incidence of aspiration pneumonia in affected animals and the fact that prednisolone administration can exacerbate muscle weakness. The use of cyclosporine and azathioprine have also been reported in the management of myasthenia gravis in dogs (Bexfield et al. 2006; Dewey et al. 1999).

Prognosis: Generally guarded, with a 1-year mortality rate of 40–60% in dogs. This is primarily because of the high incidence of megaoesophagus and recurrent aspiration pneumonia in affected animals. Prognosis can be good in cases without pharyngeal/oesophageal involvement. Prognosis is poor in fulminant cases (Dewey et al. 1997).

---

thy, junctionopathy, and myopathy can be difficult on the basis of clinical examination alone. Therefore, referral for specialist neurological assessment and advanced investigations, such as electrodiagnostics, is advised in all cases with suspected neuromuscular disease. If referral is not an option, then the focus of investigations in general practice should be to exclude systemic disease and to further investigate metabolic, infectious, or neoplastic causes for primary neuromuscular weakness.

2. Exclude systemic disease as a cause of 'secondary' neuromuscular weakness

- General physical examination, including cardiac auscultation, heart rate and rhythm, respiratory rate and rhythm, mucous membrane colour, capillary refill time, peripheral pulse assessment
- Blood pressure
- Haematology
- Serum biochemistry
- Urinalysis

3. Further investigate causes of primary neuromuscular disease

- Refer for further investigations: this may include electrodiagnostic testing (electromyography, electroneurography, repetitive nerve stimulation) +/− CSF analysis, muscle and nerve biopsy for histopathology.
- Perform further investigations in general practice.
  - Haematology, serum biochemistry, and urinalysis to further investigate metabolic/endocrine disorders.
  - Serum muscle enzymes – creatine kinase (CK), AST, and ALT. Whilst ALT is frequently included on in-house biochemistry tests, many of these panels do not include CK or AST. As ALT can also be released from damaged muscle, hepatic disease should not be considered to be the only cause for ALT elevation. Therefore, if the ALT is elevated on a basic biochemistry panel, particularly in the absence of changes to other hepatic parameters, CK and AST should be measured to further investigate the possibility of an underlying myopathy. However, a myopathy cannot be excluded on the basis of normal serum muscle enzymes as certain conditions may not result in significant muscle enzyme elevation. Mild to moderate CK elevations should also be interpreted with caution, as animals that are recumbent for reasons other than a primary myopathy may have elevated levels, particularly in large breed dogs (CK up to 5000–10 000 IU/l). Necrotising myopathies and dystrophin-deficient muscular dystrophy frequently result in very high serum muscle enzyme levels (e.g. CK >50 000– 100 000 IU/l) (Shelton 2010).
  - Total thyroid hormone (T4) and TSH levels can be run if there is a clinical suspicion for hypothyroidism in dogs. Total T4 +/− free T4 can be used to diagnose hyperthyroidism in cats.
  - Cortisol levels before and after administration of ACTH can be used to investigate hypo- and hyperadrenocorticism.

- Infectious disease testing (e.g. serological testing for *N. caninum* and *T. gondii*).
- Body cavity screening for neoplasia (e.g. thoracic radiography, abdominal ultrasonography, CT of thorax and abdomen).
- Serum nAchR antibody testing for acquired myasthenia gravis. This test will confirm a diagnosis of acquired myasthenia gravis if positive. However, a small number of affected animals may have an antibody level within the normal range (seronegative myasthenia gravis). This can be for several different reasons, including previous corticosteroid administration, the presence of antibodies targeted to a different muscle membrane protein, or if the majority of antibodies are bound to their target and unavailable for detection by the test (Shelton 2010; Shelton et al. 2001). Repeating the assay in 1–2 weeks is recommended for seronegative cases in which there is a high clinical suspicion of acquired myasthenia gravis. Carefully monitored trial treatment can be performed if the result remains negative and other possible causes for the clinical signs have been excluded.
- Muscle biopsy if a primary myopathy is highly suspected.
- Monitoring the clinical course of the disease may help to guide the most likely diagnosis, particularly in cases with a typical clinical presentation and for which further investigations are not possible (see Box 6.12.1). This is important before considering euthanasia, as some disorders may present with severe clinical signs but can show spontaneous resolution without treatment (e.g. acute canine polyradiculoneuritis). If the disease is progressive and referral or further investigations are not possible, then trial treatment for the most likely differential diagnosis may be the only option. This could include pyridostigmine for suspected acquired myasthenia gravis, or corticosteroids for suspected chronic inflammatory demyelinating polyneuropathy, idiopathic polymyositis, and some forms of motor polyneuropathy in young cats. It is vital that the owner is always made aware of the potential risks and limitations associated with this approach. Many veterinary neurologists are happy to discuss such cases over the telephone before proceeding with treatment trials.

Bibliography

6.1. Epileptic Seizures

Armaşu, M., Packer, R.M., Cook, S. et al. (2014). An exploratory study using a statistical approach as a platform for clinical reasoning in canine epilepsy. *Vet. J.* 202: 292–296.

Bailey, K.S., Dewey, C.W., Boothe, D.M. et al. (2008). Levetiracetam as an adjunct to phenobarbital treatment in cats with suspected idiopathic epilepsy. *J. Am. Vet. Med. Assoc.* 232: 867–872.

Baird-Heinz, H.E., Van Schoick, A.L., Pelsor, F.R. et al. (2012). A systematic review of the safety of potassium bromide in dogs. *J. Am. Vet. Med. Assoc.* 240: 705–715.

Barnes Heller, H. (2018). Feline epilepsy. *Vet. Clin. North Am. Small Anim. Pract.* 48: 31–43.

Barnes Heller, H., Granick, M., Van Hesteren, M., and Boothe, D.M. (2018). Serum levetiracetam concentrations and adverse events after multiple dose extended release levetiracetam administration to healthy cats. *J. Vet. Intern. Med.* 32: 1145–1148.

Beasley, M.J. and Boothe, D.M. (2015). Disposition of extended release levetiracetam in normal healthy dogs after single oral dosing. *J. Vet. Intern. Med.* 29: 1348–1353.

Berendt, M., Farquhar, R.G., Mandigers, P.J. et al. (2015). International Veterinary Epilepsy Task Force consensus report on epilepsy definition, classification and terminology in companion animals. *BMC Vet. Res.* 11: 182.

Berk, B.A., Packer, R.M.A., Law, T.H., and Volk, H.A. (2018). Investigating owner use of dietary supplements in dogs with idiopathic epilepsy. *Res. Vet. Sci.* 119: 276–284.

Bersan, E., Volk, H.A., Ros, C., and De Risio, L. (2014). Phenobarbitone-induced haematological abnormalities in idiopathic epileptic dogs: prevalence, risk factors, clinical presentation and outcome. *Vet. Rec.* 175: 247.

Bhatti, S.F., De Risio, L., Muñana, K. et al. (2015). International Veterinary Epilepsy Task Force consensus proposal: medical treatment of canine epilepsy in Europe. *BMC Vet. Res.* 11: 176.

Biddick, A.A., Bacek, L.M., and Taylor, A.R. (2018). A serious adverse event secondary to rapid intravenous levetiracetam injection in a dog. *J. Vet. Emerg. Crit. Care (San Antonio)* 28: 157–162.

Boothe, D.M., Dewey, C., and Carpenter, D.M. (2012). Comparison of phenobarbital with bromide as a first-choice antiepileptic drug for treatment of epilepsy in dogs. *J. Am. Vet. Med. Assoc.* 240: 1073–1083.

Brauer, C., Kästner, S.B., Rohn, K. et al. (2012). Electroencephalographic recordings in dogs suffering from idiopathic and symptomatic epilepsy: diagnostic value of interictal short time EEG protocols supplemented by two activation techniques. *Vet. J.* 193: 185–192.

Carnes, M.B., Axlund, T.W., and Boothe, D.M. (2011). Pharmacokinetics of levetiracetam after oral and intravenous administration of a single dose to clinically normal cats. *Am. J. Vet. Res.* 72: 1247–1252.

Chang, Y., Mellor, D.J., and Anderson, T.J. (2006). Idiopathic epilepsy in dogs: owners' perspectives on management with phenobarbitone and/or potassium bromide. *J. Small Anim. Pract.* 47: 574–581.

Charalambous, M., Brodbelt, D., and Volk, H.A. (2014). Treatment in canine epilepsy–a systematic review. *BMC Vet. Res.* 10: 257.

Charalambous, M., Shivapour, S.K., Brodbelt, D.C., and Volk, H.A. (2016). Antiepileptic drugs' tolerability and safety–a systematic review and meta-analysis of adverse effects in dogs. *BMC Vet. Res.* 12: 79.

Charalambous, M., Pakozdy, A., Bhatti, S.F.M., and Volk, H.A. (2018). Systematic review of antiepileptic drugs' safety and effectiveness in feline epilepsy. *BMC Vet. Res.* 14: 64.

Collinet, A. and Sammut, V. (2017). Suspected zonisamide-related anticonvulsant hypersensitivity syndrome in a cat. *J. Am. Vet. Med. Assoc.* 251: 1457–1461.

De Risio, L., Bhatti, S., Muñana, K. et al. (2015). International Veterinary Epilepsy Task Force consensus proposal: diagnostic approach to epilepsy in dogs. *BMC Vet. Res.* 11: 148.

Engel, O., von Klopmann, T., Maiolini, A. et al. (2017). Imepitoin is well tolerated in healthy and epileptic cats. *BMC Vet. Res.* 13: 172.

Finnerty, K.E., Barnes Heller, H.L., Mercier, M.N. et al. (2014). Evaluation of therapeutic phenobarbital concentrations and application of a classification system for seizures in cats: 30 cases (2004–2013). *J. Am. Vet. Med. Assoc.* 244: 195–199.

Forsgård, J.A., Metsähonkala, L., Kiviranta, A.M. et al. (2019). Seizure-precipitating factors in dogs with idiopathic epilepsy. *J. Vet. Intern. Med.* 33: 701–707.

Fredsø, N., Sabers, A., Toft, N. et al. (2016). A single-blinded phenobarbital-controlled trial of levetiracetam as mono-therapy in dogs with newly diagnosed epilepsy. *Vet. J.* 208: 44–49.

Fredsø, N., Toft, N., Sabers, A., and Berendt, M. (2017). A prospective observational longitudinal study of new-onset seizures and newly diagnosed epilepsy in dogs. *BMC Vet. Res.* 13: 54.

Gallucci, A., Gagliardo, T., Menchetti, M. et al. (2017). Long-term efficacy of imepitoin in the treatment of naive dogs affected by idiopathic epilepsy. *Vet. Rec.* 181: 144.

Gesell, F.K., Hoppe, S., Löscher, W., and Tipold, A. (2015). Antiepileptic drug withdrawal in dogs with epilepsy. *Front. Vet. Sci.* 2: 23.

Ghormley, T.M., Feldman, D.G., and Cook, J.R. Jr. (2015). Epilepsy in dogs five years of age and older: 99 cases (2006–2011). *J. Am. Vet. Med. Assoc.* 246: 447–450.

Hardy, B.T., Patterson, E.E., Cloyd, J.M. et al. (2012). Double-masked, placebo-controlled study of intravenous levetiracetam for the treatment of status epilepticus and acute repetitive seizures in dogs. *J. Vet. Intern. Med.* 26: 334–340.

Hülsmeyer, V.I., Fischer, A., Mandigers, P.J. et al. (2015). International Veterinary Epilepsy Task Force's current understanding of idiopathic epilepsy of genetic or suspected genetic origin in purebred dogs. *BMC Vet. Res.* 11: 175.

Kearsley-Fleet, L., O'Neill, D.G., Volk, H.A. et al. (2013). Prevalence and risk factors for canine epilepsy of unknown origin in the UK. *Vet. Rec.* 172: 338.

Kelly, D., Raimondi, F., and Shihab, N. (2017). Levetiracetam monotherapy for treatment of structural epilepsy in dogs: 19 cases (2010–2015). *Vet. Rec.* 181: 401.

Larsen, J.A., Owens, T.J., and Fascetti, A.J. (2014). Nutritional management of idiopathic epilepsy in dogs. *J. Am. Vet. Med. Assoc.* 245: 504–508.

Law, T.H., Davies, E.S., Pan, Y. et al. (2015). A randomised trial of a medium-chain TAG diet as treatment for dogs with idiopathic epilepsy. *Br. J. Nutr.* 114: 1438–1447.

Long, S., Frey, S., Freestone, D.R. et al. (2014). Placement of deep brain electrodes in the dog using the Brainsight frameless stereotactic system: a pilot feasibility study. *J. Vet. Intern. Med.* 28: 189–197.

Lowrie, M., Bessant, C., Harvey, R.J. et al. (2016). Audiogenic reflex seizures in cats. *J. Feline Med. Surg.* 18: 328–336.

Lowrie, M., Thomson, S., Bessant, C. et al. (2017). Levetiracetam in the management of feline audiogenic reflex seizures: a randomised, controlled, open-label study. *J. Feline Med. Surg.* 19: 200–206.

Martlé, V., Van Ham, L., Raedt, R. et al. (2014). Non-pharmacological treatment options for refractory epilepsy: an overview of human treatment modalities and their potential utility in dogs. *Vet. J.* 199: 332–339.

Martlé, V., Van Ham, L.M., Boon, P. et al. (2016). Vagus nerve stimulator placement in dogs: surgical implantation technique, complications, long-term follow-up, and practical considerations. *Vet. Surg.* 45: 71–78.

Muñana, K.R., Thomas, W.B., Inzana, K.D. et al. (2012). Evaluation of levetiracetam as adjunctive treatment for refractory canine epilepsy: a randomized, placebo-controlled, crossover trial. *J. Vet. Intern. Med.* 26: 341–348.

Muñana, K.R., Nettifee-Osborne, J.A., and Papich, M.G. (2015). Effect of chronic administration of phenobarbital, or bromide, on pharmacokinetics of levetiracetam in dogs with epilepsy. *J. Vet. Intern. Med.* 29: 614–619.

Muñana, K.R., Otamendi, A.J., Nettifee, J.A., and Papich, M.G. (2018). Population pharmacokinetics of extended-release levetiracetam in epileptic dogs when administered alone, with phenobarbital or zonisamide. *J. Vet. Intern. Med.* 32: 1677–1683.

Neßler, J., Rundfeldt, C., Löscher, W. et al. (2017). Clinical evaluation of a combination therapy of imepitoin with phenobarbital in dogs with refractory idiopathic epilepsy. *BMC Vet. Res.* 13: 33.

Packer, R.M. and Volk, H.A. (2015). Epilepsy beyond seizures: a review of the impact of epilepsy and its comorbidities on health-related quality of life in dogs. *Vet. Rec.* 177: 306–315.

Packer, R.M., Nye, G., Porter, S.E., and Volk, H.A. (2015). Assessment into the usage of leveti-racetam in a canine epilepsy clinic. *BMC Vet. Res.* 11: 25.

Pakozdy, A., Sarchahi, A.A., Leschnik, M. et al. (2013). Treatment and long-term follow-up of cats with suspected primary epilepsy. *J. Feline Med. Surg.* 15: 267–273.

Pakozdy, A., Halasz, P., and Klang, A. (2014). Epilepsy in cats: theory and practice. *J. Vet. Intern. Med.* 28: 255–263.

Podell, M., Volk, H.A., Berendt, M. et al. (2015, 2016). ACVIM small animal consensus statement on seizure management in dogs. *J. Vet. Intern. Med.* 30: 477–490.

Potschka, H., Fischer, A., Löscher, W. et al. (2015). International Veterinary Epilepsy Task Force consensus proposal: outcome of therapeutic interventions in canine and feline epilepsy. *BMC Vet. Res.* 11: 177.

Raimondi, F., Shihab, N., Gutierrez-Quintana, R. et al. (2017). Magnetic resonance imaging findings in epileptic cats with a normal interictal neurological examination: 188 cases. *Vet. Rec.* 180: 610.

Rossmeisl, J.H. and Inzana, K.D. (2009). Clinical signs, risk factors, and outcomes associated with bromide toxicosis (bromism) in dogs with idiopathic epilepsy. *J. Am. Vet. Med. Assoc.* 234: 1425–1431.

Royaux, E., Van Ham, L., Broeckx, B.J. et al. (2017). Phenobarbital or potassium bromide as an add-on antiepileptic drug for the management of canine idiopathic epilepsy refractory to imepitoin. *Vet. J.* 220: 51–54.

Rundfeldt, C., Tipold, A., and Löscher, W. (2015). Efficacy, safety, and tolerability of imepitoin in dogs with newly diagnosed epilepsy in a randomized controlled clinical study with long-term follow up. *BMC Vet. Res.* 11: 228.

Schwartz, M., Muñana, K.R., and Nettifee-Osborne, J. (2013). Assessment of the prevalence and clinical features of cryptogenic epilepsy in dogs: 45 cases (2003–2011). *J. Am. Vet. Med. Assoc.* 242: 651–657.

Shaw, N., Trepanier, L.A., Center, S.A., and Garland, S. (1996). High dietary chloride content associated with loss of therapeutic serum bromide concentrations in an epileptic dog. *J. Am. Vet. Med. Assoc.* 208: 234–236.

Shell, L., Scariano, R., and Rishniw, M. (2017). Features of stimulus-specific seizures in dogs with reflex epilepsy: 43 cases (2000–2014). *J. Am. Vet. Med. Assoc.* 250: 75–78.

Shihab, N., Bowen, J., and Volk, H.A. (2011). Behavioral changes in dogs associated with the development of idiopathic epilepsy. *Epilepsy Behav.* 21: 160–167.

Smith, P.M., Talbot, C.E., and Jeffery, N.D. (2008). Findings on low-field cranial MR images in epileptic dogs that lack interictal neurological deficits. *Vet. J.* 176: 320–325.

Stabile, F., Barnett, C.R., and De Risio, L. (2017). Phenobarbital administration every eight hours: improvement of seizure management in idiopathic epileptic dogs with decreased phenobarbital elimination half-life. *Vet. Rec.* 180: 178.

Stanciu, G.D., Packer, R.M.A., Pakozdy, A. et al. (2017). Clinical reasoning in feline epilepsy: which combination of clinical information is useful? *Vet. J.* 225: 9–12.

Stee, K., Martlé, V., Broeckx, B.J.G. et al. (2017). Imepitoin withdrawal in dogs with idiopathic epilepsy well-controlled with imepitoin and phenobarbital and/or potassium bromide does not increase seizure frequency. *Vet. J.* 230: 1–5.

Szelecsenyi, A.C., Giger, U., Golini, L. et al. (2017). Survival in 76 cats with epilepsy of unknown cause: a retrospective study. *Vet. Rec.* 181: 479.

Tipold, A., Keefe, T.J., Löscher, W. et al. (2015). Clinical efficacy and safety of imepitoin in comparison with phenobarbital for the control of idiopathic epilepsy in dogs. *J. Vet. Pharmacol. Ther.* 38: 160–168.

Volk, H.A., Matiasek, L.A., Luján Feliu-Pascual, A. et al. (2008). The efficacy and tolerability of levetiracetam in pharmacoresistant epileptic dogs. *Vet. J.* 176: 310–319.

Wahle, A.M., Brühschwein, A., Matiasek, K. et al. (2014). Clinical characterization of epilepsy of unknown cause in cats. *J. Vet. Intern. Med.* 28: 182–188.

Watson, F., Rusbridge, C., Packer, R.M.A. et al. (2018). A review of treatment options for behavioural manifestations of clinical anxiety as a comorbidity in dogs with idiopathic epilepsy. *Vet. J.* 238: 1–9.

Wielaender, F., James, F.M.K., Cortez, M.A. et al. (2018). Absence seizures as a feature of juvenile myoclonic epilepsy in Rhodesian Ridgeback dogs. *J. Vet. Intern. Med.* 32: 428–432.

Winter, J., Packer, R.M.A., and Volk, H.A. (2018). Preliminary assessment of cognitive impairments in canine idiopathic epilepsy. *Vet. Rec.* 182: 633.

6.2. Movement Disorders

Bhatti, S.F., Vanhaesebrouck, A.E., Van Soens, I. et al. (2011). Myokymia and neuromyotonia in 37 Jack Russell terriers. *Vet. J.* 189: 284–288.

Black, V., Garosi, L., Lowrie, M. et al. (2014). Phenotypic characterisation of canine epileptoid cramping syndrome in the border terrier. *J. Small Anim. Pract.* 55: 102–107.

De Risio, L., Bhatti, S., Muñana, K. et al. (2015). International Veterinary Epilepsy Task Force consensus proposal: diagnostic approach to epilepsy in dogs. *BMC Vet. Res.* 11: 182.

Galano, H.R., Olby, N.J., Howard, J.F. Jr., and Shelton, G.D. (2005). Myokymia and neuromyotonia in a cat. *J. Am. Vet. Med. Assoc.* 227: 1608–1612.

Garosi, L.S., Rossmeisl, J.H., de Lahunta, A. et al. (2005). Primary orthostatic tremor in Great Danes. *J. Vet. Intern. Med.* 19: 606–609.

Geiger, K.M. and Klopp, L.S. (2009). Use of a selective serotonin reuptake inhibitor for treatment of episodes of hypertonia and kyphosis in a young adult Scottish Terrier. *J. Am. Vet. Med. Assoc.* 235: 168–171.

Gill, J.L., Tsai, K.L., Krey, C. et al. (2012). A canine BCAN microdeletion associated with episodic falling syndrome. *Neurobiol. Dis.* 45: 130–136.

Gilliam, D., O'Brien, D.P., Coates, J.R. et al. (2014). A homozygous KCNJ10 mutation in Jack Russell Terriers and related breeds with spinocerebellar ataxia with myokymia, seizures, or both. *J. Vet. Intern. Med.* 28: 871–877.

Guevar, J., De Decker, S., Van Ham, L.M. et al. (2014). Idiopathic head tremor in English bulldogs. *Mov. Disord.* 29: 191–194.

Herrtage, M.E. and Palmer, A.C. (1983). Episodic falling in the cavalier King Charles spaniel. *Vet. Rec.* 112: 458–459.

Holland, C.T., Holland, J.T., and Rozmanec, M. (2010). Unilateral facial myokymia in a dog with an intracranial meningioma. *Aust. Vet. J.* 88: 357–361.

Lowrie, M. and Garosi, L. (2016a). Classification of involuntary movements in dogs: tremors and twitches. *Vet. J.* 214: 109–116.

Lowrie, M. and Garosi, L. (2016b). Natural history of canine paroxysmal movement disorders in Labrador retrievers and Jack Russell terriers. *Vet. J.* 213: 33–37.

Lowrie, M. and Garosi, L. (2017a). Classification of involuntary movements in dogs: myoclonus and myotonia. *J. Vet. Intern. Med.* 31: 979–987.

Lowrie, M. and Garosi, L. (2017b). Classification of involuntary movements in dogs: paroxysmal dyskinesias. *Vet. J.* 220: 65–71.

Lowrie, M., Garden, O.A., Hadjivassiliou, M. et al. (2015). The clinical and serological effect of a gluten-free diet in Border Terriers with epileptoid cramping syndrome. *J. Vet. Intern. Med.* 29: 1564–1568.

Lowrie, M., Bessant, C., Harvey, R.J. et al. (2016a). Audiogenic reflex seizures in cats. *J. Feline Med. Surg.* 18: 328–336.

Lowrie, M., Hadjivassiliou, M., Sanders, D.S., and Garden, O.A. (2016b). A presumptive case of gluten sensitivity in a Border terrier: a multisystem disorder? *Vet. Rec.* 179: 573.

Lowrie, M., Thomson, S., Bessant, C. et al. (2017). Levetiracetam in the management of feline audiogenic reflex seizures: a randomised, controlled, open-label study. *J. Feline Med. Surg.* 19: 200–206.

Lowrie, M., Garden, O.A., Hadjivassiliou, M. et al. (2018). Characterization of paroxysmal gluten-sensitive dyskinesia in Border terriers using serological markers. *J. Vet. Intern. Med.* 32: 775–781.

Mauler, D.A., Van Soens, I., Bhatti, S.F. et al. (2014). Idiopathic generalised tremor syndrome in two cats. *J. Feline Med. Surg.* 16: 378–380.

Packer, R.A., Patterson, E.E., Taylor, J.F. et al. (2010). Characterization and mode of inheritance of a paroxysmal dyskinesia in Chinook dogs. *J. Vet. Intern. Med.* 24: 1305–1313.

Rogatko, C.P., Glass, E.N., Kent, M. et al. (2016). Use of botulinum toxin type A for the treatment of radiation therapy-induced myokymia and neuromyotonia in a dog. *J. Am. Vet. Med. Assoc.* 248: 532–537.

Schubert, T., Clemmons, R., Miles, S., and Draper, W. (2013). The use of botulinum toxin for the treatment of generalized myoclonus in a dog. *J. Am. Anim. Hosp. Assoc.* 49: 122–127.

Swain, L., Key, G., Tauro, A. et al. (2017). Lafora disease in miniature Wirehaired Dachshunds. *PLoS One* 12 (8): e0182024.

Urkasemsin, G. and Olby, N.J. (2014). Canine paroxysmal movement disorders. *Vet. Clin. North Am. Small Anim. Pract.* 44: 1091–1102.

Urkasemsin, G. and Olby, N.J. (2015). Clinical characteristics of Scottie cramp in 31 cases. *J. Small Anim. Pract.* 56: 276–280.

Vanhaesebrouck, A.E., Van Soens, I., Poncelet, L. et al. (2010). Clinical and electrophysiological characterization of myokymia and neuromyotonia in Jack Russell Terriers. *J. Vet. Intern. Med.* 24: 882–889.

Vanhaesebrouck, A.E., Shelton, G.D., Garosi, L. et al. (2011). A novel movement disorder in related male Labrador retrievers characterized by extreme generalized muscle stiffness. *J. Vet. Intern. Med.* 25: 1089–1096.

Vanhaesebrouck, A.E., Bhatti, S.F., Franklin, R.J., and Van Ham, L. (2013). Myokymia and neuromyotonia in veterinary medicine: a comparison with peripheral nerve hyperexcitability syndrome in humans. *Vet. J.* 197: 153–162.

Wagner, S.O., Podell, M., and Fenner, W.R. (1997). Generalized tremors in dogs: 24 cases (1984–1995). *J. Am. Vet. Med. Assoc.* 211: 731–735.

Walmsley, G.L., Smith, P.M., Herrtage, M.E., and Jeffery, N.D. (2006). Facial myokymia in a puppy. *Vet. Rec.* 158: 411–412.

6.3. Altered Mentation

Brutlag, A. and Hommerding, H. (2018). Toxicology of marijuana, synthetic cannabinoids, and cannabidiol in dogs and cats. *Vet. Clin. North Am. Small Anim. Pract.* 48: 1087–1102.

Gillespie, S., Gilbert, Z., and De Decker, S. (2019). Results of oral prednisolone administration or ventriculoperitoneal shunt placement in dogs with congenital hydrocephalus: 40 cases (2005–2016). *J. Am. Vet. Med. Assoc.* 254: 835–842.

Hu, H., Barker, A., Harcourt-Brown, T. et al. (2015). Systematic review of brain tumor treatment in dogs. *J. Vet. Intern. Med.* 29: 1456–1463.

Mangat, H.S., Wu, X., Gerber et al. (2019. pii: nyz046. doi: https://doi.org/10.1093/neuros/nyz046). Hypertonic saline is superior to mannitol for the combined effect on intracranial pressure and cerebral perfusion pressure burdens in patients with severe traumatic brain injury. *Neurosurgery*. [Epub ahead of print].

Meola, S.D., Tearney, C.C., Haas, S.A. et al. (2012). Evaluation of trends in marijuana toxicosis in dogs living in a state with legalized medical marijuana: 125 dogs (2005–2010). *J. Vet. Emerg. Crit. Care (San Antonio)* 22: 690–696.

O'Neill, J., Kent, M., Glass, E.N. et al. (2013). Clinicopathologic and MRI characteristics of presumptive hypertensive encephalopathy in two cats and two dogs. *J. Am. Anim. Hosp. Assoc.* 49: 412–420.

Parratt, C.A., Firth, A.M., Boag, A.K. et al. (2018). Retrospective characterization of coma and stupor in dogs and cats presenting to a multicenter out-of-hours service (2012–2015): 386 animals. *J. Vet. Emerg. Crit. Care (San Antonio)* 28: 559–565.

Platt, S.R., Radaelli, S.T., and McDonnell, J.J. (2001). The prognostic value of the modified Glasgow Coma Scale in head trauma in dogs. *J. Vet. Intern. Med.* 15: 581–584.

Qureshi, A.I., Wilson, D.A., and Traystman, R.J. (1999). Treatment of elevated intracranial pressure in experimental intracerebral hemorrhage: comparison between mannitol and hypertonic saline. *Neurosurgery* 44: 1055–1063.

Schubert, T.A., Chidester, R.M., and Chrisman, C.L. (2011). Clinical characteristics, management and long-term outcome of suspected rapid eye movement sleep behaviour disorder in 14 dogs. *J. Small Anim. Pract.* 52: 93–100.

Shea, A., Hatch, A., De Risio, L. et al. (2018). Association between clinically probable REM sleep behavior disorder and tetanus in dogs. *J. Vet. Intern. Med.* 32: 2029–2036.

Sokhal, N., Rath, G.P., Chaturvedi, A. et al. (2017). Comparison of 20% mannitol and 3% hypertonic saline on intracranial pressure and systemic hemodynamics. *J. Clin. Neurosci.* 42: 148–154.

6.4. Blindness

Dewey, C.W. and da Costa, R.C. (2015). *Practical Guide to Canine and Feline Neurology*, 3e. Hoboken, NJ: Wiley Blackwell.

Grozdanic, S.D., Matic, M., Sakaguchi, D.S., and Kardon, R.H. (2007). Evaluation of retinal status using chromatic pupil light reflex activity in healthy and diseased canine eyes. *Invest. Ophthalmol. Vis. Sci.* 48: 5178–5183.

Heller, A.R., van der Woerdt, A., Gaarder, J.E. et al. (2017). Sudden acquired retinal degeneration in dogs: breed distribution of 495 canines. *Vet. Ophthalmol.* 20: 103–106.

Komáromy, A.M., Abrams, K.L., Heckenlively, J.R. et al. (2016). Sudden acquired retinal degeneration syndrome (SARDS) – a review and proposed strategies toward a better understanding of pathogenesis, early diagnosis, and therapy. *Vet. Ophthalmol.* 19: 319–331.

de Lahunta, A., Glass, E., and Kent, M. (2015). *Veterinary Neuroanatomy and Clinical Neurology*, 4e. St Louis, MO: Elsevier Saunders.

Mari, L., Stavinohova, R., Dominguez, E. et al. (2018). Ischemic optic neuropathy in a dog with acute bilateral blindness and primary systemic hypertension. *J. Vet. Intern. Med.* 32: 423–427.

Martin-Flores, M., Scrivani, P.V., Loew, E. et al. (2014). Maximal and submaximal mouth opening with mouth gags in cats: implications for maxillary artery blood flow. *Vet. J.* 200: 60–64.

Meekins, J.M. (2015). Acute blindness. *Top. Companion Anim. Med.* 30: 118–125.

Meekins, J.M., Guess, S.C., and Rankin, A.J. (2015). Retinopathy associated with ivermectin toxicosis in five cats. *J. Am. Vet. Med. Assoc.* 246: 1238–1241.

Montgomery, K.W., van der Woerdt, A., and Cottrill, N.B. (2008). Acute blindness in dogs: sudden acquired retinal degeneration syndrome versus neurological disease (140 cases, 2000–2006). *Vet. Ophthalmol.* 11: 314–320.

Platt, S. and Olby, N. (2013). *BSAVA Manual of Canine and Feline Neurology*, 4e. Gloucester, UK: British Small Animal Veterinary Association.

Quitt, P.R., Reese, S., Fischer, A. et al. (2019). Assessment of menace response in neurologically and ophthalmologically healthy cats. *J. Feline Med. Surg.* 21: 537–543.

Seruca, C., Ródenas, S., Leiva, M. et al. (2010). Acute postretinal blindness: ophthalmologic, neurologic, and magnetic resonance imaging findings in dogs and cats (seven cases). *Vet. Ophthalmol.* 13: 307–314.

Stiles, J., Weil, A.B., Packer, R.A., and Lantz, G.C. (2012). Post-anesthetic cortical blindness in cats: twenty cases. *Vet. J.* 193: 367–373.

Stuckey, J.A., Pearce, J.W., Giuliano, E.A. et al. (2013). Long-term outcome of sudden acquired retinal degeneration syndrome in dogs. *J. Am. Vet. Med. Assoc.* 243: 1425–1431.

6.5. Abnormalities of Pupil Size

Boydell, P. (2000a). Idiopathic Horner syndrome in the golden retriever. *J. Neuroophthalmol.* 20: 288–290.

Boydell, P. (2000b). Iatrogenic pupillary dilation resembling Pourfour du petit syndrome in three cats. *J. Small Anim. Pract.* 41: 202–203.

Boydell, P., Pike, R., Crossley, D., and Torrington, A. (1997). Horner's syndrome following intrathoracic tube placement. *J. Small Anim. Pract.* 38: 466–467.

Carpenter, J.L., King, N.W. Jr., and Abrams, K.L. (1987). Bilateral trigeminal nerve paralysis and Horner's syndrome associated with myelomonocytic neoplasia in a dog. *J. Am. Vet. Med. Assoc.* 191: 1594–1596.

Foote, B.C., Michau, T.M., Welihozkiy, A., and Stine, J.M. (2019). Retrospective analysis of ocular neuropathies in diabetic dogs following cataract surgery. *Vet. Ophthalmol.* 22: 284–293.

Grahn, B.H. and Cullen, C.L. (2004). Diagnostic ophthalmology. Iris atrophy. *Can. Vet. J.* 45: 77–78.

Guevar, J., Gutierrez-Quintana, R., Peplinski, G. et al. (2014). Cavernous sinus syndrome secondary to intracranial lymphoma in a cat. *J. Feline Med. Surg.* 16: 513–516.

Hamzianpour, N., Lam, R., Tetas, R., and Beltran, E. (2018). Clinical signs, imaging findings, and outcome in twelve cats with internal ophthalmoparesis/ophthalmoplegia. *Vet. Ophthalmol.* 21: 382–390.

Holland, C.T. (2007). Bilateral Horner's syndrome in a dog with diabetes mellitus. *Vet. Rec.* 160: 662–664.

Jones, A.M., Bentley, E., and Rylander, H. (2018). Cavernous sinus syndrome in dogs and cats: case series (2002–2015). *Open Vet. J.* 8: 186–192.

Kern, T.J., Aromando, M.C., and Erb, H.N. (1989). Horner's syndrome in dogs and cats: 100 cases (1975–1985). *J. Am. Vet. Med. Assoc.* 195: 369–373.

de Lahunta, A., Glass, E., and Kent, M. (2015). *Veterinary Neuroanatomy and Clinical Neurology*, 4e. St Louis, MO: Elsevier Saunders.

Larocca, R.D. (2000). Unilateral external and internal ophthalmoplegia caused by intracranial meningioma in a dog. *Vet. Ophthalmol.* 3: 3–9.

Melián, C., Morales, M., de los Espinosa, Monteros, A., and Peterson, M.E. (1996). Horner's syndrome associated with a functional thyroid carcinoma in a dog. *J. Small Anim. Pract.* 37: 591–593.

Morgan, R.V. and Zanotti, S.W. (1989). Horner's syndrome in dogs and cats: 49 cases (1980–1986). *J. Am. Vet. Med. Assoc.* 194: 1096–1099.

O'Neill, J.J., Kent, M., Glass, E.N. et al. (2013). Insertion of the dorsal oblique muscle in the dog: an anatomic basis for ventral strabismus associated with oculomotor nerve dysfunction. *Vet. Ophthalmol.* 16: 467–471.

Platt, S. and Olby, N. (2013). *BSAVA Manual of Canine and Feline Neurology*, 4e. Gloucester, UK: British Small Animal Veterinary Association.

Simpson, K.M., Williams, D.L., and Cherubini, G.B. (2015). Neuropharmacological lesion localization in idiopathic Horner's syndrome in Golden Retrievers and dogs of other breeds. *Vet. Ophthalmol.* 18: 1–5.

Spivack, R.E., Elkins, A.D., Moore, G.E., and Lantz, G.C. (2013). Postoperative complications following TECA-LBO in the dog and cat. *J. Am. Anim. Hosp. Assoc.* 49: 160–168.

Stephan, D.D., Vestre, W.A., Stiles, J., and Krohne, S. (2003). Changes in intraocular pressure and pupil size following intramuscular administration of hydromorphone hydrochloride and acepromazine in clinically normal dogs. *Vet. Ophthalmol.* 6: 73–76.

Tetas Pont, R., Freeman, C., Dennis, R. et al. (2017). Clinical and magnetic resonance imaging features of idiopathic oculomotor neuropathy in 14 dogs. *Vet. Radiol. Ultrasound* 58: 334–343.

Viscasillas, J., Sanchis-Mora, S., Hoy, C., and Alibhai, H. (2013). Transient Horner's syndrome after paravertebral brachial plexus blockade in a dog. *Vet. Anaesth. Analg.* 40: 104–106.

Webb, A.A., Cullen, C.L., Rose, P. et al. (2005). Intracranial meningioma causing internal ophthalmoparesis in a dog. *Vet. Ophthalmol.* 8: 421–425.

6.6. Cranial Nerve Dysfunction

Bagley, R.S., Wheeler, S.J., Klopp, L. et al. (1998). Clinical features of trigeminal nerve-sheath tumor in 10 dogs. *J. Am. Anim. Hosp. Assoc.* 34: 19–25.

Bartges, J.W. and Nielson, D.L. (1992). Reversible megaesophagus associated with atypical primary hypoadrenocorticism in a dog. *J. Am. Vet. Med. Assoc.* 201: 889–891.

Bexfield, N.H., Watson, P.J., and Herrtage, M.E. (2006). Esophageal dysmotility in young dogs. *J. Vet. Intern. Med.* 20: 1314–1318.

Blazejewski, S.W. and Shelton, G.D. (2018). Trismus, masticatory myositis and antibodies against type 2M fibers in a mixed breed cat. *JFMS Open Rep.* 4:2055116918764993.

Bookbinder, L.C., Flanders, J., Bookbinder, P.F. et al. (2016). Idiopathic canine laryngeal paralysis as one sign of a diffuse polyneuropathy: an observational study of 90 cases (2007–2013). *Vet. Surg.* 45: 254–260.

Boudrieau, R.J. and Rogers, W.A. (1985). Megaesophagus in the dog: a review of 50 cases. *J. Am. Anim. Hosp. Assoc.* 21: 33–40.

Bovens, C., Tennant, K., Reeve, J., and Murphy, K.F. (2014). Basal serum cortisol concentration as a screening test for hypoadrenocorticism in dogs. *J. Vet. Intern. Med.* 28: 1541–1545.

Braund, K.G., Steinberg, H.S., Shores, A. et al. (1989). Laryngeal paralysis in immature and mature dogs as one sign of a more diffuse polyneuropathy. *J. Am. Vet. Med. Assoc.* 194: 1735–1740.

Braund, K.G., Shores, A., Cochrane, S. et al. (1994). Laryngeal paralysis-polyneuropathy complex in young Dalmatians. *Am. J. Vet. Res.* 55: 534–542.

Cauduro, A., Paolo, F., Asperio, R.M. et al. (2013). Use of MRI for the early diagnosis of masticatory muscle myositis. *J. Am. Anim. Hosp. Assoc.* 49: 347–352.

Dewey, C.W. and da Costa, R.C. (2015). *Practical Guide to Canine and Feline Neurology*, 3e. Hoboken, NJ: Wiley Blackwell.

Dolera, M., Malfassi, L., Marcarini, S. et al. (2018). High dose hypofractionated frameless volumetric modulated arc radiotherapy is a feasible method for treating canine trigeminal nerve sheath tumors. *Vet. Radiol. Ultrasound* 59: 624–631.

Evans, J., Levesque, D., and Shelton, G.D. (2004). Canine inflammatory myopathies: a clinicopathologic review of 200 cases. *J. Vet. Intern. Med.* 18: 679–691.

Fracassi, F. and Tamborini, A. (2011). Reversible megaoesophagus associated with primary hypothyroidism in a dog. *Vet. Rec.* 329b: 168.

Gabriel, A., Poncelet, L., Van Ham, L. et al. (2006). Laryngeal paralysis-polyneuropathy complex in young related Pyrenean mountain dogs. *J. Small Anim. Pract.* 47: 144–149.

Gaynor, A.R., Shofer, F.S., and Washabau, R.J. (1997). Risk factors for acquired megaesophagus in dogs. *J. Am. Vet. Med. Assoc.* 211: 1406–1412.

Granger, N. (2011). Canine inherited motor and sensory neuropathies: an updated classification in 22 breeds and comparison to Charcot-Marie-Tooth disease. *Vet. J.* 188: 274–285.

Haines, J.M. (2019). Survey of owners on population characteristics, diagnosis, and environmental, health, and disease associations in dogs with megaesophagus. *Res. Vet. Sci.* 123: 1–6.

Hansen, K.S., Zwingenberger, A.L., Théon, A.P. et al. (2016). Treatment of MRI-diagnosed trigeminal peripheral nerve sheath tumors by stereotactic radiotherapy in dogs. *J. Vet. Intern. Med.* 30: 1112–1120.

Ito, D., Okada, M., Jeffery, N.D. et al. (2009). Symptomatic tongue atrophy due to atypical polymyositis in a Pembroke Welsh Corgi. *J. Vet. Med. Sci.* 71: 1063–1067.

Jaggy, A. and Oliver, J.E. (1994). Neurologic manifestations of thyroid disease. *Vet. Clin. North Am. Small Anim. Pract.* 24: 487–494.

Jeandel, A., Thibaud, J.L., and Blot, S. (2016). Facial and vestibular neuropathy of unknown origin in 16 dogs. *J. Small Anim. Pract.* 57: 74–78.

Jeffery, N.D., Talbot, C.E., Smith, P.M., and Bacon, N.J. (2006). Acquired idiopathic laryngeal paralysis as a prominent feature of generalised neuromuscular disease in 39 dogs. *Vet. Rec.* 158: 17.

Kent, M., Glass, E.N., de Lahunta, A. et al. (2013). Prevalence of effusion in the tympanic cavity in dogs with dysfunction of the trigeminal nerve: 18 cases (2004–2013). *J. Vet. Intern. Med.* 27: 1153–1158.

Kent, M., Talarico, L.R., Glass, E.N. et al. (2015). Denervation of the tensor veli palatini muscle and effusion in the tympanic cavity. *J. Am. Anim. Hosp. Assoc.* 51: 424–428.

Kern, T.J. and Erb, H.N. (1987). Facial neuropathy in dogs and cats: 95 cases (1975–1985). *J. Am. Vet. Med. Assoc.* 191: 1604–1609.

de Lahunta, A., Glass, E., and Kent, M. (2015). *Veterinary Neuroanatomy and Clinical Neurology*, 4e. St Louis, MO: Elsevier Saunders.

Mace, S., Shelton, G.D., and Eddlestone, S. (2012). Megaesophagus. *Compend. Contin. Educ. Vet.* 34: E1.

Macphail, C. (2014). Laryngeal disease in dogs and cats. *Vet. Clin. North Am. Small Anim. Pract.* 44: 19–31.

Mahony, O.M., Knowles, K.E., Braund, K.G. et al. (1998). Laryngeal paralysis-polyneuropathy complex in young Rottweilers. *J. Vet. Intern. Med.* 12: 330–337.

Manning, K., Birkenheuer, A.J., Briley, J. et al. (2016). Intermittent at-home suctioning of esophageal content for prevention of recurrent aspiration pneumonia in 4 dogs with megaesophagus. *J. Vet. Intern. Med.* 30: 1715–1719.

Matheis, F.L., Walser-Reinhardt, L., and Spiess, B.M. (2012). Canine neurogenic Keratoconjunctivitis sicca: 11 cases (2006–2010). *Vet. Ophthalmol.* 15: 288–290.

Mayhew, P.D., Bush, W.W., and Glass, E.N. (2002). Trigeminal neuropathy in dogs: a retrospective study of 29 cases (1991–2000). *J. Am. Anim. Hosp. Assoc.* 38: 262–270.

McBrearty, A.R., Ramsey, I.K., Courcier, E.A. et al. (2011). Clinical factors associated with death before discharge and overall survival time in dogs with generalized megaesophagus. *J. Am. Vet. Med. Assoc.* 238: 1622–1628.

Milodowski, E.J., Amengual-Batle, P., Beltran, E. et al. (2018). Clinical findings and outcome of dogs with unilateral masticatory muscle atrophy. *J. Vet. Intern. Med.* https://doi.org/10.1111/jvim.15373.

Monnet, E. (2016). Surgical treatment of laryngeal paralysis. *Vet. Clin. North Am. Small Anim. Pract.* 46: 709–717.

Nakagawa, T., Doi, A., Ohno, K. et al. (2019). Clinical features and prognosis of canine megaesophagus in Japan. *J. Vet. Med. Sci.* https://doi.org/10.1292/jvms.18-0493.

Paciello, O., Shelton, G.D., and Papparella, S. (2007). Expression of major histocompatibility complex class I and class II antigens in canine masticatory muscle myositis. *Neuromuscul. Disord.* 17: 313–320.

Pagano, T.B., Wojcik, S., Costagliola, A. et al. (2015). Age related skeletal muscle atrophy and upregulation of autophagy in dogs. *Vet. J.* 206: 54–60.

Panciera, R.J., Ritchey, J.W., Baker, J.E., and DiGregorio, M. (2002). Trigeminal and polyradiculoneuritis in a dog presenting with masticatory muscle atrophy and Horner's syndrome. *Vet. Pathol.* 39: 146–149.

Parzefall, B., Fischer, A., Blutke, A. et al. (2011). Naturally-occurring canine herpesvirus-1 infection of the vestibular labyrinth and ganglion of dogs. *Vet. J.* 189: 100–102.

Pfaff, A.M., March, P.A., and Fishman, C. (2000). Acute bilateral trigeminal neuropathy associated with nervous system lymphosarcoma in a dog. *J. Am. Anim. Hosp. Assoc.* 36: 57–61.

von Pfeil, D.J.F., Zellner, E., Fritz, M.C. et al. (2018). Congenital laryngeal paralysis in Alaskan huskies: 25 cases (2009–2014). *J. Am. Vet. Med. Assoc.* 253: 1057–1065.

Pitcher, G.D. and Hahn, C.N. (2007). Atypical masticatory muscle myositis in three cavalier King Charles spaniel littermates. *J. Small Anim. Pract.* 48: 226–228.

Platt, S. and Olby, N. (2013). *BSAVA Manual of Canine and Feline Neurology*, 4e. Gloucester, UK: British Small Animal Veterinary Association.

Quintavalla, F., Menozzi, A., Pozzoli, C. et al. (2017). Sildenafil improves clinical signs and radiographic features in dogs with congenital idiopathic megaoesophagus: a randomised controlled trial. *Vet. Rec.* 180: 404.

Reiter, A.M. and Schwarz, T. (2007). Computed tomographic appearance of masticatory myositis in dogs: 7 cases (1999–2006). *J. Am. Vet. Med. Assoc.* 231: 924–930.

Roynard, P., Behr, S., Barone, G. et al. (2012). Idiopathic hypertrophic pachymeningitis in six dogs: MRI, CSF and histological findings, treatment and outcome. *J. Small Anim. Pract.* 53: 543–548.

Schmidt, R.F., Yick, F., Boghani, Z. et al. (2013). Malignant peripheral nerve sheath tumors of the trigeminal nerve: a systematic review of 36 cases. *Neurosurg. Focus.* 34: E5.

Schultz, R.M., Tucker, R.L., Gavin, P.R. et al. (2007). Magnetic resonance imaging of acquired trigeminal nerve disorders in six dogs. *Vet. Radiol. Ultrasound* 48: 101–104.

Shelton, G.D., Cardinet, G.H. 3rd, and Bandman, E. (1987). Canine masticatory muscle disorders: a study of 29 cases. *Muscle Nerve* 10: 753–766.

Shelton, G.D., Podell, M., Poncelet, L. et al. (2003). Inherited polyneuropathy in Leonberger dogs: a mixed or intermediate form of Charcot-Marie-Tooth disease? *Muscle Nerve* 27: 471–477.

Smith, P.M., Gonçalves, R., and McConnell, J.F. (2012). Sensitivity and specificity of MRI for detecting facial nerve abnormalities in dogs with facial neuropathy. *Vet. Rec.* 171: 349.

Strøm, P.C., Marks, S.L., Rivera, J.A., and Shelton, G.D. (2018). Dysphagia secondary to focal inflammatory myopathy and consequent dorsiflexion of the tongue in a dog. *J. Small Anim. Pract.* 59: 714–718.

Swift, K.E., McGrath, S., Nolan, M.W. et al. (2017). Clinical and imaging findings, treatments, and outcomes in 27 dogs with imaging diagnosed trigeminal nerve sheath tumors: a multicenter study. *Vet. Radiol. Ultrasound* 58: 679–689.

Tauro, A., Addicott, D., Foale, R.D. et al. (2015). Clinical features of idiopathic inflammatory polymyopathy in the Hungarian Vizsla. *BMC Vet. Res.* 11: 97.

Thieman, K.M., Krahwinkel, D.J., Sims, M.H., and Shelton, G.D. (2010). Histopathological confirmation of polyneuropathy in 11 dogs with laryngeal paralysis. *J. Am. Anim. Hosp. Assoc.* 46: 161–167.

Toyoda, K., Uchida, K., Matsuki, N. et al. (2010). Inflammatory myopathy with severe tongue atrophy in Pembroke Welsh Corgi dogs. *J. Vet. Diagn. Investig.* 22: 876–885.

Vamvakidis, C.D., Koutinas, A.F., Kanakoudis, G. et al. (2000). Masticatory and skeletal muscle myositis in canine leishmaniasis (*Leishmania infantum*). *Vet. Rec.* 146: 698–703.

Varejão, A.S., Muñoz, A., and Lorenzo, V. (2006). Magnetic resonance imaging of the intratemporal facial nerve in idiopathic facial paralysis in the dog. *Vet. Radiol. Ultrasound* 47: 328–333.

Wessmann, A., Hennessey, A., Goncalves, R. et al. (2013). The association of middle ear effusion with trigeminal nerve mass lesions in dogs. *Vet. Rec.* 173: 449.

Whitley, N.T. (1995). Megaoesophagus and glucocorticoid-deficient hypoadrenocorticism in a dog. *J. Small Anim. Pract.* 36: 132–135.

Wilson, D. and Monnet, E. (2016). Risk factors for the development of aspiration pneumonia after unilateral arytenoid lateralization in dogs with laryngeal paralysis: 232 cases (1987–2012). *J. Am. Vet. Med. Assoc.* 248: 188–194.

Wray, J.D. and Sparkes, A.H. (2006). Use of radiographic measurements in distinguishing myasthenia gravis from other causes of canine megaoesophagus. *J. Small Anim. Pract.* 47: 256–263.

Yam, P.S., Shelton, G.D., and Simpson, J.W. (1996). Megaoesophagus secondary to acquired myasthenia gravis. *J. Small Anim. Pract.* 37: 179–183.

6.7. Vestibular Syndrome

Dewey, C.W. and da Costa, R.C. (2015). *Practical Guide to Canine and Feline Neurology*, 3e. Hoboken, NJ: Wiley Blackwell.

Garosi, L.S., Dennis, R., and Penderis, J. (2001). Results of magnetic resonance imaging in dogs with vestibular disorders: 85 cases (1996–1999). *J. Am. Vet. Med. Assoc.* 218: 385–391.

Garosi, L.S., Lowrie, M.L., and Swinbourne, N.F. (2012). Neurological manifestations of ear disease in dogs and cats. *Vet. Clin. North Am. Small Anim. Pract.* 42: 1143–1160.

Jeandel, A., Thibaud, J.L., and Blot, S. (2016). Facial and vestibular neuropathy of unknown origin in 16 dogs. *J. Small Anim. Pract.* 57: 74–78.

Kent, M., Platt, S.R., and Schatzberg, S.J. (2010). The neurology of balance: function and dysfunction of the vestibular system in dogs and cats. *Vet. J.* 185: 247–258.

Lowrie, M. (2012a). Vestibular disease: anatomy, physiology, and clinical signs. *Compend. Contin. Educ. Vet.* 34: E1.

Lowrie, M. (2012b). Vestibular disease: diseases causing vestibular signs. *Compend. Contin. Educ. Vet.* 34: E2.

Marks, S.L., Lipsitz, D., Vernau, K.M. et al. (2011). Reversible encephalopathy secondary to thiamine deficiency in 3 cats ingesting commercial diets. *J. Vet. Intern. Med.* 25: 949–953.

Skelly, B.J. and Franklin, R.J. (2002). Recognition and diagnosis of lysosomal storage diseases in the cat and dog. *J. Vet. Intern. Med.* 16: 133–141.

6.8. Cerebellar Dysfunction

Altay, U.M., Skerritt, G.C., Hilbe, M. et al. (2011). Feline cerebrovascular disease: clinical and histopathologic findings in 16 cats. *J. Am. Anim. Hosp. Assoc.* 47: 89–97.

Bertalan, A., Glass, E.N., Kent, M. et al. (2014). Late-onset cerebellar abiotrophy in a Labrador retriever. *Aust. Vet. J.* 92: 339–342.

Boudreau, C.E. (2018). An update on cerebrovascular disease in dogs and cats. *Vet. Clin. North Am. Small Anim. Pract.* 48: 45–62.

Brown, C.A., Munday, J.S., Mathur, S., and Brown, S.A. (2005). Hypertensive encephalopathy in cats with reduced renal function. *Vet. Pathol.* 42: 642–649.

Cardy, T.J., Lam, R., Peters, L.M. et al. (2017). Successful medical management of a domestic longhair cat with subdural intracranial empyema and multifocal pneumonia. *J. Vet. Emerg. Crit. Care (San Antonio)* 27: 238–242.

Cherubini, G.B., Rusbridge, C., Singh, B.P. et al. (2007). Rostral cerebellar arterial infarct in two cats. *J. Feline Med. Surg.* 9: 246–253.

Chrisman, C.L., Cork, L.C., and Gamble, D.A. (1984). Neuroaxonal dystrophy of Rottweiler dogs. *J. Am. Vet. Med. Assoc.* 184: 464–467.

Cornelis, I., Van Ham, L., Gielen, I. et al. (2019). Clinical presentation, diagnostic findings, prognostic factors, treatment and outcome in dogs with meningoencephalomyelitis of unknown origin: a review. *Vet. J.* 244: 37–44.

Dewey, C.W. and da Costa, R.C. (2015). *Practical Guide to Canine and Feline Neurology*, 3e. Hoboken, NJ: Wiley Blackwell.

Evans, J., Levesque, D., Knowles, K. et al. (2003). Diazepam as a treatment for metronidazole toxicosis in dogs: a retrospective study of 21 cases. *J. Vet. Intern. Med.* 17: 304–310.

Garosi, L., McConnell, J.E., Platt, S.R. et al. (2005). Results of diagnostic investigations and long-term outcome of 33 dogs with brain infarction (2000–2004). *J. Vet. Intern. Med.* 19: 725–731.

Garosi, L., McConnell, J.F., Platt, S.R. et al. (2006). Clinical and topographic magnetic resonance characteristics of suspected brain infarction in 40 dogs. *J. Vet. Intern. Med.* 20: 311–321.

Garosi, L., Dawson, A., Couturier, J. et al. (2010). Necrotizing cerebellitis and cerebellar atrophy caused by Neospora caninum infection: magnetic resonance imaging and clinicopathologic findings in seven dogs. *J. Vet. Intern. Med.* 24: 571–578.

Hahn, K., Rohdin, C., Jagannathan, V. et al. (2015). TECPR2 associated neuroaxonal dystrophy in Spanish water dogs. *PLoS One* 10: e0141824.

Henke, D., Böttcher, P., Doherr, M.G. et al. (2008). Computer-assisted magnetic resonance imaging brain morphometry in American Staffordshire Terriers with cerebellar cortical degeneration. *J. Vet. Intern. Med.* 22: 969–975.

Hoon-Hanks, L.L., McGrath, S., Tyler, K.L. et al. (2018). Metagenomic investigation of idiopathic meningoencephalomyelitis in dogs. *J. Vet. Intern. Med.* 32: 324–330.

Inada, S., Mochizuki, M., Izumo, S. et al. (1996). Study of hereditary cerebellar degeneration in cats. *Am. J. Vet. Res.* 57: 296–301.

Ives, E.J., MacKillop, E., and Olby, N.J. (2018). Saccadic oscillations in 4 dogs and 1 cat. *J. Vet. Intern. Med.* 32: 1392–1396.

Kent, M., Glass, E.N., Haley, A.C. et al. (2014). Ischemic stroke in greyhounds: 21 cases (2007–2013). *J. Am. Vet. Med. Assoc.* 245: 113–117.

Kwiatkowska, M., Pomianowski, A., Adamiak, Z., and Bocheńska, A. (2013). Magnetic resonance imaging and brainstem auditory evoked responses in the diagnosis of cerebellar cortical degeneration in american staffordshire terriers. *Acta Vet. Hung.* 61: 9–18.

de Lahunta, A. (1980). Diseases of the cerebellum. *Vet. Clin. North Am. Small Anim. Pract.* 10: 91–101.

de Lahunta, A. and Averill, D.R. Jr. (1976). Hereditary cerebellar cortical and extrapyramidal nuclear abiotrophy in Kerry Blue Terriers. *J. Am. Vet. Med. Assoc.* 168: 1119–1124.

de Lahunta, A., Glass, E., and Kent, M. (2015). *Veterinary Neuroanatomy and Clinical Neurology*, 4e. St Louis, MO: Elsevier Saunders.

Lowrie, M. and Garosi, L. (2016). Classification of involuntary movements in dogs: tremors and twitches. *Vet. J.* 214: 109–116.

Lowrie, M., De Risio, L., Dennis, R. et al. (2012). Concurrent medical conditions and long-term outcome in dogs with nontraumatic intracranial hemorrhage. *Vet. Radiol. Ultrasound* 53: 381–388.

Lucot, K.L., Dickinson, P.J., Finno, C.J. et al. (2018). A missense mutation in the vacuolar protein sorting 11 (VPS11) gene is associated with neuroaxonal dystrophy in Rottweiler dogs. *G3 (Bethesda)* 8: 2773–2780.

Martin-Vaquero, P., da Costa, R.C., and Daniels, J.B. (2011). Presumptive meningoencephalitis secondary to extension of otitis media/interna caused by Streptococcus equi subspecies zooepidemicus in a cat. *J. Feline Med. Surg.* 13: 606–609.

Mauler, D.A., Van Soens, I., Bhatti, S.F. et al. (2014). Idiopathic generalised tremor syndrome in two cats. *J. Feline Med. Surg.* 16: 378–380.

McConnell, J.F., Garosi, L., and Platt, S.R. (2005). Magnetic resonance imaging findings of presumed cerebellar cerebrovascular accident in twelve dogs. *Vet. Radiol. Ultrasound* 46: 1–10.

Negrin, A., Gaitero, L., and Añor, S. (2009). Presumptive caudal cerebellar artery infarct in a dog: clinical and MRI findings. *J. Small Anim. Pract.* 50: 615–618.

Negrin, A., Taeymans, O.N.J., Spencer, S.E., and Cherubini, G.B. (2018). Presumed caudal cerebellar artery infarction in three cats: neurological signs, MRI findings, and outcome. *Front. Vet. Sci.* 5: 155.

Nibe, K., Kita, C., Morozumi, M. et al. (2007). Clinicopathological features of canine neuroaxonal dystrophy and cerebellar cortical abiotrophy in Papillon and Papillon-related dogs. *J. Vet. Med. Sci.* 69: 1047–1052.

Nibe, K., Nakayama, H., and Uchida, K. (2010). Comparative study of cerebellar degeneration in canine neuroaxonal dystrophy, cerebellar cortical abiotrophy, and neuronal ceroid-lipofuscinosis. *J. Vet. Med. Sci.* 72: 1495–1499.

Olby, N., Blot, S., Thibaud, J.L. et al. (2004). Cerebellar cortical degeneration in adult American Staffordshire Terriers. *J. Vet. Intern. Med.* 18: 201–208.

O'Neill, J., Kent, M., Glass, E.N., and Platt, S.R. (2013). Clinicopathologic and MRI characteristics of presumptive hypertensive encephalopathy in two cats and two dogs. *J. Am. Anim. Hosp. Assoc.* 49: 412–420.

Parzefall, B., Driver, C.J., Benigni, L., and Davies, E. (2014). Magnetic resonance imaging characteristics in four dogs with central nervous system neosporosis. *Vet. Radiol. Ultrasound* 55: 539–546.

Platt, S. and Olby, N. (2013). *BSAVA Manual of Canine and Feline Neurology*, 4e. Gloucester, UK: British Small Animal Veterinary Association.

Platt, S., Hicks, J., and Matiasek, L. (2016). Intracranial intra-arachnoid diverticula and cyst-like abnormalities of the brain. *Vet. Clin. North Am. Small Anim. Pract.* 46: 253–263.

Poncelet, L., Héraud, C., Springinsfeld, M. et al. (2013). Identification of feline panleukopenia virus proteins expressed in Purkinje cell nuclei of cats with cerebellar hypoplasia. *Vet. J.* 196: 381–387.

Sewell, A.C., Haskins, M.E., and Giger, U. (2012). Dried blood spots for the enzymatic diagnosis of lysosomal storage diseases in dogs and cats. *Vet. Clin. Pathol.* 41: 548–557.

Sisó, S., Ferrer, I., and Pumarola, M. (2001). Juvenile neuroaxonal dystrophy in a Rottweiler: accumulation of synaptic proteins in dystrophic axons. *Acta Neuropathol.* 102: 501–504.

Skelly, B.J. and Franklin, R.J. (2002). Recognition and diagnosis of lysosomal storage diseases in the cat and dog. *J. Vet. Intern. Med.* 16: 133–141.

Steinberg, T., Matiasek, K., Brühschwein, A., and Fischer, A. (2007). Imaging diagnosis–intracranial epidermoid cyst in a Doberman Pinscher. *Vet. Radiol. Ultrasound* 48: 250–253.

Stuetzer, B. and Hartmann, K. (2014). Feline parvovirus infection and associated diseases. *Vet. J.* 201: 150–155.

Sturges, B.K., Dickinson, P.J., Kortz, G.D. et al. (2006). Clinical signs, magnetic resonance imaging features, and outcome after surgical and medical treatment of otogenic intracranial infection in 11 cats and 4 dogs. *J. Vet. Intern. Med.* 20: 648–656.

Tauro, A., Beltran, E., Cherubini, G.B. et al. (2018). Metronidazole-induced neurotoxicity in 26 dogs. *Aust. Vet. J.* 96: 495–501.

Thomsen, B., Garosi, L., Skerritt, G. et al. (2016). Neurological signs in 23 dogs with suspected rostral cerebellar ischaemic stroke. *Acta Vet. Scand.* 58: 40.

Urkasemsin, G., Linder, K.E., Bell, J.S. et al. (2010). Hereditary cerebellar degeneration in Scottish terriers. *J. Vet. Intern. Med.* 24: 565–570.

Wagner, S.O., Podell, M., and Fenner, W.R. (1997). Generalized tremors in dogs: 24 cases (1984–1995). *J. Am. Vet. Med. Assoc.* 211: 731–735.

Whittaker, D.E., Drees, R., and Beltran, E.M.R.I. (2018). Clinical characteristics of suspected cerebrovascular accident in nine cats. *J. Feline Med. Surg.* 20: 674–684.

6.9. Neck and/or Spinal Pain

Bathen-Noethen, A., Carlson, R., Menzel, D. et al. (2008). Concentrations of acute-phase proteins in dogs with steroid responsive meningitis-arteritis. *J. Vet. Intern. Med.* 22: 1149–1156.

Brisson, B.A. (2010). Intervertebral disc disease in dogs. *Vet. Clin. North Am. Small Anim. Pract.* 40: 829–858.

Coelho, A.M., Cherubini, G., De Stefani, A. et al. (2019). Serological prevalence of toxoplasmosis and neosporosis in dogs diagnosed with suspected meningoencephalitis in the UK. *J. Small Anim. Pract.* 60: 44–50.

Cummings, K.R., Vilaplana Grosso, F., Moore, G.E. et al. (2018). Objective measurements of the atlantoaxial joint on radiographs performed without flexion can increase the confidence of diagnosis of atlantoaxial instability in toy breed dogs. *Vet. Radiol. Ultrasound* 59: 667–676.

De Strobel, F., Paluš, V., Vettorato, E. et al. (2019). Cervical hyperaesthesia in dogs: an epidemiological retrospective study of 185 cases. *J. Small Anim. Pract.* 60: 404–410.

Girod, M., Allerton, F., Gommeren, K. et al. (2016). Evaluation of the effect of oral omeprazole on canine cerebrospinal fluid production: a pilot study. *Vet. J.* 209: 119–124.

Graham, G.G., Davies, M.J., Day, R.O. et al. (2013). The modern pharmacology of paracetamol: therapeutic actions, mechanism of action, metabolism, toxicity and recent pharmacological findings. *Inflammopharmacology* 21: 201–232.

Hechler, A.C. and Moore, S.A. (2018). Understanding and treating Chiari-like malformation and syringomyelia in dogs. *Top. Companion Anim. Med.* 33: 1–11.

Kiviranta, A.M., Rusbridge, C., Laitinen-Vapaavuori, O. et al. (2017). Syringomyelia and craniocervical junction abnormalities in Chihuahuas. *J. Vet. Intern. Med.* 31: 1771–1781.

Lowrie, M., Penderis, J., McLaughlin, M. et al. (2009). Steroid responsive meningitis-arteritis: a prospective study of potential disease markers, prednisolone treatment, and long-term outcome in 20 dogs (2006–2008). *J. Vet. Intern. Med.* 23: 862–870.

Plessas, I.N., Rusbridge, C., Driver, C.J. et al. (2012). Long-term outcome of Cavalier King Charles spaniel dogs with clinical signs associated with Chiari-like malformation and syringomyelia. *Vet. Rec.* 171: 501.

Rusbridge, C., McFadyen, A.K., and Knower, S.P. (2019). Behavioral and clinical signs of Chiari-like malformation-associated pain and syringomyelia in Cavalier King Charles spaniels. *J. Vet. Intern. Med.* 33: 2138–2150.

Schueler, R.O., White, G., Schueler, R.L. et al. (2018). Canine pancreatic lipase immunoreactivity concentrations associated with intervertebral disc disease in 84 dogs. *J. Small Anim. Pract.* 59: 305–310.

Schulze, S., Refai, M., Deutschland, M. et al. (2018). Prevalence of syringomyelia in clinically unaffected Cavalier King Charles spaniels in Germany (2006–2016). *Tierarztl. Prax. Ausg. K Kleintiere Heimtiere* 46: 157–162.

Slanina, M.C. (2016). Atlantoaxial instability. *Vet. Clin. North Am. Small Anim. Pract.* 46: 265–275.

Tipold, A. and Schatzberg, S.J. (2010). An update on steroid responsive meningitis-arteritis. *J. Small Anim. Pract.* 51: 150–154.

Tipold, A. and Stein, V.M. (2010). Inflammatory diseases of the spine in small animals. *Vet. Clin. North Am. Small Anim. Pract.* 40: 871–879.

Webb, A.A., Taylor, S.M., and Muir, G.D. (2002). Steroid-responsive meningitis-arteritis in dogs with noninfectious, nonerosive, idiopathic, immune-mediated polyarthritis. *J. Vet. Intern. Med.* 16: 269–273.

6.10. Paresis, Paralysis, and Proprioceptive Ataxia

Bennaim, M., Porato, M., Jarleton, A. et al. (2017). Preliminary evaluation of the effects of photobiomodulation therapy and physical rehabilitation on early postoperative recovery of dogs undergoing hemilaminectomy for treatment of thoracolumbar intervertebral disk disease. *Am. J. Vet. Res.* 78 (2): 195–206.

Bergknut, N., Egenvall, A., Hagman, R. et al. (2012). Incidence of intervertebral disk degeneration–related diseases and associated mortality rates in dogs. *J. Am. Vet. Med. Assoc.* 240 (11): 1300–1309.

Brown, E.A., Dickinson, P.J., Mansour, T. et al. (2017). FGF4 retrogene on CFA12 is responsible for chondrodystrophy and intervertebral disc disease in dogs. *Proc. Natl. Acad. Sci. U. S. A.* 114 (43): 11476–11481.

Bubenik, L. and Hosgood, G. (2008). Urinary tract infection in dogs with thoracolumbar intervertebral disc herniation and urinary tract dysfunction managed by manual expression, indwelling catheterization or intermittent catheterization. *Vet. Surg.* 37 (8): 791–800.

Bubenik, L.J., Hosgood, G.L., Waldron, D.R. et al. (2007). Frequency of urinary tract infection in catheterized dogs and comparison of bacterial culture and susceptibility testing results for catheterized and noncatheterized dogs with urinary tract infections. *J. Am. Vet. Med. Assoc.* 231 (6): 893–899.

Cardy, T.J., De Decker, S., Kenny, P.J., and Volk, H.A. (2015). Clinical reasoning in canine spinal disease: what combination of clinical information is useful? *Vet. Rec.* 177 (7): 171.

Crawford, A.H. and De Decker, S. (2017). Clinical presentation and outcome of dogs treated medically or surgically for thoracolumbar intervertebral disc protrusion. *Vet. Rec.* 180 (23): 569.

Da Costa, R.C. and Parent, J.M. (2007). One-year clinical and magnetic resonance imaging follow-up of Doberman Pinschers with cervical spondylomyelopathy treated medically or surgically. *J. Am. Vet. Med. Assoc.* 231 (2): 243–250.

De Decker, S., Bhatti, S.F., Duchateau, L. et al. (2009). Clinical evaluation of 51 dogs treated conservatively for disc-associated wobbler syndrome. *J. Small Anim. Pract.* 50 (3): 136–142.

De Risio, L.A. (2015). Review of fibrocartilaginous embolic myelopathy and different types of peracute non-compressive intervertebral disk extrusions in dogs and cats. *Front. Vet. Sci.* 2: 24.

De Risio, L., Adams, V., Dennis, R. et al. (2008). Association of clinical and magnetic resonance imaging findings with outcome in dogs suspected to have ischemic myelopathy: 50 cases (2000–2006). *J. Am. Vet. Med. Assoc.* 233: 129–135.

Doran, C., Platt, S.R., and Garosi, L.S. (2019). Long-term imaging follow-up of a conservatively managed presumptive osseous cervical stenotic myelopathy in a puppy. *J. Small Anim. Pract.* 60: 198.

Drum, M.G. (2010). Physical rehabilitation of the canine neurologic patient. *Vet. Clin. North Am. Small Anim. Pract.* 40 (1): 181–193.

Fenn, J., Drees, R., Volk, H.A., and De Decker, S. (2016). Comparison of clinical signs and outcomes between dogs with presumptive ischemic myelopathy and dogs with acute noncompressive nucleus pulposus extrusion. *J. Am. Vet. Med. Assoc.* 249 (7): 767–775.

Forterre, F., Konar, M., Tomek, A. et al. (2008). Accuracy of the withdrawal reflex for localization of the site of cervical disk herniation in dogs: 35 cases (2004–2007). *J. Am. Vet. Med. Assoc.* 232: 559–563.

Freeman, P. and Jeffery, N.D. (2017). Re-opening the window on fenestration as a treatment for acute thoracolumbar intervertebral disc herniation in dogs. *J. Small Anim. Pract.* 58 (4): 199–204.

Full, A.M., Heller, H.L., and Mercier, M. (2016). Prevalence, clinical presentation, prognosis, and outcome of 17 dogs with spinal shock and acute thoracolumbar spinal cord disease. *J. Vet. Emerg. Crit. Care (San Antonio)* 26 (3): 412–418.

Gonçalves, R., Penderis, J., Chang, Y.P. et al. (2008). Clinical and neurological characteristics of aortic thromboembolism in dogs. *J. Small Anim. Pract.* 49 (4): 178–184.

Hansen, T., Smolders, L.A., Tryfonidou, M.A. et al. (2017). The myth of fibroid degeneration in the canine intervertebral disc: a histopathological comparison of intervertebral disc degeneration in chondrodystrophic and nonchondrodystrophic dogs. *Vet. Pathol.* 54 (6): 945–952.

Hayashi, A.M., Matera, J.M., and Fonseca Pinto, A.C. (2007). Evaluation of electroacupuncture treatment for thoracolumbar intervertebral disk disease in dogs. *J. Am. Vet. Med. Assoc.* 231 (6): 913–918.

Janssens, L., Beosier, Y., and Daems, R. (2009). Lumbosacral degenerative stenosis in the dog. The results of epidural infiltration with methylprednisolone acetate: a retrospective study. *Vet. Comp. Orthop. Traumatol.* 22 (6): 486–491.

Jeffery, N.D. and Freeman, P.M. (2018). The role of fenestration in management of Type I thoracolumbar disk degeneration. *Vet. Clin. North Am. Small Anim. Pract.* 48 (1): 187–200.

Jeffery, N.D., Barker, A.K., Hu, H.Z. et al. (2016). Factors associated with recovery from paraplegia in dogs with loss of pain perception in the pelvic limbs following intervertebral disk herniation. *J. Am. Vet. Med. Assoc.* 248 (4): 386–394.

Jeffery, N.D., Harcourt-Brown, T.R., Barker, A.K. et al. (2018). Choices and decisions in decompressive surgery for thoracolumbar intervertebral disk herniation. *Vet. Clin. North Am. Small Anim. Pract.* 48 (1): 169–186.

Joaquim, J.G., Luna, S.P., Brondani, J.T. et al. (2010). Comparison of decompressive surgery, electroacupuncture, and decompressive surgery followed by electroacupuncture for the treatment of dogs with intervertebral disk disease with long-standing severe neurologic deficits. *J. Am. Vet. Med. Assoc.* 236 (11): 1225–1229.

Kathmann, I., Cizinauskas, S., Doherr, M.G. et al. (2006). Daily controlled physiotherapy increases survival time in dogs with suspected degenerative myelopathy. *J. Vet. Intern. Med.* 20: 927–932.

Levine, J.M., Levine, G.J., Johnson, S.I. et al. (2007). Evaluation of the success of medical management for presumptive thoracolumbar intervertebral disk herniation in dogs. *Vet. Surg.* 36 (5): 482–491.

Mari, L., Behr, S., Shea, A. et al. (2017). Outcome comparison in dogs with a presumptive diagnosis of thoracolumbar fibrocartilaginous embolic myelopathy and acute non-compressive nucleus pulposus extrusion. *Vet. Rec.* 181 (11): 293.

Marschall, J., Carpenter, C.R., Fowler, S. et al. (2013). Antibiotic prophylaxis for urinary tract infections after removal of urinary catheter: meta-analysis. *BMJ* f3147: 346.

Mauler, D.A., De Decker, S., De Risio, L. et al. (2014). Signalment, clinical presentation, and diagnostic findings in 122 dogs with spinal arachnoid diverticula. *J. Vet. Intern. Med.* 28 (1): 175–181.

Nessler, J., Flieshardt, C., Tünsmeyer, J. et al. (2018). Comparison of surgical and conservative treatment of hydrated nucleus pulposus extrusion in dogs. *J. Vet. Intern. Med.* 32 (6): 1989–1995.

Olby, N.J., MacKillop, E., Cerda-Gonzalez, S. et al. (2010). Prevalence of urinary tract infection in dogs after surgery for thoracolumbar intervertebral disc extrusion. *J. Vet. Intern. Med.* 24 (5): 1106–1111.

Olby, N.J., Lim, J.H., Wagner, N. et al. (2019). Time course and prognostic value of serum GFAP, pNFH, and S100β concentrations in dogs with complete spinal cord injury because of intervertebral disc extrusion. *J. Vet. Intern. Med.* 33 (2): 726–734.

Palamara, J.D., Bonczynski, J.J., Berg, J.M. et al. (2016). Perioperative cefovecin to reduce the incidence of urinary tract infection in dogs undergoing hemilaminectomy. *J. Am. Anim. Hosp. Assoc.* 52 (5): 297–304.

Skytte, D. and Schmökel, H. (2018). Relationship of preoperative neurologic score with intervals to regaining micturition and ambulation following surgical treatment of thoracolumbar disk herniation in dogs. *J. Am. Vet. Med. Assoc.* 253: 196–200.

Sullivan, L.A., Campbell, V.L., and Onuma, S.C. (2010). Evaluation of open versus closed urine collection systems and development of nosocomial bacteriuria in dogs. *J. Am. Vet. Med. Assoc.* 237 (2): 187–190.

Zidan, N., Sims, C., Fenn, J. et al. (2018). A randomized, blinded, prospective clinical trial of postoperative rehabilitation in dogs after surgical decompression of acute thoracolumbar intervertebral disc herniation. J. Vet. Intern. Med. 32 (3) : 1133–1144.

6.11. Monoparesis and Lameness

Griffiths, I.R., Duncan, I.D., and Lawson, D.D. (1974). Avulsion of the brachial plexus–2. Clinical aspects. *J. Small Anim. Pract.* 15: 177–183.

Janssens, L., Beosier, Y., and Daems, R. (2009). Lumbosacral degenerative stenosis in the dog. The results of epidural infiltration with methylprednisolone acetate: a retrospective study. *Vet. Comp. Orthop. Traumatol.* 22: 486–491.

Lacassagne, K., Hearon, K., Berg, J. et al. (2018). Canine spinal meningiomas and nerve sheath tumours in 34 dogs (2008–2016): distribution and long-term outcome based upon histopathology and treatment modality. *Vet. Comp. Oncol.* 16: 344–351.

Ródenas, S., Summers, B.A., Saveraid, T. et al. (2013). Chronic hypertrophic ganglioneuritis mimicking spinal nerve neoplasia: clinical, imaging, pathologic findings, and outcome after surgical treatment. *Vet. Surg.* 42: 91–98.

Van Stee, L., Boston, S., Teske, E. et al. (2017). Compartmental resection of peripheral nerve tumours with limb preservation in 16 dogs (1995–2011). *Vet. J.* 226: 40–45.

6.12. Neuromuscular Weakness

Aleman, M., Dickinson, P.J., Williams, D.C. et al. (2014). Electrophysiologic confirmation of heterogenous motor polyneuropathy in young cats. *J. Vet. Intern. Med.* 28: 1789–1798.

Añor, S. (2014). Acute lower motor neuron tetraparesis. *Vet. Clin. North Am. Small Anim. Pract.* 44: 1201–1222.

Bensfield, A.C., Evans, J., Pesayco, J.P. et al. (2011). Recurrent demyelination and remyelination in 37 young Bengal cats with polyneuropathy. *J. Vet. Intern. Med.* 25: 882–889.

Bexfield, N.H., Watson, P.J., and Herrtage, M.E. (2006). Management of myasthenia gravis using cyclosporine in 2 dogs. *J. Vet. Intern. Med.* 20: 1487–1490.

Dewey, C.W. and da Costa, R.C. (2015). *Practical Guide to Canine and Feline Neurology*, 3e. Hoboken, NJ: Wiley Blackwell.

Dewey, C.W., Bailey, C.S., Shelton, G.D. et al. (1997). Clinical forms of acquired myasthenia gravis in dogs: 25 cases (1988–1995). *J. Vet. Intern. Med.* 11: 50–57.

Dewey, C.W., Coates, J.R., Ducoté, J.M. et al. (1999). Azathioprine therapy for acquired myasthenia gravis in five dogs. *J. Am. Anim. Hosp. Assoc.* 35: 396–402.

Evans, J., Levesque, D., and Shelton, G.D. (2004). Canine inflammatory myopathies: a clinicopathologic review of 200 cases. *J. Vet. Intern. Med.* 18: 679–691.

Farrow, B.R., Murrell, W.G., Revington, M.L. et al. (1983). Type C botulism in young dogs. *Aust. Vet. J.* 60: 374–377.

Giannuzzi, A.P., Ricciardi, M., De Simone, A., and Gernone, F. (2017). Neurological manifestations in dogs naturally infected by *Leishmania infantum*: descriptions of 10 cases and a review of the literature. *J. Small Anim. Pract.* 58: 125–138.

Glass, E.N. and Kent, M. (2002). The clinical examination for neuromuscular disease. *Vet. Clin. North Am. Small Anim. Pract.* 32: 1–29.

Hague, D.W., Humphries, H.D., Mitchell, M.A., and S.G.D. (2015). Risk factors and outcomes in cats with acquired myasthenia gravis (2001–2012). *J. Vet. Intern. Med.* 29: 1307–1312.

Hirschvogel, K., Jurina, K., Steinberg, T.A. et al. (2012). Clinical course of acute canine polyra-diculoneuritis following treatment with human IV immunoglobulin. *J. Am. Anim. Hosp. Assoc.* 48: 299–309.

Holt, N., Murray, M., Cuddon, P.A., and Lappin, M.R. (2011). Seroprevalence of various infectious agents in dogs with suspected acute canine polyradiculoneuritis. *J. Vet. Intern. Med.* 25: 261–266.

Khorzad, R., Whelan, M., Sisson, A., and Shelton, G.D. (2011). Myasthenia gravis in dogs with an emphasis on treatment and critical care management. *J. Vet. Emerg. Crit. Care (San Antonio)* 21: 193–208.

King, L.G. and Vite, C.H. (1998). Acute fulminating myasthenia gravis in five dogs. *J. Am. Vet. Med. Assoc.* 212: 830–834.

de Lahunta, A., Glass, E., and Kent, M. (2015). *Veterinary Neuroanatomy and Clinical Neurology*, 4e. St Louis, MO: Elsevier Saunders.

Laws, E.J., Harcourt-Brown, T.R., Granger, N., and Rose, J.H. (2017). An exploratory study into factors influencing development of acute canine polyradiculoneuritis in the UK. *J. Small Anim. Pract.* 58: 437–443.

Platt, S. and Olby, N. (2013). *BSAVA Manual of Canine and Feline Neurology*, 4e. Gloucester, UK: British Small Animal Veterinary Association.

Podell, M. (2002). Inflammatory myopathies. *Vet. Clin. North Am. Small Anim. Pract.* 32: 147–167.

Robat, C.S., Cesario, L., Gaeta, R. et al. (2013). Clinical features, treatment options, and outcome in dogs with thymoma: 116 cases (1999–2010). *J. Am. Vet. Med. Assoc.* 243: 1448–1454.

Rupp, A., Galban-Horcajo, F., Bianchi, E. et al. (2013). Anti-GM2 ganglioside antibodies are a biomarker for acute canine polyradiculoneuritis. *J. Peripher. Nerv. Syst.* 18: 75–88.

Shelton, G.D. (2002). Myasthenia gravis and disorders of neuromuscular transmission. *Vet. Clin. North Am. Small Anim. Pract.* 32: 189–206.

Shelton, G.D. (2010). Routine and specialized laboratory testing for the diagnosis of neuromuscular diseases in dogs and cats. *Vet. Clin. Pathol.* 39: 278–295.

Shelton, G.D., Schule, A., and Kass, P.H. (1997). Risk factors for acquired myasthenia gravis in dogs: 1,154 cases (1991–1995). *J. Am. Vet. Med. Assoc.* 211: 1428–1431.

Shelton, G.D., Skeie, G.O., Kass, P.H., and Aarli, J.A. (2001). Titin and ryanodine receptor autoantibodies in dogs with thymoma and late-onset myasthenia gravis. *Vet. Immunol. Immunopathol.* 78: 97–105.

Tauro, A., Addicott, D., Foale, R.D. et al. (2015). Clinical features of idiopathic inflammatory polymyopathy in the Hungarian Vizsla. *BMC Vet. Res.* 11: 97.

Chapter 7 Neurological Emergencies

Edward Ives and Paul M. Freeman

This chapter will summarise a logical approach to the following emergency presentations, with a focus on management in general practice:

- head trauma and traumatic brain injury (TBI)
- status epilepticus and acute repetitive seizures
- acute spinal cord injury.

Having confidence in how to approach these cases is vital, as many animals may be unfit to travel to a referral centre at the time of presentation and the initial management is often most important to optimise the prognosis. However, this also means that such cases can be incredibly rewarding for vets and nurses to manage in general practice. As for many aspects of veterinary medicine, a 'back-to-basics' approach is recommended, and the focus should be on life-threatening injuries and systemic stabilisation before considering further investigations or complex treatments. This is to ensure that the injured brain or spinal cord is provided with adequate perfusion of oxygenated blood at all times.

7.1 Head Trauma in Dogs and Cats

Edward Ives

Head trauma is a relatively common presentation in general practice, with the most frequently reported causes including road traffic accidents, bites, kicks, and falls. Fortunately, many animals will only require basic supportive care together with

---

A Practical Approach to Neurology for the Small Animal Practitioner, First Edition. Paul M. Freeman and Edward Ives.
© 2020 John Wiley & Sons Ltd. Published 2020 by John Wiley & Sons Ltd.
Companion Website: www.wiley.com/go/freeman/neurology

management of superficial wounds, and ocular, jaw, or dental injuries. However, head trauma may also result in potentially fatal, structural or physiological disruption of the brain, termed traumatic brain injury (TBI). Early recognition and management of TBI is vital to give the best chance of a successful outcome. Affected animals may appear severely affected at the time of initial presentation and it is easy to assume that the prognosis will be poor. However, with appropriate stabilisation and supportive care many animals will show a remarkable ability to compensate for even severe TBI and can recover to have a good quality of life.

Head trauma can result in two forms of brain injury.

1. Primary injury
   This is the direct physical disruption of the brain and its associated tissues that occurs at the time of trauma. Examples of primary injury include:
   • Contusion or laceration of the brain parenchyma.
   • Skull fractures – skull fractures are commonly observed following head trauma but are not always associated with TBI. This is dependent on the region of the skull affected and the extent of skull fragment displacement.
   • Rupture of intracranial blood vessels resulting in haemorrhage and haematoma formation.
   Expanding haematomas or depressed skull fractures that are compressing the brain parenchyma may benefit from surgical management. However, in the majority of cases the primary brain injury cannot be prevented or directly treated. If this injury has not resulted in death at the time of trauma, then its main significance in terms of clinical management is in the initiation of a complex cascade of biochemical processes, termed 'secondary injury'.

2. Secondary injury
   Secondary injury occurs over minutes to days following primary injury and has the potential to result in a catastrophic, expanding focus of tissue damage and cell death. Therefore, the prevention and treatment of secondary injury forms a vital part of TBI management.

The main drivers of secondary injury include:

• Release of excitatory neurotransmitters (e.g. glutamate) from damaged regions of the brain, resulting in an increased cerebral metabolic activity, energy depletion, and failure of ion homeostasis via ATP-dependent cell membrane ion pumps. The subsequent influx of positively charged ions, such as sodium and calcium, results in a vicious cycle of further depolarisation, cellular swelling (cytotoxic oedema), activation of destructive intracellular enzymes, and programmed cell death (apoptosis).
• Local production of reactive oxygen species (ROS) secondary to reduced tissue perfusion, increased iron levels following haemorrhage, and local tissue acidosis all contribute towards further damage to the lipid-rich neuronal cell membranes.

- Release of inflammatory cytokines from injured tissues results in disruption to the blood–brain barrier, local nitric oxide production, chemotaxis, and accumulation of inflammatory cells. Nitric oxide is a potent vasodilator and the subsequent increase in intracranial blood volume can perpetuate any elevation of intracranial pressure (ICP).

Head trauma is frequently accompanied by systemic changes such as hypotension, hypoxaemia, hypercapnia, and derangements in electrolyte and glucose levels. These changes will exacerbate secondary injury by compromising cerebral perfusion and oxygen delivery, thus further driving ischaemia, excitotoxicity, energy depletion, and cell death. It is for this reason that systemic stabilisation forms such an important part of TBI management in humans and animals.

7.1.1 Intracranial Pressure and Cerebral Perfusion

The cranial vault can be thought of as a closed box constrained by a rigid skull. The contents of this box include three basic compartments:

- brain parenchyma – c.80% of intracranial volume
- blood – c.10% of intracranial volume, with venous blood being the majority
- cerebrospinal fluid (CSF) – c.10% of intracranial volume.

There is a constant low pressure of 5–12 mmHg within this box that is exerted by the tissues and fluids contained within it. This is the intracranial pressure (ICP), against which the mean arterial blood pressure (MABP) must pump to provide the brain with an adequate supply of oxygen and nutrients. Thus, the cerebral perfusion pressure (CPP) can be defined as the MABP minus the ICP.

It is important that the ICP is kept tightly regulated at all times to ensure that there is an optimal environment for the brain to function. According to the principles of intracranial compliance and the Monrie–Kellie doctrine, an increase in the volume of one compartment (e.g. brain, blood, or CSF), or the appearance of a new substance within this closed box (e.g. tumour, haematoma, skull fragment), must be met by an equal and opposite decrease in the volume of another compartment. This is to ensure that the ICP remains constant and usually involves compensatory shunting of venous blood or CSF out of the intracranial vault. If this compensatory capacity is overwhelmed, then even a small additional increase in volume will result in an exponentially large increase in ICP. The oedema, haemorrhage, and other changes that accompany primary and secondary brain injury can rapidly overwhelm this compensatory mechanism. If the ICP rises to over 20 mmHg then this can result in death secondary to reduced cerebral perfusion, brain herniation, brainstem compression, and cardiorespiratory failure.

Regulatory mechanisms also exist to ensure adequate cerebral blood flow (CBF) in the face of fluctuations in MABP and cerebral oxygen and carbon dioxide levels.

1. Pressure autoregulation

   In the normal animal, the CBF is kept constant over a wide range of MABPs (50–150 mmHg) by altering the cerebral vascular resistance; vasoconstriction in response to increased CPP and vasodilation in response to reduced CPP. This regulatory mechanism can fail following TBI, meaning that CBF changes in a more linear relationship with MABP. This can result in cerebral ischaemia if the CBF becomes inadequate to maintain cerebral oxygen demand in the face of systemic hypotension.

2. Chemical autoregulation

   The processes of chemical autoregulation alter the cerebral vascular resistance to optimise CBF in response to changes in cerebral oxygen and carbon dioxide levels.
   - Cerebral arterial vasodilation to increase CBF in response to hypercapnia, hypoxaemia, increases in cerebral metabolic rate, or the release of vasoactive substances (e.g. nitric oxide). CBF increases in a linear relationship with $p_a(CO_2)$ levels between 20 and 80 mmHg.
   - Cerebral arterial vasoconstriction in response to hypocapnia.

As previously discussed, systemic derangements are commonly observed in trauma cases, including hypoxaemia and hypercapnia secondary to thoracic injuries and hypoventilation. In contrast to pressure autoregulation, chemical autoregulation may be maintained following TBI and this can be counterproductive as the systemic derangements will stimulate cerebral arterial vasodilation. This will result in an increased intracranial blood volume which has the potential to exacerbate ICP elevation.

Whilst these processes may appear complex, their primary significance is to reinforce the vital importance of systemic stabilisation and the maintenance of appropriate blood pressure and oxygen and carbon dioxide levels in animals following TBI.

7.1.2 Management of Head Trauma in Dogs and Cats

A logical approach to any case presenting with a history of head trauma, or a clinical examination compatible with it, can be divided into the following considerations:

1. Triage and general assessment
2. Systemic stabilisation, including seizure management if applicable
3. Neurological assessment
4. Management of increased ICP
5. Analgesia and sedation
6. Supportive care and nutrition

Successful management of a trauma case often requires multiple tasks being performed at the same time. Recruiting help from veterinary nurses and other practitioners as soon as possible after presentation means that a stressful situation can appear more manageable and ensures optimal care of the animal.

1. Triage and general assessment

The initial assessment of any trauma patient should focus on the 'ABC' of emergency care and identification of any life-threatening injuries before a neurological examination is performed.

Airway: Endotracheal intubation or tracheostomy may be required if the airway is not patent.

Breathing: Endotracheal intubation and manual or mechanical ventilation is required if the animal presents with apnoea. Assessment and monitoring of respiratory function should include:

- thoracic auscultation
- respiratory rate and effort
- saturation of peripheral oxygen [$Sp(O_2)$] by pulse oximetry
- end-tidal carbon dioxide [$Et(CO_2)$] by capnography.

Thoracic focused assessment with sonography for trauma (TFAST) can be performed to assess for pneumothorax, pleural effusion (e.g. haemothorax), or pulmonary contusion. Systemic stabilisation should be prioritised over diagnostic imaging unless there is a clinical suspicion of pneumothorax or significant pleural effusion that may require emergency drainage to ensure adequate ventilation.

Circulation: Animals will often present in hypovolaemic shock following trauma. It is essential that this is recognised and addressed as soon as possible to establish normovolaemia, restore cerebral perfusion, and minimise the extent of secondary brain injury. Basic assessment should include:

- pulse rate and peripheral pulse quality
- mucous membrane colour and capillary refill time
- blood pressure
- electrocardiography (ECG) – thoracic trauma concurrent with head trauma may result in traumatic myocarditis and subsequent cardiac arrhythmia.

Readers are referred to the many excellent texts on veterinary emergency and critical care for a more in-depth discussion on triage of a trauma patient and methods of cardiopulmonary resuscitation.

Head trauma may be accompanied by injury to other body regions and the initial assessment should include identification of both life-threatening injuries and those that are likely to require further treatment (e.g. long bone fractures). This is very important so that the owner can be informed regarding the potential long-term prognosis, including anticipated surgeries that may be required and their associated costs.

- Assessment for sites of external haemorrhage or wounds requiring cleaning and dressing.
- Limb palpation to assess for fractures – open fractures may require emergency management to minimise the risk of infection and fixation failure. Closed fractures do not usually require urgent fixation and can be initially managed using support dressings.
- Abdominal palpation for body wall rupture and bladder integrity.

Thoracic radiography, abdominal radiography, abdominal focused assessment with sonography for trauma (AFAST), TFAST, and/or whole body computed tomography (CT) can be performed following systemic stabilisation to further assess for concurrent injuries to other body regions.

2. Systemic stabilisation and seizure management
a. Seizure management
If an animal presents in a state of generalised seizure activity, then this should be managed as a priority in order to minimise the potential for exacerbating ICP elevation (Box 7.1). The approach to seizure management following head trauma is the same as for any animal presenting in status epilepticus and is summarised in Section 7.2 'Status Epilepticus and Acute Repetitive Seizures'. It is important to note that systemic stabilisation should always be continued between drug doses whilst attempts are made to control the seizure activity.

Box 7.1 Post-traumatic Epilepsy

Seizures following head injury can be classified as either early (<7 days) or late (>7 days). If an animal presents in a state of generalised seizure activity or suffers a seizure at any point during management of TBI, then stopping the seizure is a priority to avoid the detrimental effects on the brain and other organs. The prophylactic use of antiepileptic medications before potential seizure development remains controversial in human medicine and has not been shown to reduce the incidence of seizures occurring more than 7 days after injury. It is currently not recommended to start antiepileptic medications in every animal with known head trauma, and consideration should also be made to the potential cardiorespiratory effects associated with their use. However, owners should be warned that an estimated 6–10% of dogs suffering head trauma may develop seizures in later life, a condition termed post-traumatic epilepsy (Friedenburg et al. 2012; Steinmetz et al. 2013).

---

b. Systemic stabilisation

Systemic stabilisation is the most important factor determining the outcome following TBI in humans and animals, with both hypoxaemia and hypovolaemia strongly correlated with elevated ICP and increased mortality in human patients. The focus of stabilisation is to establish adequate oxygenation, ventilation, and normovolaemia.

i. Oxygenation

Oxygen delivery to the brain is vital to prevent cerebral ischaemia and to mitigate secondary brain injury. The mortality rate in humans with documented hypoxia after TBI is twice that of patients without hypoxia. Oxygen should be delivered by flow-by, with or without a mask. Nasal oxygen prongs or cannulas should be used with care as they may stimulate sneezing, which can further increase ICP. The use of an oxygen cage is not advised as their use would preclude the frequent monitoring required in these cases. As previously mentioned, intubation may be required in apnoeic or comatose animals.

Goals for oxygenation are:

- normal mucous membrane colour, respiratory rate, and pattern
- $Sp(O_2)$ of >95% (reflecting a $p_a(O_2)$ of >80 mmHg)
- $p_a(O_2)$ of >80–90 mmHg.

ii. Ventilation

Adequate ventilation is required for both oxygenation of the blood and carbon dioxide exchange. The $p_a(CO_2)$ is a potent regulator of CBF, with hypercapnia resulting in cerebral arterial vasodilation, increased cerebral blood volume, and possible exacerbation of ICP elevation. Conversely, hypocapnia results in cerebral arterial vasoconstriction, reduced CBF, and the potential for cerebral ischaemia. Airway obstruction, thoracic injury or pain, damage to the brainstem respiratory centres, or the cardiorespiratory depressive effects of sedative and antiepileptic medications may all contribute towards hypoventilation in trauma cases. The goal of ventilation in these cases (whether spontaneous, manual, or mechanical) is to maintain a normal $p_a(CO_2)$ level of 35–40 mmHg. If arterial blood gas analysis is not available, then venous CO_2 levels or $Et(CO_2)$ levels can be monitored; venous CO_2 is usually around 5 mmHg higher than $p_a(CO_2)$, and $Et(CO_2)$ tends to underestimate the actual $p_a(CO_2)$ level.

Deliberate hyperventilation in an attempt to reduce the ICP by lowering the $p_a(CO_2)$ and inducing cerebral arterial vasoconstriction has been suggested in both humans and animals following TBI. However, this is not currently recommended due to the risk of exacerbating cellular ischaemia and it is advised that the $p_a(CO_2)$ level is maintained above 35 mmHg in these cases.

iii. Achieve intravenous access

Intravenous access by placement of one or more wide-bore intravenous cannulas is essential to allow fluid resuscitation and administration of medications.

iv. Establish a minimum database

A reasonable minimum database would comprise a packed cell volume (PCV), total protein (TP), blood glucose, urea, electrolyte levels, and urine specific gravity. Blood can be collected at the time of intravenous catheter placement. Sampling from the jugular veins should be avoided if possible, as jugular occlusion could reduce venous drainage from the head and elevate ICP.

v. Fluid therapy

The goal of fluid therapy is the rapid restoration of circulating fluid volume to ensure an adequate CBF and oxygen delivery to vital organs. The benefits obtained by restoration of cerebral perfusion are widely regarded to outweigh the potential risks of exacerbating cerebral oedema by fluid administration; a 150% increase in mortality has been reported for human TBI patients with a systolic blood pressure <90 mmHg (Chestnut et al. 1993).

The choice of fluid to use following head trauma remains controversial and will also depend upon availability in general practice. However, regardless of the fluid used, vital parameters should be assessed regularly and the fluids titrated to avoid volume overload. The goal should be to achieve a systolic blood pressure of 100–120 mmHg.

- *Isotonic crystalloids* – Boluses of 15–20 ml/kg (dog) or 10–15 ml/kg (cat) of 0.9% sodium chloride until there is normalisation of the heart rate, pulse quality, capillary refill time, mucous membrane colour, and blood pressure (MABP 80–100 mmHg).
- *Hypertonic saline* (7.5% sodium chloride) – Smaller volumes of this hypertonic solution may be used to produce a rapid rise in blood osmolarity, drawing fluid into the circulation from the interstitial and intracellular compartments. This volume-expanding effect occurs within minutes and lasts for 15–75 minutes before redistribution to other fluid compartments occurs. The recommended dose is 4 ml/kg of 7.5% sodium chloride administered over 3–5 minutes. The administration of isotonic crystalloids following the use of hypertonic saline is essential to prevent tissue dehydration, provide maintenance fluid requirements, and correct for on-going losses.
- *Colloids* – It has been suggested that colloids may act synergistically with hypertonic solutions for restoring blood volume, and that co-administration prolongs the volume-expanding effects. However, a Cochrane database systematic review failed to show a benefit of colloids over crystalloids for fluid resuscitation in critically ill humans, including those with TBI (Lewis et al. 2018). The availability of colloids in veterinary general practice may also limit their use in

animals and hypertonic saline has other potential benefits in the management of ICP elevation following head trauma, as discussed below.

vi. Positioning
To aid venous drainage from the head and avoid increases in cerebral blood volume that could exacerbate raised ICP, the animal's head should be midline and elevated by 10–30°. A tilted, rigid board can be useful as it avoids neck kinking and potential jugular compression. Jugular blood sampling, jugular catheter placement, and constrictive collars or neck dressings should also be avoided in these cases.

3. Neurological assessment
Neurological assessment should ideally be performed once normotension, appropriate oxygenation, and ventilation are achieved. Many animals may appear severely affected when they present in hypotensive shock, but the level of mentation and neurological function will be significantly improved following systemic stabilisation and fluid resuscitation. The potential influence of analgesic or sedative medications on the interpretation of the neurological examination should also be considered, but never at the expense of leaving an animal in discomfort. Frequent reassessment and recording of trends are vital to guide the response to treatment and potential prognosis. Repeat assessment is recommended every 30–60 minutes until the animal appears stable to ensure prompt recognition of animals that are deteriorating in spite of treatment.

The use of a scoring system allows for a more objective assessment of neurologic dysfunction, aids in the consistency of monitoring clinical progression, and assists in case handover between the staff responsible for animal care. The use of two different scoring systems has been reported for head trauma in veterinary medicine:

a. Modified Glasgow Coma Scale (MGCS)
b. Animal trauma triage (ATT) score.

a. Modified Glasgow Coma Scale (MGCS)
The MGCS focuses on assessment of three broad categories of neurologic function: level of consciousness, voluntary motor activity, and brainstem reflexes (Figure 7.1). Each category is graded from 1 to 6 to give a total score from 3 (most severely affected) to 18 (normal). From a neuroanatomical perspective, changes in this score broadly reflect alterations in brainstem and diffuse cerebrocortical function. As the ICP rises, herniation of the forebrain underneath the tentorium cerebelli and/or herniation of the cerebellum through the foramen magnum can result in progressive compression of the brainstem. Direct trauma to the brainstem, bilateral or global cerebral abnormalities, and intraparenchymal haemorrhage can also result in loss of neurologic functions and a lower MGCS.

	Score
Motor activity	
Normal gait and spinal reflexes	6
Hemiparesis, tetraparesis, or decerebrate activity	5
Recumbent, intermittent extensor rigidity	4
Recumbent, constant extensor rigidity	3
Recumbent, constant extensor rigidity with opisthotonus	2
Recumbent, hypotonia, depressed or absent spinal reflexes	1
Brainstem reflexes	
Normal PLR and oculocephalic (vestibulo-ocular) reflexes	6
Slow PLR and normal to reduced oculocephalic (vestibulo-ocular) reflexes	5
Bilateral unresponsive miosis with normal to reduced oculocephalic (vestibulo-ocular) reflexes	4
Pinpoint pupils with reduced to absent oculocephalic (vestibulo-ocular) reflexes	3
Unilateral, unresponsive mydriasis with reduced/absent oculocephalic (vestibulo-ocular) reflexes	2
Bilateral unresponsive mydriasis with reduced/absent oculocephalic (vestibulo-ocular) reflexes	1
Level of consciousness	
Occasional periods of alertness and responsive to environment	6
Depression or delirium, capable of responding but response may be inappropriate	5
Semi-comatose, responsive to visual stimuli	4
Semi-comatose, responsive to auditory stimuli	3
Semi-comatose, responsive only to repeated noxious stimuli	2
Comatose, unresponsive to repeated noxious stimuli	1

Figure 7.1 The modified Glasgow Coma Scale (MGCS).

A recent study examined the MGCS as a predictor of mortality outcome (death or euthanasia) in over 3500 injured dogs (Ash et al. 2018). The MGCS showed a good performance for trauma cases as a whole, and particularly for head trauma cases. A previous study also demonstrated that survival to 48 hours from head trauma was correlated with MGCS on admission, with a score of 8 approximating a 50% chance of survival (Platt et al. 2001). This study did not look at survival beyond 48 hours or the quality of life/functional outcome of animals that did survive. Until further studies are performed, the MGCS may be better used to monitor clinical progression rather than to accurately guide prognosis; however, animals presenting in a coma with unresponsive pupils have a guarded prognosis. Limitations of the MGCS that need to be considered are that it remains a subjective scoring system that is ordinal and not linear. This means that a change in score from one point to another should not be interpreted as an equal change in underlying pathology. It is also important to consider the influence of injuries to other body systems. Limb or spinal injuries may greatly influence the motor score, and ocular injuries may result in a 'falsely' decreased score for brainstem reflexes as they can interfere with accurate assessment of pupil size (e.g. miosis as a result of traumatic uveitis).

b. Animal trauma triage (ATT) score

In contrast to the MGCS, this scoring system focuses on a broader, systemic assessment, with six categories being scored from 0 (normal or slight injury) to 3 (severe injury): perfusion, cardiac, respiratory, eye/muscle/skin, skeletal, neurological. In the same multi-centre study that looked at the MGCS in over 3500 dogs following trauma, the ATT score showed a linear relationship with mortality risk (Ash et al. 2018). When assessment was restricted to the 341 dogs with head injury, the ATT score out-performed the MGCS as a predictor of mortality (death or euthanasia). This may be related to the fact that it provides a more global assessment of the animal, which will reflect the systemic abnormalities that both exacerbate secondary brain injury and could influence the decision for euthanasia in the veterinary setting. A refined ATT score focusing only on perfusion, respiratory, and neurological categories still provided a good objective predictor of mortality risk in this study.

4. Management of increased intracranial pressure

If there is a concern from the neurological assessment regarding persistently increased ICP in spite of systemic stabilisation, then further management is required to reduce the ICP. This most commonly involves the administration of hyperosmolar agents, such as mannitol or hypertonic saline. The theory behind

---

Box 7.2 The Cushing Reflex

If the ICP rises to the point at which cerebral perfusion is compromised, then elevated $p_a(CO_2)$ levels will trigger a reflex increase in arterial blood pressure in an attempt to maintain cerebral perfusion. This increase in MABP (often in the region of >160–180 mmHg) triggers a baroreceptor reflex, with resultant marked bradycardia (e.g. 40–60 beats per minute). This combination of systemic hypertension and bradycardia is known as the cerebral ischaemic response or 'Cushing reflex'. This reflex will only be seen in animals with significant ICP elevation and will therefore always be accompanied by other indicators of elevated ICP (e.g. reduced level of mentation, recumbency, pupil abnormalities, loss of gag reflex). A dog that is bright and alert, walking normally, and has a normal cranial nerve examination should not immediately be assumed to have a Cushing reflex if the blood pressure is elevated and the heart rate is lower than expected. Other possible causes for this combination of parameters, such as the effects of previously administered medications (e.g. opiates, dexmedetomidine), should be considered in these cases. Management of animals with a high suspicion of a true Cushing reflex should focus on aggressive management of elevated ICP. The use of agents to increase the heart rate (e.g. atropine or glycopyrrolate) is not recommended as the bradycardia is protective and should normalise once the ICP is reduced by other means.

the use of these fluids is to increase the osmotic gradient across the blood–brain barrier and shift water from the interstitial space into the intravascular space, thus reducing cerebral oedema and the ICP. An increase in the circulating fluid volume will also decrease the blood viscosity, which improves cerebral perfusion and oxygen delivery. This decrease in viscosity also triggers cerebral vasoconstriction, resulting in a reduced intracranial blood volume and ICP. In euvolaemic animals that fail to respond to one of mannitol or hypertonic saline, the use of the other agent should be considered.

- Mannitol: 0.5–1 g/kg given IV over 15–20 minutes
  Mannitol is an osmotic diuretic that can be used to reduce ICP by a combination of reduced blood viscosity and by drawing extracellular fluid from normal and damaged brain tissue into the peripheral circulation. The reduction in blood viscosity persists for approximately 75 minutes, and the altered osmotic gradient across the blood–brain barrier lasts approximately 5–8 hours. The diuretic effect of mannitol is a concern in hypotensive animals and its use should be reserved for animals that are clinically deteriorating in spite of volume resuscitation. In animals that are in hypovolaemic shock, such as at the time of initial presentation, hypertonic saline is a more appropriate fluid choice. The concurrent administration of furosemide and mannitol is not currently recommended given the risk of further worsening hypovolaemia. Previous concerns regarding the use of mannitol in animals with suspected cerebral haemorrhage have not been supported by good clinical evidence and should not influence the decision to use this agent. The benefits of mannitol often outweigh the potential risks in animals with elevated ICP; however, these risks include exacerbation of hypovolaemia, electrolyte abnormalities (hyponatraemia, hypochloraemia, hyperkalaemia), acidosis, renal compromise, volume overload, and pulmonary oedema. It is essential that mannitol administration is followed by appropriate rates of isotonic crystalloids to avoid dehydration.
- Hypertonic saline: 4 ml/kg of 7.5% solution given IV over 3–5 minutes
  As previously discussed, hypertonic saline is a useful first-line fluid for the restoration of circulating fluid volume following trauma. This expansion of plasma volume increases the MABP, decreases blood viscosity, and improves cerebral perfusion and oxygen delivery. The intact blood–brain barrier is relatively impermeable to sodium and chloride, and water will follow the higher intravascular concentrations of these ions down an osmotic gradient away from the interstitial and intracellular spaces. This results in a decreased brain water content and a reduced ICP. Other suggested benefits of hypertonic saline include reduction in cerebrovascular endothelial oedema that improves CBF, and immunomodulatory effects that decrease brain excitotoxicity by promoting glutamate re-uptake. The use of hypertonic saline should be avoided in cases with systemic dehydration, hypernatraemia, or chronic

hyponatraemia. It is also essential that administration is followed by appropriate rates of isotonic crystalloids to avoid dehydration.

5. Analgesia and sedation

The provision of analgesia is vital for any animal following trauma, and this is particularly relevant in head trauma as pain and anxiety may increase the ICP. Opiates are the most commonly used analgesics in critically ill cases (e.g. methadone 0.1–0.3 mg/kg every 4–6 hours, butorphanol 0.1–0.3 mg/kg every 1–2 hours). The dose should be carefully titrated to achieve adequate analgesia whilst avoiding hypotension and respiratory depression. If available, short-acting agents such as fentanyl can be very effective when given as constant rate infusions (fentanyl 2–6 µg/kg/hour). The use of non-steroidal anti-inflammatory drugs (NSAIDs) should ideally be delayed until euvolaemia is established and renal perfusion is not compromised.

Sedatives, such as midazolam, are widely used in human medicine following severe head trauma, with the aim of maintaining a normal ICP by reducing the cerebral metabolic rate. They can also be useful adjuncts to opiates by providing anxiolysis with minimal cardiovascular and respiratory effects. However, neurological status becomes more difficult to interpret as the level of sedation increases. This complicates the monitoring of clinical progression and response to treatment in heavily sedated patients. Clinical decision-making in human medicine relies heavily upon direct ICP monitoring. The high cost of this equipment currently limits its widespread use in veterinary medicine, thus complicating the routine use of many sedative protocols; however, direct ICP monitoring in animals may become more common in the future.

The role of ketamine and alpha-2 agonists to provide sedation, anxiolysis, and/or analgesia in dogs and cats with head trauma remains uncertain, with mixed evidence for their potential benefit in human medicine. Until further studies are performed, the use of these agents should be avoided unless other sedatives or analgesics with fewer potential adverse effects are not available.

6. Supportive care and nutrition

Dogs and cats may be recumbent following head trauma and require intensive nursing to avoid further complications such as aspiration pneumonia, decubital ulcers, and corneal ulcers. Nursing considerations should include:

- Frequent turning and the provision of soft, clean, dry bedding.
- Physiotherapy to maintain joint mobility and avoid contractures.
- Placement of a urinary catheter to allow monitoring of fluid 'ins-and-outs' and to relieve anxiety or discomfort that could be associated with a need to urinate. Intermittent catheterisation or manual bladder expression can also be performed to reduce the risk of urinary tract infections associated with the prolonged use of indwelling catheters.

- Gastric ulcer prophylaxis to reduce the incidence of stress ulceration and gastric bleeding that has been associated with TBI in humans (e.g. omeprazole, famotidine, sucralfate).
- Maintenance of a normal body temperature (37–38.5 °C) to avoid increases in cerebral metabolic rate and ICP associated with hyperthermia.
- Nutrition and maintenance of normoglycaemia – early nutritional support is essential to maintain gastrointestinal health and to manage the trauma-induced hypermetabolic state. If an animal cannot protect their airway to allow enteral feeding, then a feeding tube can be placed to allow early feeding. Nasogastric tube placement has the advantage of not requiring anaesthesia but should be placed carefully to avoid sneezing, coughing, or gagging that may increase ICP. Animals should be systemically stable before being anaesthetised for the surgical placement of oesophagostomy feeding tubes. This is to avoid exacerbation of secondary injury associated with the influence of anaesthetic agents on blood pressure and ICP, with inhalational agents contraindicated in animals with increased ICP. Total intravenous anaesthesia, using agents such as propofol, can be performed in these cases; however, careful dosing and monitoring is still required to avoid hypotension and hypoventilation. Medications that promote gastric motility, such as metoclopramide, may be useful to manage the delayed gastric emptying that can be seen in trauma cases, thereby improving tolerance of enteral feeding and reducing the risk of aspiration pneumonia.

7.1.3 The Role of Corticosteroids in Head Trauma

A large randomised, placebo-controlled trial of intravenous corticosteroid administration to humans with TBI demonstrated an increased mortality in the corticosteroid group (Edwards et al. 2005). It is now widely accepted that the use of corticosteroids, particularly high intravenous doses of methylprednisolone sodium succinate (MPSS), is contraindicated in the management of head trauma in humans and animals.

7.1.4 Diagnostic Imaging

Diagnostic imaging in head trauma cases should initially focus on the identification of polytrauma and any injuries that may require urgent attention. As previously discussed, thoracic and abdominal radiography, TFAST and AFAST, or whole-body CT can be performed in the conscious animal, or under the influence of light sedation once normovolaemia and adequate oxygenation/ventilation have been established. Spinal radiographs can be taken to assess for injuries that may influence both the safe handling of the patient and interpretation of the neurological examination. It is not uncommon for patients with head trauma to have concurrent spinal injuries (e.g. cervical fractures), therefore all patients with known trauma should be handled with care and ideally not sedated until the presence of an unstable spinal injury is excluded. Radiography of the skull can be useful to assess for mandibular fractures that may require further treatment but is of limited value in the recognition of fractures involving other bones of the skull or in the assessment of intracranial structures.

Advanced imaging of the head can be performed to identify skull fractures and regions of haemorrhage and to assess the brain parenchyma itself. Computed tomography (CT) is the initial modality of choice as it is faster and lower in cost compared to magnetic resonance imaging (MRI), and does not usually require general anaesthesia (Figure 7.2). A study evaluating the CT findings in 27 dogs with head trauma identified cranial vault fractures and/or parenchymal abnormalities in 89% of these dogs (Chai et al. 2017). The presence of haemorrhage and ventricular asymmetry were negatively associated with short-term (10 days) and long-term (>6 months) survival. A study of 50 dogs that had an MRI scan within 14 days of head trauma (median 1 day) reported a significant association between the MRI findings (midline shift, parenchymal lesions, brain herniation, skull fractures) and both the clinical status at presentation (MGCS) and prognosis (Beltran et al. 2014). The results of recent studies appear to indicate a potential role of advanced imaging in guiding the prognosis for dogs and cats with TBI. However, in light of the fact that surgical management may not be an option for many owners, and that some animals with significant injury can still go on to have a good functional outcome, whether the findings of advanced imaging significantly influence the management choices in the majority of cases remains uncertain.

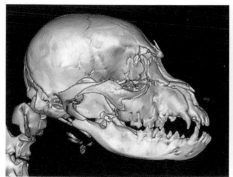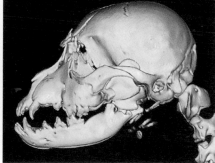

Figure 7.2 Left and right lateral views of a three-dimensional CT reconstruction of the skull of a 1-year-old terrier dog that was bitten on the head by another dog. There are multiple skull fractures involving parietal and frontal bones, with impingement of some of the skull fragments into the cranial vault. These fragments were compressing the olfactory lobes, with associated parenchymal oedema, intracranial haemorrhage, and secondary frontal lobe shift. Other injuries observed on the CT scan included fracture of the cribriform plate, traumatic pneumocephalus, bilateral frontal sinus fractures with associated sinusitis/haemorrhage, bilateral comminuted nasal fractures with associated bleeding within the nasal cavities, and complete, transverse, mildly displaced fractures of the rami of both mandibles.

7.1.5 Prognosis

The reported mortality rate in dogs following head trauma is around 20%. Poor prognostic indicators reported in the literature include a higher ATT score, decreased MGCS (<11), poor perfusion, and the need for intubation or hypertonic saline administration (Sharma and Holowaychuk 2015). As previously discussed, the findings of both CT and MRI have also been suggested to guide prognosis in dogs with TBI (Beltran et al. 2014; Chai et al. 2017; Yanai et al. 2015).

In summary, the management of animals presenting with head trauma should focus on initial triage for life-threatening injuries, systemic stabilisation, and frequent monitoring of neurological status. Rapid recognition of those animals that are not responding to normalisation of vital parameters allows for the instigation of further treatments in an attempt to reduce the ICP. A treatment algorithm for head trauma cases can be found in Figure 7.3.

Box 7.3 Hormonal Abnormalities Following Head Trauma

Together with the possibility of acquiring post-traumatic epilepsy, hypothalamic–anterior pituitary hormone deficiencies have also been reported in dogs following TBI (Murtagh et al. 2015). This can include decreased IGF-1, total thyroid hormone, and basal cortisol concentrations. Therefore, animals should be monitored for clinical signs that could indicate a hormonal abnormality following head trauma and their owners warned of these possible sequelae.

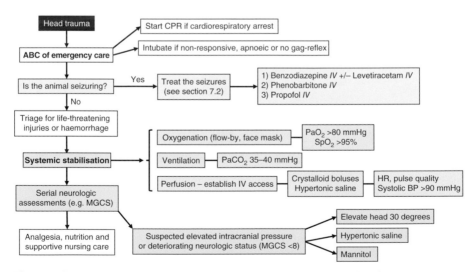

Figure 7.3 A summary of the clinical approach to an animal following head trauma.

7.2   Status Epilepticus and Acute Repetitive Seizures

Edward Ives

An epileptic seizure is a stressful event for the owner of a dog or cat, particularly if their animal has no previous history of seizures. They are therefore a common reason for out-of-hours telephone advice calls and emergency appointments. The majority of epileptic seizures are fortunately self-limiting and do not require emergency treatment (further discussion on the approach to seizures can be found in Chapter 6). In a minority of cases, the seizure activity is not self-limiting or may recur a short time after the last event. This can have deleterious effects on the central nervous system (CNS) and other organs, therefore prompt recognition and treatment of prolonged or recurrent seizure activity is essential.

7.2.1   What Is Status Epilepticus?

Status epilepticus is the term used to describe a state of continuous seizure activity that is not self-limiting. Irreversible neuronal damage may occur after 20–30 minutes and previous definitions of status epilepticus were based upon this finding. However, this definition has been modified to account for the fact that emergency management should be instituted as soon as possible, before irreversible neuronal damage occurs. Status epilepticus is now widely defined as either:

- continuous seizure activity for longer than 5 minutes
- or two or more seizures over a 30 minute period without recovery of consciousness between.

Acute repetitive seizures (cluster seizures) also represent a neurological emergency and are defined as the occurrence of two or more isolated seizures within a 24-hour period, with a recovery of consciousness between events.

7.2.2   Why Does Status Epilepticus Occur?

An epileptic seizure results from excessive and hypersynchronous neuronal activity in the cerebral cortex. The pathophysiology underlying why the excessive neuronal activity fails to stop in cases of status epilepticus is incompletely understood but is likely to depend upon genetic factors and the cause of the seizure itself. Possible mechanisms may include:

- Failure of inhibition of neuronal excitation resulting from alterations in the expression, location, or number of receptors for the inhibitory neurotransmitter gamma-aminobutyric acid (GABA).

- Excessive neuronal excitation mediated by excitatory neurotransmitters such as glutamate, aspartate, and acetylcholine.

7.2.3 How Common Is Status Epilepticus in Veterinary Medicine?

Status epilepticus may be the first manifestation of seizure activity in dogs and cats, particularly following toxin exposure. It is more commonly reported secondary to structural brain disease and metabolic-toxic disorders; however, one study reported that 59% of dogs with idiopathic epilepsy had one or more episodes of status epilepticus in their lifetime (Saito et al. 2001). This may occur even if the animal's epilepsy has been well-controlled on antiepileptic medications prior to this event.

Acute repetitive seizures have been reported to affect 38–77% of dogs with idiopathic epilepsy, with certain breeds (e.g. German Shepherd Dog) and dogs of a younger age at seizure onset more likely to be affected (Monteiro et al. 2012; Packer et al. 2016). These dogs may have a reduced likelihood of achieving seizure freedom and a decreased survival time from diagnosis.

7.2.4 Why Is Emergency Treatment of Status Epilepticus Required?

Similar to the management of TBI, the emergency treatment of status epilepticus is essential to reduce the risk of irreversible neuronal injury and to manage the severe systemic effects associated with prolonged seizure activity. In the early stages, increased skeletal muscle activity and autonomic stimulation leads to a combination of hypertension, tachycardia, hyperglycaemia, and hyperthermia. As compensatory processes start to fail, and the body is unable to meet the increased cerebral metabolic demand, death may result from cardiac arrhythmias, rhabdomyolysis, acute renal tubular necrosis, hypoglycaemia, acidosis, hyperkalaemia, hypoxaemia, and hypotension. Early, aggressive treatment is therefore important and studies in human medicine have demonstrated that whilst mortality rates are primarily dependent on the underlying cause, they are also influenced by seizure duration prior to treatment. A mortality rate of 25% was reported in a retrospective study of 156 dogs with status epilepticus or cluster seizures, with a worse prognosis if seizure control was lost after 6 hours of hospitalisation (Bateman and Parent 1999).

7.2.5 Clinical Approach to Status Epilepticus/Acute Repetitive Seizures

The clinical approach to the management of a dog or cat presenting for status epilepticus, or with a history of multiple seizures in the preceding 24 hours, can be divided into the following considerations and is summarised in Figure 7.4.

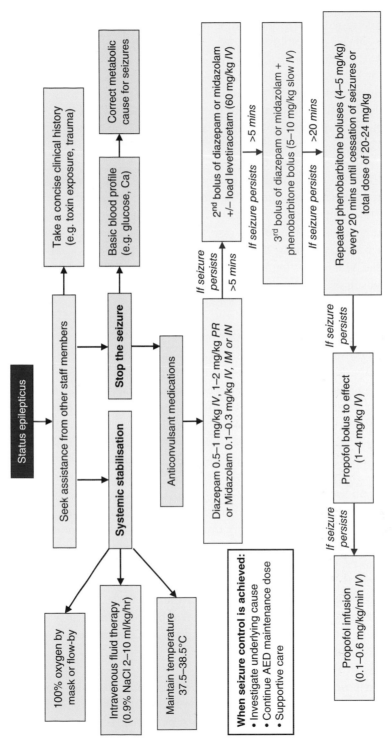

Figure 7.4 The clinical approach to an animal presenting in status epilepticus.

1. Is this an epileptic seizure?
2. Seek assistance from other staff members
3. Take a concise clinical history
4. Systemic stabilisation
5. Stop the seizure activity
6. Nursing care of a hospitalised animal
7. Identify the underlying cause for the seizure activity
8. Introduce or continue maintenance antiepileptic drug therapy

1. Is this an epileptic seizure?

Owners may report that their pet is having an epileptic seizure when in reality the event represents an alternative cause for collapse or involuntary motor activity. Differentiating these 'seizure mimics' from a true epileptic seizure is important to ensure appropriate case management. Potential seizure mimics include syncope, vestibular disorders, paroxysmal dyskinesias ('movement disorders', see Video 10), neuromuscular disease, or neck pain with associated muscle spasms (see Video 8). Further discussion regarding mimics of epileptic seizures can be found in Chapters 1 and 6.

2. Seek assistance from other staff members

It is extremely difficult to provide the care required for an animal in status epilepticus without assistance. The placement of intravenous catheters, blood sampling, and provision of oxygen ideally requires at least two trained members of staff and is further complicated by the continuous muscle activity and limb movements associated with on-going seizure activity. The exact time at either the onset of seizure activity (if observed) or when treatment was started should be recorded to assist in the planning and timing of interventions.

3. Take a concise clinical history

During the initial assessment and stabilisation, another veterinarian or nurse should take a concise clinical history from the owner. This is important as it may guide possible differential diagnoses and the choice of appropriate medications and drug doses. Questions should focus on:

- known or suspected toxin exposure (e.g. metaldehyde in slug pellets, mycotoxins in mouldy food, topical application of permethrin in cats)
- the current seizure history – onset, duration, and appearance
- previous diagnoses of a seizure disorder (e.g. idiopathic epilepsy, meningoencephalitis, intracranial neoplasia)
- concurrent medical conditions (e.g. diabetes mellitus, hepatic disease)
- current medications and doses, including both antiepileptic medications and other medications (e.g. insulin, antibiotics, parasiticides)
- any medications administered in the last 24 hours (e.g. rectal Diazepam prior to presentation).

4. Systemic stabilisation

The approach to systemic stabilisation of animals in status epilepticus is very similar to that described for head trauma and should start with assessment of the airway, breathing, and circulation. A face mask can be used to administer 100% oxygen and intravenous access should be acquired as soon as possible to allow for drug administration and fluid therapy. The following parameters should be recorded and monitored, with the aim of maintaining parameters within the normal range (e.g. $Sp(O_2) > 95\%$, $p_a(O_2) > 80\,mmHg$, MABP 80–100 mmHg):

• heart rate, pulse quality, mucous membrane colour, capillary refill time
• respiratory rate and effort
• $Sp(O_2)$ by pulse oximetry
• systolic blood pressure
• cardiac rhythm by electrocardiography.

Hyperthermia is a common consequence of prolonged seizure activity. The temperature should therefore be monitored, and passive cooling started if the temperature exceeds 39.5 °C (aiming for 37.5–38.5 °C).

Intravenous fluid therapy is essential to manage the systemic effects of seizure activity and to optimise cerebral blood flow (CBF). Isotonic crystalloids, such as 0.9% sodium chloride, can be started at 2–10 ml/kg/hour or be given as intravenous boluses of 10–15 ml/kg, with the aim of restoring and maintaining an adequate arterial blood pressure (MABP 80–100 mmHg).

5. Stop the seizure activity

At the same time as systemic stabilisation, the priority of treatment should be to stop any on-going seizure activity. This may be achieved by:

a. either correcting an underlying metabolic cause for the seizure activity
b. or administration of anticonvulsant medications.

a. Correcting a metabolic cause for seizure activity

Rectifying a metabolic derangement, if present, will often be the most rapid and effective way of stopping any associated seizure activity. A baseline blood sample should always be taken at the time of presentation and can usually be achieved when the intravenous catheter is placed. A minimum database should comprise a PCV, total solids, urea, calcium, glucose, and electrolytes (sodium, chloride, and potassium). Serum ammonia can also be useful in cases with suspected hepatic dysfunction (e.g. congenital portosystemic shunt). Surplus blood can be collected for additional testing after emergency management, such as serum bile acids or antiepileptic drug serum levels if the dog is already receiving treatment (e.g. phenobarbitone or potassium bromide).

The two most common metabolic abnormalities that can result in acute seizure activity are hypocalcaemia (e.g. post-partum eclampsia, hypoparathyroidism) and hypoglycaemia (e.g. insulin overdose, insulinoma, xylitol toxicity). The clinical history may raise the index of suspicion for these conditions and confirming normoglycaemia, at a minimum, is vital before focusing on anticonvulsant therapy.

i. Hypoglycaemia

Seizure activity may occur at serum levels <2–2.5 mmol/l.

Correction: A bolus of 0.5–1 ml/kg 50% glucose solution should be administered by intravenous injection. Dilution with an equal volume of saline is recommended to reduce the risk of phlebitis associated with this hyperosmolar solution. This can be followed by a 5% dextrose solution to meet the maintenance fluid and glucose requirements.

ii. Hypocalcaemia

Dependent on ionised calcium levels, neurological signs such as muscle tremors/fasciculations, cramping, pain, facial pruritus, and seizures may be observed at serum total calcium levels <1.9 mmol/l.

Correction: A bolus of 1 ml/kg 10% calcium gluconate solution should be administered by intravenous injection over 20 minutes. Care should be taken regarding perivascular injection as tissue necrosis and skin sloughing can occur.

It is important to monitor the heart rate and rhythm during administration for possible bradycardia.

b. Administration of anticonvulsant medications
i. Acute repetitive seizures

If an animal presents with a history of two or more generalised seizures over the last 24 hours but has recovered by the time of presentation, then the emergency administration of anticonvulsant medications may not be required. It remains important to take a detailed clinical history, determine whether the previous events are likely to have represented epileptic seizures, and ensure that systemic parameters are stable. An intravenous catheter should be placed as soon as possible to allow for the prompt administration of medications in the event of further seizures. A blood sample should also be taken to investigate possible extra-cranial causes for the previous events. If there is a recurrence of seizure activity during the hospitalisation period, then the approach described below for status epilepticus should be followed.

If no apparent cause for the acute repetitive seizures is identified from the clinical history and blood tests, then the option of referring the animal for further investigations should be discussed with the owner. Toxin exposure is a common cause for status epilepticus but would be less likely to result in multiple isolated seizures with full recovery between, unless there is repeat exposure over a short period of time. In animals receiving treatment for previously diagnosed idiopathic epilepsy, blood should also be taken to determine the current serum drug levels. Consideration can then be given as to whether the dose(s) need to be increased, or whether an additional maintenance drug should be started.

Some dogs with idiopathic epilepsy may show a tendency for recurrent clusters of acute repetitive seizures, separated by a normal inter-ictal period. The use of levetiracetam as a pulse therapy, in addition to other maintenance drugs, has been suggested in these cases, with the aim of reducing the total number of seizures in each cluster:

• 60 mg/kg single oral loading dose of levetiracetam after recovery from the first observed seizure, followed by 20–30 mg/kg every 8 hours for 2–3 days.

ii. Status epilepticus

There is a lack consensus regarding the optimal protocol for the medical management of status epilepticus in both humans and veterinary medicine. It is unlikely that a single protocol would be appropriate for all patients, given differences in underlying seizure aetiology, the potential influence of concurrent medical conditions (e.g. hepatic or renal dysfunction), and the variability in whether a patient is already receiving antiepileptic medications. The use of electroencephalography (EEG) to record cerebrocortical neuronal activity is common for therapeutic decision-making in human medicine, such as when weaning or introducing agents used for seizure control. The use of EEG in veterinary medicine is currently limited to specialist centres and defined therapeutic end points remain controversial in human medicine, particularly in relation to patient outcome.

First-line drugs:

• Diazepam
• Midazolam

Most protocols involve the first-line administration of a lipophilic anticonvulsant medication to rapidly cross the blood–brain barrier and stop seizure activity. The most frequently used drugs in veterinary medicine are the benzodiazepines diazepam and midazolam. If intravenous access is not available, then they may be administered by intramuscular injection, intranasal, or per rectum dependent on the medication.

Diazepam can be administered by intravenous injection (0.5–1 mg/kg) or by the per rectum or intranasal routes (1–2 mg/kg). Intramuscular injection results in local tissue irritation and should be avoided.

Midazolam can be administered by the intravenous, intramuscular, or intranasal routes (0.1–0.3 mg/kg). Midazolam results in less CNS and respiratory depression compared to diazepam, and a recent study demonstrated superior efficacy of intranasal midazolam (administered using a mucosal atomisation device) when compared to rectal diazepam for the management of status epilepticus in dogs (Charalambous et al. 2017).

Repeated bolus administration of benzodiazepines may result in drug accumulation within the CNS and the potential for detrimental cardiorespiratory depression. An interval of 3–5 minutes is recommended between boluses to give time for the medication to achieve adequate CNS concentrations. This avoids the potential for unnecessary repeated administration. If there is continuous seizure activity (or rapid seizure recurrence) following the use of two or three benzodiazepine boluses, then it is important that further seizures are not managed with repeated boluses of benzodiazepines alone. Administration of an antiepileptic medication with a longer half-life, that can also be used as daily maintenance therapy, should always be introduced at this time to improve seizure control.

Second-line drugs:

- Levetiracetam
- Phenobarbitone

Levetiracetam is a novel anticonvulsant medication that is not currently licensed for use in dogs or cats. The primary anticonvulsant effect is thought to result from binding to the synaptic vesicle protein 2A (SVP2A), resulting in decreased release of glutamate from the pre-synaptic membrane. Multiple other mechanisms of action have also been suggested, and the fact that these differ to those of benzodiazepines and barbiturates make it an attractive choice in the emergency management of prolonged or recurrent seizures. Levetiracetam may also have both neuroprotective properties and influence the complex process of seizure generation (epileptogenesis), reducing the likelihood of further seizures developing.

Levetiracetam can be administered by the intravenous, subcutaneous, intramuscular, oral, or rectal routes. It has minimal hepatic metabolism, few reported adverse effects, and shows minimal interaction with other medications. The minimal hepatic metabolism means that its use should be considered in animals with known or suspected hepatic dysfunction. The availability and high cost of the intravenous formulation may limit its use in general practice; however, it appears to be a safe and potentially effective second-line agent for status epilepticus. A randomised, double-masked, placebo-controlled prospective study of 19 dogs with status epilepticus or acute repetitive seizures demonstrated that dogs receiving intravenous levetiracetam after a single dose of diazepam required significantly fewer further boluses of diazepam compared to those receiving placebo (Hardy et al. 2012). A greater proportion of dogs receiving levetiracetam (56%) compared to placebo (10%) showed no further seizure activity but this did not reach statistical significance. A recent case report described a fatal adverse event following the rapid intravenous administration of undiluted levetiracetam

(60 mg/kg) to a dog (Biddick et al. 2018). It is therefore advised to dilute the solution 1 : 10 with saline and to administer by slow intravenous injection.

A suggested protocol for the use of levetiracetam in the emergency management of status epilepticus is as follows:

- 60 mg/kg single intravenous dose if seizure activity persists for >5 minutes after a single bolus of diazepam or midazolam
- followed by 20–30 mg/kg IV or per os every 8 hours.

Phenobarbitone is a barbiturate that acts at a different binding site on the GABA-A receptor to benzodiazepines. It is widely used in veterinary medicine for the emergency management of seizures that are not responding to benzodiazepines alone. It can be administered by the intravenous or intramuscular routes, with higher 'loading' doses used to more rapidly achieve therapeutic serum concentrations. The majority of intravenous formulations require diluting 1 : 10 with saline and should be administered by slow intravenous injection. Phenobarbitone takes 20–30 minutes to distribute to the brain following administration and animals should be monitored closely for hypotension and cardiorespiratory depression following intravenous injection, particularly after concurrent benzodiazepine administration. Intravenous fluid therapy and the provision of intubation and ventilation should therefore be available.

The following protocol can be used for animals that have not responded to the administration of benzodiazepines +/– levetiracetam:

- 5–10 mg/kg intravenous bolus if seizure activity persists for >5 minutes after a single bolus of benzodiazepine
- repeated 4–5 mg/kg intravenous boluses every 20 minutes until cessation of seizure activity is observed, or a total dose of 20–24 mg/kg is reached
- continue as a maintenance therapy at 2–3 mg/kg IV or per os every 12 hours.

The total loading dose may also be calculated in dogs not currently receiving phenobarbitone according to the following formula, with a target serum concentration of 25 µg/ml being a reasonable goal:

$$\text{loading dose (mg)} = \text{body weight (kg)} \times 0.8 \times \text{target serum concentration} (\mu g / ml)$$

Third-line drugs:

- Propofol
- Other agents with a potential role in the control of persistent seizure activity

If seizures persist following two or three boluses of diazepam/midazolam, levetiracetam administration (if available), and intravenous loading of phenobarbitone, then it can be assumed that the animal has been in a state of continuous seizure activity for at least 25–30 minutes. Treatment options at this stage include use of a benzodiazepine constant rate infusion (e.g. midazolam at 0.2 mg/kg/hour) or introduction of a new agent, with propofol being the most widely used in veterinary medicine.

Propofol is an alkylphenol that has multiple potential anticonvulsant mechanisms, including acting as a GABA-A agonist, modulation of calcium channels, and inhibition of excitatory glutamate receptors. In animals that are not responding to the protocols described above, or for which phenobarbitone use is contraindicated, then the following dosing schedule can be considered:

- 1–4 mg/kg intravenous bolus to effect
- followed by a constant rate infusion of 0.1–0.6 mg/kg/minute for a minimum of 6–24 hours.
- If seizures are subsequently controlled, then the dose should be tapered by 25% every 6 hours, unless EEG is available to monitor for epileptiform activity.

Propofol formulations that do not contain the preservative benzoyl alcohol should be used for constant rate infusions, and Heinz body formation can complicate the use of propofol infusions in cats. Vital parameters should be constantly monitored, with provision for intubation and ventilation available at all times. All animals should receive oxygen by flow-by or face mask if not intubated, together with regular monitoring of heart rate, pulse quality, respiratory rate and effort, pulse oximetry, temperature, and blood pressure. Corneal lubrication should be provided regularly, and animals should be turned every 1–2 hours if unable to do so themselves.

During recovery from a seizure, and particularly following propofol administration, tonicity or movements such as paddling can be observed that are difficult to distinguish from a recurrence of seizure activity. This may result in the inappropriate administration of medications to an animal that would have otherwise continued to recover. These movements will often lack the sustained tonicity and involuntary, rhythmic nature of a true seizure recurrence.

If status epilepticus is refractory to benzodiazepines, phenobarbitone, levetiracetam, and propofol, then the prognosis is unfortunately likely to be poor. The evidence to support the use of other agents is currently lacking in veterinary medicine but further options could include the following.

- Inhalational anaesthetic agents (e.g. isoflurane, sevoflurane)
  The use of inhalational anaesthetic agents is reserved for refractory status epilepticus in humans and, until further evidence is available, the same should apply for veterinary medicine. Exacerbation of ICP elevation and the hypotensive effects of these agents are significant concerns. Isoflurane may

be preferred over sevoflurane, as the latter undergoes greater metabolism, increasing the risk of organ damage and resulting in the production of epileptogenic metabolites. The prolonged use of inhalational anaesthesia in human patients with refractory status epilepticus (e.g. over 7 days) is unlikely to be feasible in veterinary medicine.

- Ketamine
  Ketamine is a glutamate receptor antagonist with conflicting evidence regarding its use for refractory status epilepticus in humans. It has been shown to have neuroprotective effects in rodent models of status epilepticus and may assist in suppression of epileptiform activity on EEG. However, concerns regarding its use include exacerbation of elevated ICP and the potential to cause neuronal damage and cerebral atrophy in humans. A single case report in veterinary medicine described the use of two intravenous boluses of ketamine (5 mg/kg), followed by a constant rate infusion (5 mg/kg/hour) in a dog with inflammatory brain disease and seizures that were inadequately controlled with diazepam, phenobarbitone, and propofol (Serrano et al. 2006). The dog survived to discharge but was subsequently euthanised due to persistent neurological deficits. No evidence of NMDA-antagonist neurotoxicity was observed at post-mortem in this case.

- Dexmedetomidine
  The use of dexmedetomidine as a possible anticonvulsant medication is mainly limited to experimental models and a single conference presentation describing its use as an adjunctive medication in the management of status epilepticus in dogs. The evidence to support its use is currently weak and the potential anticonvulsant effects are likely to be dependent on the species and dose used. Epileptic seizures have also been described in a neonatal child following the administration of dexmedetomidine, suspected to be related to reduction in the anticonvulsant activity of neurons located in the locus coeruleus (Kubota et al. 2013). The routine use of dexmedetomidine in the management of status epilepticus in dogs and cats is currently not recommended; however, intramuscular administration could be considered to assist with intravenous catheter placement in animals with severe involuntary motor activity, or for the management of severe tremors without loss of consciousness (e.g. tremorgenic mycotoxicosis).

- Imepitoin
  The use of imepitoin is not currently recommended in the management of acute repetitive seizures or status epilepticus. Animals that are already receiving the medication as maintenance therapy should be continued on the current dosing regime, if oral administration is possible.

- Potassium bromide
  The limited availability of intravenous formulations of potassium bromide restricts its use for the emergency management of seizures. Potassium

bromide undergoes renal excretion and can therefore be a useful drug in dogs with hepatic dysfunction. It should be used with caution in dogs with renal disease and should not be used in cats due to the potential to cause severe bronchial inflammation. The long half-life of potassium bromide means that loading is required to more rapidly achieve therapeutic serum concentrations. This can be performed per rectum (100 mg/kg every 6 hours for 24 hours) if oral loading is not possible.

6. Nursing care of a hospitalised animal

The nursing care and monitoring required during and after the emergency management of seizures will depend upon the degree of neurological compromise, the systemic stability of the animal, and the requirement for continued use of sedative or anaesthetic medications to control seizure activity. Intensive care may be required in many cases and this can be costly for the owner, involving 24-hour nursing of an animal that is not fit for transport to a dedicated referral centre or out-of-hours provider.

The following factors should be considered in all cases:

- Provision of clean, soft, dry bedding and turning every 2–4 hours.
- Ocular lubrication to avoid corneal ulceration, particularly in deeply sedated or anaesthetised animals.
- Intermittent bladder expression or placement of an in-dwelling urinary catheter.
- Frequent monitoring of heart rate, pulse quality, mucous membrane colour, capillary refill time, respiratory rate and pattern, body temperature, pulse oximetry, blood pressure +/− end-tidal CO_2 for intubated animals.
- Monitoring of blood glucose and electrolytes, with supplementation of intravenous fluid therapy as required.
- Nutritional support for anorexic patients, with consideration regarding the increased risk of aspiration pneumonia in recumbent or sedated animals that cannot protect their airway.
- Provision of analgesia if there is a concurrent painful condition, or if the animal appears in discomfort.
- Frequent neurological assessment, particularly in animals with an unidentified cause for seizure activity. An objective scoring system such as the MGCS can be used to assist in monitoring of trends and allow prompt recognition of a deterioration in clinical status.

7. Identify the underlying cause for the seizure activity

The decision to perform further investigations should be made once an animal is stable and the seizure activity is well-controlled. This will depend on the clinical history and owner factors. The underlying cause will already be known, or highly suspected, in animals with a history of head trauma, observed toxin exposure, or a consistent metabolic abnormality on blood testing. An underlying structural cause for status epilepticus or acute repetitive seizures should always be considered if there are persistent neurological deficits beyond the post-ictal period, even in animals with a prior history of idiopathic epilepsy. Further diagnostic investigations should be recommended in these cases, which will usually involve referral to a specialist centre for MRI of the brain and cerebrospinal fluid analysis (see Chapter 6).

If referral is not an option following careful discussion with the owner, then maintenance antiepileptic drug therapy should be started or continued. The most appropriate diagnostic investigations to perform in general practice will be dependent on the clinical history and signalment of the animal:

- A portosystemic shunt may be suspected in a 6-month-old Yorkshire Terrier with a history of seizures, lethargy after eating, stunted growth, and gastrointestinal signs. Bile acid stimulation testing, serum ammonia, and abdominal ultrasound would be most appropriate in this case.
- Inflammatory brain disease (e.g. meningoencephalitis of unknown origin) may be suspected in a young or middle aged, small breed dog (e.g. Chihuahua or Pug) with persistent inter-ictal neurological deficits that are consistent with a multifocal intracranial, or forebrain, neuroanatomic localisation. If referral is not an option and the animal is deteriorating clinically, then a trial of immunosuppressive prednisolone (1 mg/kg twice daily) could be considered. This should only follow discussion with the owner regarding the clinical suspicion, and the risks and limitations of this approach if there is a different underlying cause.
- Intracranial neoplasia would be highly suspected in an older large breed dog (e.g. Boxer) that presents in status epilepticus or shows an acute onset of frequent generalised seizures, particularly if asymmetric inter-ictal neurological deficits are identified. If referral is not an option, then palliative medical management using a maintenance antiepileptic medication and an anti-inflammatory dose of prednisolone (0.5 mg/kg once daily) could be considered in this case.
- Idiopathic epilepsy would be the most likely diagnosis in a 2-year-old Labrador Retriever or Border Collie that has no history of toxin exposure, has a normal inter-ictal neurological examination, and normal haematology and serum biochemistry. Close monitoring of clinical progression and use of a maintenance antiepileptic drug alone would not be inappropriate in this instance. An alternative diagnosis should always be investigated if the subsequent clinical course is inconsistent with a diagnosis of idiopathic epilepsy, particularly the appearance of inter-ictal neurological deficits.

8. Introduce or continue maintenance antiepileptic drug therapy

Oral maintenance antiepileptic drug therapy should be started/continued in all animals presenting for acute repetitive seizures or status epilepticus until a definitive cause for the seizure activity is identified. The decision can then be made as to whether long-term medical management is required. This may not be required in animals for which an identified metabolic abnormality has been corrected (e.g. hypoglycaemia), or if there was a known history of toxin exposure. A retrospective study on 20 dogs with prolonged status epilepticus secondary to intoxication (13/20 dogs having a seizure duration longer than 12 hours), reported that no dogs had further seizures and suggested that long-term treatment might not be needed after short-term control of status epilepticus (Jull et al. 2011).

7.3 Acute Spinal Cord Injury

Paul M. Freeman

7.3.1 Causes of Spinal Cord Injury

There are many potential causes of significant spinal cord injury, including vascular disorders (e.g. fibrocartilaginous embolism), sterile inflammatory disorders (e.g. meningomyelitis of unknown origin), infectious disease (e.g. spinal empyema), injury associated with congenital anomalies (e.g. atlantoaxial instability), acute intervertebral disc extrusion, or even acute deterioration of chronic intervertebral disc protrusion. The diagnostic approach and management of these conditions has already been discussed in Chapter 6, and this chapter therefore focuses primarily on acute spinal cord injury that may result from vertebral fracture and/or luxation. However, it should be remembered that any animal presenting with an acute onset of severe paraparesis/paraplegia, or severe tetraparesis/tetraplegia, should be considered as a potential neurological emergency. Although this section is concerned largely with traumatic spinal cord injury, mention will be made of other conditions when appropriate, and the guidelines for patient evaluation and management are applicable whatever the cause of spinal cord injury.

7.3.2 Pathophysiology of Acute Spinal Cord Injury

The spinal cord may be injured in a variety of ways, and several different mechanisms may be involved in the same case.

Contusion: Contusion or bruising of the spinal cord is caused by direct impact leading to rupture of the microvasculature. This can be through intrinsic trauma, such as from the explosive extrusion of an intervertebral disc, through to external impact such as in a road traffic accident. Contusion causes release of local inflammatory mediators, cytotoxic substances, and excitatory neurotransmitters that induce a chain of secondary events leading to ischaemia and energy depletion within cells. This in turn can lead to the development of cytotoxic oedema due to a failure of the energy-dependent sodium channels in the neuronal cell walls, accumulation of intracellular sodium ions, and subsequent swelling of cells. This is a pre-morbid process, ultimately ending in cell necrosis and apoptosis which may continue for several days.

Compression: Acute spinal cord compression may be caused by herniated intervertebral disc material, haemorrhage, or by an unstable vertebral fracture/luxation. The spinal cord is able to tolerate a high degree of compression, especially if it occurs slowly, but acute compression is less well tolerated and may be a further cause of contusion through crushing of microvasculature. In addition, compression may impede blood flow to the spinal cord parenchyma and further increase the ischaemia which results from severe contusion. Compression can mechanically disrupt and distort axons, myelin sheaths, and neuronal cell bodies; if severe enough, this too may lead to irreversible cellular changes and cell death. Chronic compression leads to demyelination and axonal loss, and this should also be considered when planning treatment following vertebral fracture or luxation.

Laceration: Physical disruption of spinal cord tissue is most commonly caused by vertebral fracture/luxation, or external factors such as gunshot. The axons may be torn, myelin sheaths disrupted, and cell bodies may be crushed. Complete physical disruption of the spinal cord may be caused by a severe, traumatic vertebral fracture/luxation, and this is likely to be irreversible even after months or years.

7.3.3 Patient Assessment

Most vertebral fractures and luxations are associated with road traffic accidents, especially in the dog. Cats may present more commonly with either an unknown history or a history of falling from a height. Therefore, it is common to find concomitant injuries to many other body systems, some of which may be immediately life-threatening. As for head trauma, patient assessment should always begin with the 'ABC' of airway, breathing, and circulation. The initial assessment should focus on the vital physiological and cardiovascular parameters, since many patients presenting with spinal cord injury following external trauma will also be suffering from hypovolaemic shock or blood loss. Although these issues should be considered first, extreme care should be taken when moving an animal that has been involved in a road traffic accident as vertebral instability may be present. If it is necessary to move the patient, then attempts should be made to provide some kind of external support, and the use of a firm stretcher is advisable. The need to support the circulatory system and to ensure that there is a good airway and breathing are of paramount importance in all cases. Therefore, if the animal has to be moved in order to provide essential life support, then of course this takes priority over any suspected spinal cord injury. Furthermore, physiological stabilisation is very important in protecting the spinal cord from further damage in acute severe spinal cord injury.

Baseline heart rate and rhythm, breathing rate and quality, and rectal temperature should be recorded. In cervical spinal cord injury, the breathing may be affected by damage to the upper motor neurons from the respiratory centres in the brainstem. Various other mechanisms may also influence the breathing, such as diaphragmatic rupture, rib fractures, and pneumothorax. Thoracic radiography may therefore need to be performed rapidly and pneumothorax addressed if present. If there is airway compromise or persistent breathing difficulty, then intubation and ventilation may be required.

The mean arterial blood pressure (MABP) and, if possible, blood gas measurement should be performed. Pulse oximetry should be used to monitor the $Sp(O_2)$. Maintenance of adequate systemic blood pressure and blood oxygen saturation are the mainstays of neuroprotection in cases of acute CNS injury (see below and Section 7.1 'Head Trauma in Dogs and Cats').

Neurological examination

A neurological assessment should be performed as soon as the patient is stable. An attempt should be made to anatomically localise the region of suspected injury, since this will guide imaging and therapy. In some instances of severe trauma, it may not be possible to effectively evaluate the level of mentation, and the possibility of brain trauma rather than spinal cord injury may exist (see Section 7.1 'Head Trauma in Dogs and Cats'). However, in most cases it will be clear that one is dealing with spinal cord injury alone.

Important tests to perform include evaluation of the spinal reflexes (e.g. flexor withdrawal reflex) in all limbs and the cutaneous trunci reflex. In cases of tetraparesis or tetraplegia, then a distinction needs to be made between a lesion affecting the C1–C5 spinal cord segments and a lesion affecting C6–T2 segments. This may be best evaluated using the flexor withdrawal reflexes in the thoracic limbs, although interpretation may be difficult and unreliable. Other possible indicators of a C6–T2 lesion would include Horner syndrome and absence of the cutaneous trunci reflex at any level of stimulation. Ultimately, it may not be possible or overly important to differentiate between a C1–C5 and C6–T2 lesion, since this is unlikely to make a significant difference to imaging requirements in most dogs and cats. However, a more cranial cervical injury can be more immediately life-threatening than a caudal cervical injury due to potential disruption of phrenic nerve and diaphragmatic function, and the need to provide external support may be more critical in this region due to the inherent instability compared to the caudal cervical spine.

Several studies have found that the thoracolumbar region is the most common location for vertebral fractures and luxations, followed by the lumbar and lumbosacral regions. The cervical vertebral column is the least common region to be affected, and in one study no cats were found with fracture or luxation in the cervical vertebral column (Bali et al. 2009).

Care should be taken not to misinterpret the Schiff–Sherrington posture as an indicator of tetraparesis (see Chapters 3 and 4). This rigid extension of the thoracic limbs in conjunction with paraplegia can be seen in acute severe thoracolumbar spinal cord injuries. It is caused by disruption of inhibitory *ascending* interneurons (Border cells) which normally serve to inhibit extensor muscle tone in the thoracic limbs as part of the mechanism of thoracic and pelvic limb coordination (see Figure 6.10.1 in Section 6.10 'Paresis, Paralysis, and Proprioceptive Ataxia' and Video 23).

An animal presenting with suspected Schiff–Sherrington posture must also be distinguished from an animal that has suffered a brain injury and is presenting in a decerebrate or decerebellate posture; more detail of these presentations and how to distinguish them may be found in Chapter 3. For this reason, it is important to perform a full neurological examination whenever possible, in order that potentially confusing signs may be correctly interpreted. A patient with severe tetraparesis or tetraplegia may have normal *or* reduced spinal reflexes depending on the precise location of the injury, but the postural reactions and voluntary motor function will always be affected in both the thoracic and pelvic limbs. In contrast, an animal with paraplegia and Schiff–Sherrington posture will have normal spinal reflexes, normal postural reactions, and good voluntary movement in the thoracic limbs. However, assessing this may not be easy if there is doubt about spinal stability. Therefore, the clinician must perform the neurological examination carefully and systematically in order to arrive at the correct conclusion and neuroanatomic localisation.

In cases of paraplegia, it should be apparent that the thoracic limbs are normal (except in the cases of Schiff–Sherrington posture described above). The pelvic limb flexor withdrawal reflexes and the patellar reflexes may assist in differentiating between a lesion affecting the T3–L3 spinal cord segments (normal reflexes) from one affecting the L4–S3 spinal cord segments (reduced reflexes). Again, this may be difficult and can be complicated by the phenomenon known as spinal shock, which results in a counterintuitive weakness of the pelvic limb withdrawal reflexes secondary to an acute upper motor neuron lesion (see Chapter 4). Therefore, when presented with an animal that is paraplegic and appears to have reduced pelvic limb spinal reflexes, a careful examination of the cutaneous trunci reflex should always be performed in order to ensure that the lesion is not mistakenly localised to the L4–S3 segments rather than the T3–L3 segments. In genuine lower motor neuron lesions (L4–S3 segments), the cutaneous trunci reflex should be intact and there may also be loss of tail tone and perineal reflex.

The most important prognostic indicator in acute spinal cord injury is the presence or absence of deep pain perception in the distal limbs (see Chapter 3 and Video 15). As previously stated, it is unusual for an animal to be presented with absent deep pain perception in all four limbs since most such animals will have died as a result of such a severe cervical spinal cord injury. If absent deep pain perception in all four limbs is suspected, the clinician must be certain that the test is being performed correctly and that the animal's responses are not being affected by shock or analgesic medication.

In acute thoracolumbar spinal cord injuries, the absence of pelvic limb deep pain perception is the only factor that has been shown to have prognostic value. In cases of Hansen type 1 intervertebral disc extrusion, the prognosis for recovery in dogs with absent pelvic limb deep pain perception is around 55% with surgical treatment. In cases of vertebral fracture/luxation and traumatic spinal cord injury, the prognosis is believed to be much worse and therefore euthanasia should be considered. However, caution should be exercised in the interpretation of deep pain perception testing at the time of presentation, and dogs or cats that present with absent deep pain perception should always be considered candidates for potential referral as soon as they are stable. Furthermore, it may be prudent to delay any decision to perform euthanasia for at least 24 hours following an acute injury, since the effects of initial shock may lead to confusing neurological signs including, on occasion, the apparent absence of deep pain perception which subsequently returns once the animal has been stabilised.

Recently, a study has shown the potential prognostic value of a serum glial fibrillary acidic protein (GFAP) test in predicting recovery in deep pain-negative dogs caused by acute intervertebral disc extrusion (Olby et al. 2019). Should this test become commercially available, it may prove a useful addition to patient assessment and prediction of potential recovery. So far, no work has been published regarding the utility of this test in cases of vertebral fracture and luxation.

7.3.4 Management of Acute Spinal Cord Injury

Aside from the general management factors discussed above, there are some specific considerations for limiting the effects of spinal cord injury. At present, there is little that can be done to prevent the effects of contusion. The primary goal of treatment is to maintain blood flow to the injured spinal cord and there is convincing evidence in the human literature that hypotension plays a role in secondary spinal cord injury. Therefore, ensuring that the mean arterial pressure is maintained within normal limits is vital. Monitoring the blood pressure and the appropriate use of fluid therapy, including volume expanders such as hypertonic saline where necessary, is one of the few ways to tackle the effects of ischaemia and secondary spinal cord damage.

Maintaining oxygenation is the other significant factor which can be influenced by good patient management. This ensures that the spinal cord is supplied with adequate energy to minimise the effects of ischaemia. Blood gas monitoring is ideal, but when not available, pulse oximetry is valuable. The use of flow-by oxygen therapy or, in some situations, intubation and ventilation may be appropriate.

1. Pharmacological agents

High dose corticosteroid therapy was once favoured in the treatment of human spinal cord injury but has fallen out of use due to more recent work showing a possible detrimental effect. Currently, there is no evidence to support the use of corticosteroids in acute severe spinal cord injury in cats and dogs. Their use is associated with significant morbidity, and they are of limited or no value in reducing the cytotoxic oedema which predominates in such injury, as opposed to the vasogenic oedema associated with neoplasia and chronic compressive spinal cord lesions.

Other potentially beneficial agents, such as polyethylene glycol (PEG), are undergoing clinical trials but as yet there is no evidence for the efficacy of any such compounds. Therefore, the focus should be on ensuring appropriate analgesia in cases of spinal cord trauma, since the pain associated with such injuries may be significant. Opioids such as methadone may be used, providing care is taken over any possible respiratory depressive effects. Intravenous paracetamol may also be considered. NSAIDs, such as meloxicam or carprofen, may also be appropriate, although their use should be avoided in hypovolaemic animals as they may have significant gastrointestinal and renal side-effects in such situations.

2. Diagnostic investigations

Survey radiographs of the entire spine should be taken as soon as the patient is stable. If possible, general anaesthesia should be avoided due to the potential loss of the spinal stabilising effect of muscular spasm. Sedation with a combination of an α2 agonist such as medetomidine in combination with an opioid analgesic is preferred. Radiographs should be taken by centring on the region of suspected injury based on the neurological examination, and orthogonal views are mandatory for identifying vertebral fracture/luxation (see Figure 7.5). Identification of

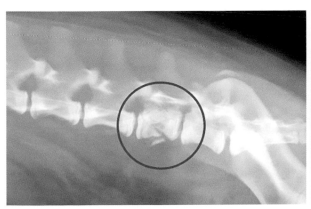
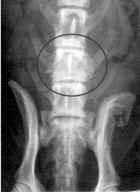

Figure 7.5 Radiographs of a comminuted fracture of the L6 vertebra; it can be seen that the fracture is much more obvious on the lateral view than on the ventrodorsal view; care should always be taken when reviewing radiographs of animals suffering with suspected vertebral trauma and it is important, if possible, to ensure that orthogonal views are available in such cases.

a potentially unstable fracture or luxation is an indication for surgical referral if possible.

Assessment of spinal radiographs requires an understanding of normal vertebral column anatomy, as well as the ligamentous structures and mechanisms involved in vertebral column stability. The vertebral column is made up of functional units consisting of an adjacent pair of vertebrae, the intervertebral disc lying between them, the articular facet joints on each side, and the joint capsule and ligaments which connect the vertebrae. Three-dimensional imaging using computed tomography (CT) can provide additional information regarding vertebral fracture/luxation and is particularly beneficial in cases where there is doubt about the presence of a fracture(s), or when assessment of stability is difficult. It is also very beneficial for surgical planning if surgical stabilisation is considered. Furthermore, one study found that the sensitivity of survey radiography for identifying vertebral fractures/luxations was only around 75% compared to CT as the gold standard (Kinns et al. 2006). Therefore, practitioners should always be aware of the potential to miss a fracture or luxation on plain radiography alone.

3. Management of vertebral fracture/luxation

If a vertebral fracture and/or luxation is present, referral for surgical decompression and stabilisation may be necessary for recovery. A three-compartment model has been proposed for vertebral trauma, with the dorsal spine, dorsal arch, and articular facet joints forming the dorsal compartment, the ventral pedicle, dorsal annulus fibrosus, and dorsal part of the vertebral body forming the middle compartment, and the ventral part of the vertebral body and remainder of the intervertebral disc forming the ventral compartment (see Figure 7.6). It is proposed that if damage is limited to a single compartment, then the fracture should be stable and may be managed conservatively. Damage to two or more compartments, however, will be unstable and require surgical stabilisation.

For most cases of vertebral fracture/luxation, surgical stabilisation and/or decompression is likely to give the best prognosis for recovery. Surgical treat-

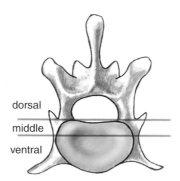

Figure 7.6 Illustration to show the proposed three-compartment model used in the assessment of vertebral column stability associated with spinal fractures.

ment methods are beyond the scope of this text but for the practitioner faced with a case of vertebral fracture/luxation, there are some situations where non-surgical management may be appropriate, or for cases when referral for surgical management is not an option. If only a single compartment is affected, deep pain perception is preserved, and referral is not an option, then either external splinting or strict cage rest may allow fracture healing to occur. This applies to fractures of any region of the vertebral column, including the thoracic and lumbar regions. However, any suggestion of instability or significant vertebral displacement that is causing disruption of the vertebral canal would be contraindications for a conservative approach. As already stated, thoracic and lumbar vertebral fractures/luxations that are accompanied by a loss of pelvic limb deep pain perception carry an extremely poor prognosis. If this neurological finding is confirmed by repeated assessment following systemic stabilisation, then serious consideration should be given to euthanasia of such severely affected animals. Furthermore, if external splinting or cage confinement is initially applied but the animal shows further neurological deterioration, then this implies potential instability and referral for surgical treatment should again be considered.

In terms of conservative management techniques, mid-cervical fracture/luxations are probably best suited to external splinting since it may be possible to simply wrap the neck in a well-padded bandage in order to provide some support to these injuries. Even in the case of a fracture of the dens of C2, conservative management may be successful with this approach. However, persistent pain may make this very difficult even in small and toy breeds. More caudal cervical injuries are more difficult to stabilise in this way, and great care must be taken to avoid compromise to the airway. If a padded bandage or splint is applied to the neck whilst an animal is anaesthetised or heavily sedated, then the animal must be very carefully observed during recovery to ensure that there is no airway compromise.

External splinting of thoracic and lumbar vertebral fracture/luxations is more difficult to achieve effectively and attempts often end in disappointment. Further problems associated with soft tissue necrosis and pressure sores can also be common. Strict cage confinement may be a better option with injuries in this location. For caudal lumbar and lumbosacral injuries, it must be remembered that the spinal cord ends at approximately the L5–L6 level in dogs and L6–L7 in cats, so injuries caudal to this will cause damage to the cauda equina rather than the spinal cord itself. This has implications for prognosis, given that recovery after nerve root or peripheral nerve injury is usually better than after spinal cord injury. Therefore, the prognosis is generally better with injuries at the caudal lumbar and lumbosacral level than in the more cranial lumbar and thoracolumbar regions. Conservative management of vertebral fracture/luxations at this level is also likely to have a better prognosis, although the pain associated with spinal nerve compression may be significant and a reason to consider surgical treatment.

4. Care of animals recovering from spinal cord trauma

The major considerations for the management of animals recovering from spinal cord injury are providing adequate analgesia, minimising the risks of recumbency (e.g. pressure sores and pneumonia), and management of the urinary bladder. As discussed above, opioids such as methadone and morphine are likely to be required in the early stages, alongside a NSAID +/− paracetamol. Gabapentin may be a useful additional analgesic, although is only available as an oral formulation. Regular assessment for pain and adaptation of the analgesic protocol in order to most appropriately manage the individual is also important to reduce the potentially detrimental effects associated particularly with opioids.

Avoiding the risks of prolonged recumbency requires regular moving and turning, with the use of slings and lifting aids where necessary. Regular turning of recumbent patients (every 2–4 hours) can help to avoid pressure sores, as well as reduce the risk of lung congestion and potential pneumonia. The use of well-padded beds for recumbent animals can further reduce the risk of decubitus ulcers, and some form of plastic padded mattress covered by a soft stay-dry bedding such as 'Vet-Bed' can be very effective. Care with nutrition is also important. Animals should be fed in sternal recumbency, or preferably helped into a sitting or standing position if possible, and great care taken to avoid any potential aspiration of food or water. If anorexia is prolonged, or face/jaw injuries make eating impossible, consideration should be given to the placement of a feeding tube.

Management of bladder emptying problems may be achieved in a number of ways. Manual expression may be possible in some situations, particularly in the case of the so-called 'lower motor neuron' bladder which is seen following damage to the S1–S3 spinal cord segments or nerve roots. In such cases, there is loss of sphincter and detrusor muscle tone and manual expression may be relatively easy. However, there is often significant urine leakage which can lead to urine scalding and exacerbate problems of soft-tissue management associated with recumbency.

Placement of an indwelling urinary catheter is likely to be the best way to manage many cases with an 'upper motor neuron' bladder, as observed in spinal cord lesions cranial to the L4 spinal segments (i.e. the majority of cervical, thoracolumbar, and lumbar spinal injuries). In such cases, there is often strong urethral sphincter tone which makes manual bladder expression difficult, and many animals become very resistant to attempts to express their bladder. For the reasons stated above, the author may also use an indwelling urinary catheter in cases with a lower motor neuron bladder, especially in the early stages of rehabilitation; this can simplify case management and reduce animal distress associated with frequent bladder expression. It is always important to monitor the urine output, as urinary catheters can become kinked or blocked. Inevitably with time there is a significant risk of developing a urinary tract infection if an indwelling urinary catheter is placed, although one study found that this risk was no greater than with either manual expression or repetitive rigid catheterisation (Bubenik and Hosgood 2008).

7.3.5 Summary

In summary, acute severe spinal cord injury will usually present as either paraplegia or tetraplegia, depending on the location of the injury, and a focused neurological examination should be performed in order to establish the most likely location of the lesion. The spine should be supported whilst the patient is assessed, and careful consideration should be given to the rest of the body as animals with spinal cord trauma commonly will have traumatic injuries elsewhere.

The presence or absence of deep pain perception in the paralysed limbs remains the most important prognostic indicator, but care should be taken when interpreting this test in a shocked animal at the time of presentation. Once the animal is stable, survey radiographs should be taken of the region of suspected trauma in order to identify any potential instability of the vertebral column. Referral should always be offered if vertebral fracture/luxation is diagnosed or suspected, but an animal that has truly lost deep pain perception in the pelvic limbs as a result of external spinal cord trauma unfortunately has a very guarded prognosis for recovery even with surgical treatment.

Bibliography

7.1. Head Trauma in Dogs and Cats

Ash, K., Hayes, G.M., Goggs, R., and Sumner, J.P. (2018). Performance evaluation and validation of the animal trauma triage score and modified Glasgow Coma Scale with suggested category adjustment in dogs: a VetCOT registry study. *J. Vet. Emerg. Crit. Care (San Antonio)* 28: 192–200.

Beltran, E., Platt, S.R., McConnell, J.F. et al. (2014). Prognostic value of early magnetic resonance imaging in dogs after traumatic brain injury: 50 cases. *J. Vet. Intern. Med.* 24: 1256–1262.

Burgess, S., Abu-Laban, R.B., Slavik, R.S. et al. (2016). A systematic review of randomized controlled trials comparing hypertonic sodium solutions and mannitol for traumatic brain injury: implications for emergency department management. *Ann. Pharmacother.* 50: 291–300.

Caine, A., Brash, R., De Risio, L. et al. (2019). Magnetic resonance imaging in 30 cats with traumatic brain injury. *J. Feline Med. Surg.* 21: 1111–1119.

Chai, O., Peery, D., Bdolah-Abram, T. et al. (2017). Computed tomographic findings in dogs with head trauma and development of a novel prognostic computed tomography-based scoring system. *Am. J. Vet. Res.* 78: 1085–1090.

Chestnut, R.M., Marshall, L.F., Klauber, M.R. et al. (1993). The role of secondary brain injury in determining outcome from severe head injury. *J. Trauma* 34: 216–222.

Coles, J.P., Fryer, T.D., Coleman, M.R. et al. (2007). Hyperventilation following head injury: effect on ischemic burden and cerebral oxidative metabolism. *Crit. Care Med.* 35: 568–578.

Edwards, P., Arango, M., Balica, L. et al. (2005). Final results of the MRC CRASH, a randomized placebo-controlled trial of intravenous corticosteroid in adults with head injury – outcomes at 6 months. *Lancet* 365: 1957–1959.

Friedenburg, S.G., Butler, A.L., Wei, L. et al. (2012). Seizures following head trauma in dogs: 259 cases (1999–2009). *J. Am. Vet. Med. Assoc.* 241: 1479–1483.

Kuo, K.W., Bacek, L.M., and Taylor, A.R. (2018). Head trauma. *Vet. Clin. North Am. Small Anim. Pract.* 48: 111–128.

Lewis, S.R., Pritchard, M.W., Evans, D.J. et al. (2018). Colloids versus crystalloids for fluid resuscitation in critically ill people. *Cochrane Database Syst. Rev.* (8) Art. No.: CD000567.

Li, M., Chen, T., Chen, S.D. et al. (2015). Comparison of equimolar doses of mannitol and hypertonic saline for the treatment of elevated intracranial pressure after traumatic brain injury: a systematic review and meta-analysis. *Medicine (Baltimore)* 94: 736.

Murtagh, K., Arrol, L., Goncalves, R. et al. (2015). Hypothalamic-anterior pituitary hormone deficiencies following traumatic brain injury in dogs. *Vet. Rec.* 176: 20–25.

Platt, S. and Olby, N. (2013). *BSAVA Manual of Canine and Feline Neurology*, 4e. Gloucester, UK: British Small Animal Veterinary Association.

Platt, S.R., Radaelli, S.T., and McDonell, J.J. (2001). The prognostic value of the modified Glasgow Coma Scale in head trauma in dogs. *J. Vet. Intern. Med.* 15: 581–584.

Sande, A. and West, C. (2010). Traumatic brain injury: a review of pathophysiology and management. *J. Vet. Emerg. Crit. Care (San Antonio)* 20: 177–190.

Sharma, D. and Holowaychuk, M. (2015). Retrospective evaluation of prognostic indicators in dogs with head trauma: 72 cases (January–March 2011). *J. Vet. Emerg. Crit. Care (San Antonio)* 25: 631–639.

Steinmetz, S., Tipold, A., and Löscher, W. (2013). Epilepsy after head injury in dogs: a natural model of posttraumatic epilepsy. *Epilepsia* 54: 580–588.

Stocchetti, N., Maas, A.I., Chieregato, A., and van der Plas, A.A. (2005). Hyperventilation in head injury: a review. *Chest* 127: 1812–1827.

Syring, R.S., Otto, C.M., and Drobatz, K.J. (2001). Hyperglycaemia in dogs and cats with head trauma: 122 cases (1997–1999). *J. Am. Vet. Med. Assoc.* 218: 1124–1129.

Todd, M.M., Cutkomp, J., and Brian, J.E. (2006). Influence of mannitol and furosemide, alone and in combination, on brain water content after fluid percussion injury. *Anesthesiology* 105: 1176–1181.

Wang, X., Arima, H., Yang, J. et al. (2015). Mannitol and outcome in intracerebral hemorrhage: propensity score and multivariable intensive blood pressure reduction in acute cerebral hemorrhage Trial 2 results. *Stroke* 46: 2762–2767.

Yanai, H., Tapia-Nieto, R., Cherubini, G.B., and Caine, A. (2015). Results of magnetic resonance imaging performed within 48 hours after head trauma in dogs and association with outcome: 18 cases (2007–2012). *J. Am. Vet. Med. Assoc.* 246: 1222–1229.

Yozova, I.D., Howard, J., Henke, D. et al. (2017). Comparison of the effects of 7.2% hypertonic saline and 20% mannitol on whole blood coagulation and platelet function in dogs with suspected intracranial hypertension – a pilot study. *BMC Vet. Res.* 13: 185.

7.2. Status Epilepticus and Acute Repetitive Seizures

Bateman, S.W. and Parent, J.M. (1999). Clinical findings, treatment, and outcome of dogs with status epilepticus or cluster seizures: 156 cases (1990–1995). *J. Am. Vet. Med. Assoc.* 215: 1463–1468.

Biddick, A.A., Bacek, L.M., and Taylor, A.R. (2018). A serious adverse event secondary to rapid intravenous levetiracetam injection in a dog. *J. Vet. Emerg. Crit. Care (San Antonio)* 28: 157–162.

Blades Golubovic, S. and Rossmeisl, J.H. Jr. (2017). Status epilepticus in dogs and cats, part 1: etiopathogenesis, epidemiology, and diagnosis. *J. Vet. Emerg. Crit. Care (San Antonio)* 27: 278–287.

Blades Golubovic, S. and Rossmeisl, J.H. Jr. (2017). Status epilepticus in dogs and cats, part 2: treatment, monitoring and prognosis. *J. Vet. Emerg. Crit. Care (San Antonio)* 27: 288–300.

Charalambous, M., Bhatti, S.F.M., Van Ham, L. et al. (2017). Intranasal midazolam versus rectal diazepam for the management of canine status epilepticus: a multicenter randomized parallel-group clinical trial. *J. Vet. Intern. Med.* 31: 1149–1158.

Drislane, F.W., Blum, A.S., Lopez, M.R. et al. (2009). Duration of refractory status epilepticus and outcome: loss of prognostic utility after several hours. *Epilepsia* 50: 1566–1571.

Fang, Y. and Wang, X. (2015). Ketamine for the treatment of refractory status epilepticus. *Seizure* 30: 14–20.

Hardy, B.T., Patterson, E.E., Cloyd, J.M. et al. (2012). Double-masked, placebo-controlled study of intravenous levetiracetam for the treatment of status epilepticus and acute repetitive seizures in dogs. *J. Vet. Intern. Med.* 26: 334–340.

Jull, P., Risio, L.D., Horton, C., and Volk, H.A. (2011). Effect of prolonged status epilepticus as a result of intoxication on epileptogenesis in a UK canine population. *Vet. Rec.* 169: 361.

Kan, M.C., Wang, W.P., Yao, G.D. et al. (2013). Anticonvulsant effect of dexmedetomidine in a rat model of self-sustaining status epilepticus with prolonged amygdala stimulation. *Neurosci. Lett.* 543: 17–21.

Kapur, J. (2018). Role of NMDA receptors in the pathophysiology and treatment of status epilepticus. *Epilepsia Open* 3: 165–168.

Keros, S., Buraniqi, E., Alex, B. et al. (2017). Increasing ketamine use for refractory status epilepticus in US pediatric hospitals. *J. Child Neurol.* 32: 638–646.

Kubota, T., Fukasawa, T., Kitamura, E. et al. (2013). Epileptic seizures induced by dexmedetomidine in a neonate. *Brain Dev.* 35: 360–362.

Kwiatkowska, M., Tipold, A., Huenerfauth, E., and Pomianowski, A. (2018). Clinical risk factors for early seizure recurrence in dogs hospitalized for seizure evaluation. *J. Vet. Intern. Med.* 32: 757–763.

McCarren, H.S., Arbutus, J.A., Ardinger, C. et al. (2018). Dexmedetomidine stops benzodiazepine-refractory nerve agent-induced status epilepticus. *Epilepsy Res.* 141: 1–12.

Monteiro, R., Adams, V., Keys, D., and Platt, S.R. (2012). Canine idiopathic epilepsy: prevalence, risk factors and outcome associated with cluster seizures and status epilepticus. *J. Small Anim. Pract.* 53: 526–530.

Packer, R.M., Shihab, N.K., Torres, B.B., and Volk, H.A. (2016). Risk factors for cluster seizures in canine idiopathic epilepsy. *Res. Vet. Sci.* 105: 136–138.

Patterson, E.N. (2014). Status epilepticus and cluster seizures. *Vet. Clin. North Am. Small Anim. Pract.* 44: 1103–1112.

Platt, S.R. and Haag, M. (2002). Canine status epilepticus: a retrospective study of 50 cases. *J. Small Anim. Pract.* 43: 151–153.

Platt, S. and Olby, N. (2013). *BSAVA Manual of Canine and Feline Neurology*, 4e. Gloucester, UK: British Small Animal Veterinary Association.

Podell, M. (1995). The use of diazepam per rectum at home for the acute management of cluster seizures in dogs. *J. Vet. Intern. Med.* 9: 68–74.

Saito, M., Munana, K.R., Sharp, N.J.H. et al. (2001). Risk factors for development of status epilepticus in dogs with idiopathic epilepsy and effects of status epilepticus on outcome and survival time: 32 cases (1990–1996). *J. Am. Vet. Med. Assoc.* 219: 618–623.

Schwartz, M., Muñana, K.R., Nettifee-Osborne, J.A. et al. (2013). The pharmacokinetics of midazolam after intravenous, intramuscular, and rectal administration in healthy dogs. *J. Vet. Pharmacol. Ther.* 36: 471–477.

Serrano, S., Hughes, D., and Chandler, K. (2006). Use of ketamine for the management of refractory status epilepticus in a dog. *J. Vet. Intern. Med.* 20: 194–197.

Talke, P., Stapelfeldt, C., and Garcia, P. (2007). Dexmedetomidine does not reduce epileptiform discharges in adults with epilepsy. *J. Neurosurg. Anesthesiol.* 19: 195–199.

Xu, K.L., Liu, X.Q., Yao, Y.L. et al. (2018). Effect of dexmedetomidine on rats with convulsive status epilepticus and association with activation of cholinergic anti-inflammatory pathway. *Biochem. Biophys. Res. Commun.* 495: 421–426.

7.3. Acute Spinal Cord Injury

Ahuja, C.S., Schroeder, G.D., Vaccaro, A.R. et al. (2017). Spinal cord injury – what are the controversies? *J. Orthop. Trauma* 31: S7–S13.

Alkabie, S. and Boileau, A.J. (2016). The role of therapeutic hypothermia after traumatic spinal cord injury – a systematic review. *World Neurosurg.* 86: 432–449.

Bali, M.S., Lang, J., Jaggy, A. et al. (2009). Comparative study of vertebral fractures and luxations in dogs and cats. *Vet. Comp. Orthop. Traumatol.* 22: 47–53.

Bruce, C.W., Brisson, B.A., and Gyselinck, K. (2008). Spinal fracture and luxation in dogs and cats: a retrospective evaluation of 95 cases. *Vet. Comp. Orthop. Traumatol.* 21: 280–284.

Bubenik, L. and Hosgood, G. (2008). Urinary tract infection in dogs with thoracolumbar intervertebral disc herniation and urinary bladder dysfunction managed by manual expression, indwelling catheterization or intermittent catheterization. *Vet. Surg.* 37: 791–800.

Dixon, A. and Fauber, A.E. (2017). Effect of anesthesia-associated hypotension on neurologic outcome in dogs undergoing hemilaminectomy because of acute, severe thoracolumbar intervertebral disk herniation: 56 cases (2007–2013). *J. Am. Vet. Med. Assoc.* 250: 417–423.

Fenn, J., Laber, E., Williams, K. et al. (2017). Associations between anesthetic variables and functional outcome in dogs with thoracolumbar intervertebral disk extrusion undergoing decompressive hemilaminectomy. *J. Vet. Intern. Med.* 31: 814–824.

Granger, N. and Carwardine, D. (2014). Acute spinal cord injury: tetraplegia and paraplegia in small animals. *Vet. Clin. North Am. Small Anim. Pract.* 44: 1131–1156.

Jeffery, N.D. (2010). Vertebral fracture and luxation in small animals. *Vet. Clin. North Am. Small Anim. Pract.* 40: 809–828.

Kinns, J., Mai, W., Seiler, G. et al. (2006). Radiographic sensitivity and negative predictive value for acute canine spinal trauma. *Vet. Radiol. Ultrasound* 47: 563–570.

Kube, S.A. and Olby, N.J. (2008). Managing acute spinal cord injuries. *Compend. Contin. Educ. Vet.* 30: 496–504.

Olby, N., Levine, J., Harris, T. et al. (2003). Long-term functional outcome of dogs with severe injuries of the thoracolumbar spinal cord: 87 cases (1996–2001). *J. Am. Vet. Med. Assoc.* 222: 762–769.

Olby, N.J., Muguet-Chanoit, A.C., Lim, J.H. et al. (2016). A placebo-controlled, prospective, randomized clinical trial of polyethylene glycol and methylprednisolone sodium succinate in dogs with intervertebral disk herniation. *J. Vet. Intern. Med.* 30: 206–214.

Olby, N.J., Lim, J.H., Wagner, N. et al. (2019). Time course and prognostic value of serum GFAP, pNFH, and S100β concentrations in dogs with complete spinal cord injury because of intervertebral disc extrusion. *J. Vet. Intern. Med.* 33: 726–734.

Rouanet, C., Reges, D., Rocha, E. et al. (2017). Traumatic spinal cord injury: current concepts and treatment update. *Arq. Neuropsiquiatr.* 75: 387–393.

Smith, P.M. and Jeffery, N.D. (2005). Spinal shock--comparative aspects and clinical relevance. *J. Vet. Intern. Med.* 19: 788–793.

Index

Page locators in **bold** indicate tables. Page locators in *italics* indicate figures.

A Practical Approach to Neurology for the Small Animal Practitioner, First Edition. Paul M. Freeman and Edward Ives.
© 2020 John Wiley & Sons Ltd. Published 2020 by John Wiley & Sons Ltd.
Companion Website: www.wiley.com/go/freeman/neurology